Suicidal Behaviors: Prevention, Intervention and Postvention

Suicidal Behaviors: Prevention, Intervention and Postvention

Guest Editors

Irene Caro-Cañizares
María Cantero-García
Eva Izquierdo-Sotorrío

MDPI

Basel • Beijing • Wuhan • Barcelona • Belgrade • Novi Sad • Cluj • Manchester

Guest Editors
Irene Caro-Cañizares
Psychology and Health
Sciences School
Universidad a Distancia de
Madrid (UDIMA)
Collado Villalba
Spain

María Cantero-García
Psychology and Health
Sciences School
Universidad a Distancia de
Madrid (UDIMA)
Collado Villalba
Spain

Eva Izquierdo-Sotorrío
Psychology and Health
Sciences School
Universidad a Distancia de
Madrid (UDIMA)
Collado Villalba
Spain

Editorial Office
MDPI AG
Grosspeteranlage 5
4052 Basel, Switzerland

This is a reprint of the Special Issue, published open access by the journal *Behavioral Sciences* (ISSN 2076-328X), freely accessible at: https://www.mdpi.com/journal/behavsci/special_issues/C99S021UL5.

For citation purposes, cite each article independently as indicated on the article page online and as indicated below:

Lastname, A.A.; Lastname, B.B. Article Title. *Journal Name* **Year**, *Volume Number*, Page Range.

ISBN 978-3-7258-6998-5 (Hbk)
ISBN 978-3-7258-6999-2 (PDF)
https://doi.org/10.3390/books978-3-7258-6999-2

Contents

About the Editors

Irene Caro-Cañizares

Irene Caro-Cañizares holds a PhD in Clinical Psychology. She has worked for over ten years as a clinical psychologist in outpatient clinics. She currently combines her university teaching at UDIMA with research. In recent years, she has focused her research on the study of emotional dysregulation in children and adolescents, suicidal behavior and self-harm in young adults, and the study of dual pathology in pregnant women. Along with Dr. Eva Izquierdo, she coordinates the HOPES Research Group (GI-23/3, Health Outcomes from Psychology and Education for Suicide Prevention).

María Cantero-García

María Cantero-García holds a PhD in Clinical and Health Psychology. She is an Associate Professor at UDIMA, where she combines teaching with research. Her work focuses on clinical and health psychology, with particular emphasis on psycho-oncology, psychological well-being in health contexts, and comprehensive care for patients and their families. She is the Coordinator of the Research Group PsyCaRe (GI-25/3, Psychology of Health, Humanization of Care and Resilience) and Director of the Chair of Digital Transformation in Health Management, from which she promotes innovation and digitalization processes in healthcare systems.

Eva Izquierdo-Sotorrío

Eva Izquierdo-Sotorrío holds a PhD in Psychology and is the Dean of the Faculty of Psychology and Health Sciences at UDIMA. She has extensive academic and research experience in the field of clinical and health psychology, with a particular focus on psychological assessment, suicide prevention, and gender perspectives in health. Her research addresses issues such as risk and protective factors in suicidal behavior, and the impact of gender and violence on mental health. Together with Dr. Irene Caro, she coordinates the HOPES Research Group (GI-23/3, *Health Outcomes from Psychology and Education for Suicide Prevention*).

Preface

We all know that suicide is a global problem, with the World Health Organization (WHO) reporting that approximately 700,000 people die by suicide every year. This alarming figure is compounded by other manifestations of suicidal behavior, such as suicidal ideation and suicide attempts, which are far more prevalent in the population and cause profound suffering. Suicidal behaviors (SBs) therefore represent serious psychosocial and public health issues worldwide, with undeniable consequences for the individual, their family, and society. Yet political, social, and healthcare responses are often hindered by stigma and by a reluctance to address the problem directly. Although progress has been made in identifying risk factors, understanding the multidimensional and existential nature of suicidal behavior remains a challenge. Key aspects such as the relative weight of different risk factors, the role of protective factors, the influence of interpersonal, psychosocial, and contextual variables, and the mechanisms underlying the onset of suicidal ideation and its transition to suicidal acts still require further study. Exploring these issues in greater depth will contribute to the development of more effective universal, selective, and indicated prevention strategies, while also enabling more personalized approaches to intervention and postvention.

The aim of this Special Issue is to enhance our understanding of suicidal behaviors (SBs) and their risk and protective factors, while highlighting innovative proposals for intervention, prevention, and postvention.

Irene Caro-Cañizares, María Cantero-García, and Eva Izquierdo-Sotorrío
Guest Editors

behavioral sciences

MDPI

Article

Identification and Analysis of Critical Suicide Sites and Factors in Castilla-La Mancha (2020–2024): Forensic and Healthcare Collaboration for Prevention

Beatriz Vallejo-Sánchez [1,2,3,4,*], Natalia Solano-Pinto [2,5], Ana Huertes-Del Arco [4,6], Valeriano Muñoz [7], Mónica Casillas [8], Carolina Arroyo [9] and Fernando Moreno [10]

1 Central Services of the Castilla-La Mancha Health Service (SESCAM), 45007 Toledo, Spain
2 Health, Education and Society Research Group, Health Research Institute of Castilla La Mancha (IDISCAM), 45071 Toledo, Spain; natalia.solano@uclm.es
3 Faculty of Languages and Education, Nebrija University, 28043 Madrid, Spain
4 School of Health Sciences and Education, Open University of Madrid (UDIMA), 28400 Madrid, Spain; ana.huertes@udima.es
5 Department of Psychology, University of Castilla La Mancha, 45071 Toledo, Spain
6 Department of Personality, Assessment and Psychological Treatments, Faculty of Psychology, National University of Distance Education (UNED), 28040 Madrid, Spain
7 Forensic Pathology Section, Institute of Legal Medicine and Forensic Sciences of Toledo, 45003 Toledo, Spain; valeriano.munoz@justicia.es
8 Pathology Service, Institute of Legal Medicine and Forensic Sciences of Albacete, Cuenca, and Guadalajara, 02001 Albacete, Spain; monica.casillas@justicia.es
9 Institute of Legal Medicine and Forensic Sciences of Toledo, 45003 Toledo, Spain; carolina.arroyo@justicia.es
10 Clinical Service, Institute of Legal Medicine and Forensic Sciences of Albacete, Cuenca, and Guadalajara, 02001 Albacete, Spain; fernando.moreno@justicia.es
* Correspondence: bvallejo@sescam.jccm.es or beatriz.vallejo@udima.es

Abstract

Suicide is a major public health concern worldwide, and identifying the spatial patterns associated with its occurrence is essential for designing effective preventive strategies. This study aimed to identify and characterize suicide locations in two provinces of Castilla-La Mancha, Spain, using a descriptive and retrospective analysis of 421 cases recorded by the Institutes of Legal Medicine and Forensic Sciences of Toledo and Albacete between 2020 and 2024. Locations were classified as critical or non-critical based on recurrence and public accessibility, and logistic regression was used to explore predictors of suicide in public settings. Results showed that 82% of cases involved men, yielding a 5:1 male-to-female ratio that exceeds the national average; the mean age was 56.6 years, and hanging was the most frequent method (56.1%). Most suicides occurred in private environments, and only one location met the criteria for a critical site. These findings indicate that spatial clustering plays a minimal role in the regional suicide burden and that prevention efforts should prioritize means restriction and early detection in private settings, along with broader measures for dispersed public cases rather than hotspot-focused interventions. The study underscores the importance of systematically incorporating spatial information into forensic records to improve regional suicide surveillance and inform more targeted, context-sensitive prevention policies.

Keywords: suicide prevention and control; risk factors; forensic medicine; epidemiological surveillance; public health; descriptive epidemiology

 https://doi.org/10.3390/bs16010007

1. Introduction

Suicide is one of the leading causes of preventable death worldwide, with more than 700,000 deaths annually (World Health Organization, 2025). Within this global phenomenon, there is a particular subset of deaths that occur in specific public places known as "hotspots," or locations with a high incidence of suicide. These are defined as locations that have a disproportionate number of suicides compared to other environments (Joyner et al., 2025). Some authors establish as a criterion the location's having more than one suicide or serious attempt documented in a five-year period, along with additional conditions such as public or semi-public access, availability of a highly lethal method, relative isolation that would hinder early intervention, or local recognition as a recurring location for suicides (Owens et al., 2015; Pirkis et al., 2015; Too et al., 2024). Other authors, however, adopt different criteria for suicide hotspots, such as having a rate of at least 0.5 suicides per year over a decade (Hemmer et al., 2017). Critical sites often include infrastructure such as bridges, cliffs, railways, subway stations, tall buildings, or coastal areas, where the method used frequently results in death. The choice of these locations may be motivated by their reputation, personal significance, or association with previous deaths, even when people must travel from distant areas (Joyner et al., 2025).

The relevance of public locations is notable due to the high social, emotional, and media impact they generate. These events are often more visible to the community, affecting witnesses, family members, and emergency personnel (Giupponi et al., 2019; National Institute for Mental Health in England, 2006), and can trigger an imitation or contagion effect (known as the "Werther effect"), especially when the media reports in detail on the location or characteristics of the critical site (Marzano et al., 2025). In addition to the human consequences, these episodes have economic, legal, and logistical repercussions for the institutions responsible (Jain et al., 2024).

According to Merli and Costanza (2024), the percentage of suicides occurring at such locations varies with the context. For example, jumping from a great height accounts for fewer than 10% of total suicides, although this figure can increase substantially in places with easy access. Studies conducted at specific locations in New York found that the percentage increased to 24%; in Hong Kong, to 45%; in Singapore, to 60%; and in San Francisco, to 70%. Recently, Shin et al. (2025), in an analysis of 42,656 suicide cases, noted that 25.2% had occurred in public places.

Prevention strategies at critical sites have been based on four strategic axes (Cox et al., 2013; Joyner et al., 2025; Owens et al., 2009): (a) restricting access to lethal means through physical barriers that block access to the critical site, nets to cushion and/or prevent falls, or platform doors that open only to allow access to trains; (b) facilitating third-party intervention through surveillance, patrols, or security cameras; (c) encouraging people to seek help through crisis hotlines or preventive signage that may deter suicidal intent; and (d) responsible communication, promoting a responsible change in narrative in the coverage of suicide.

Scientific evidence supports the effectiveness of these interventions. Systematic review studies and meta-analyses (LeFevre, 2014; Too et al., 2025) indicate that measures to restrict access to lethal methods can reduce suicide deaths by up to 91–93%; in certain cases, implementing barriers has even eliminated cases entirely. These figures are supported by confirmation that people who wish to die by suicide but encounter restrictions at their chosen location do not repeat the attempt elsewhere (Cox et al., 2013; Pirkis et al., 2015; Too et al., 2025). An example of a critical site in the United States is the Golden Gate Bridge in San Francisco, where the installation of preventive nets reduced suicides by more than 80% (Mackenzie et al., 2016). At elevated sites in Switzerland, the placement of barriers achieved a 69% reduction and that of nets a 77% reduction (Hemmer et al., 2017). In Asia,

https://doi.org/10.3390/bs16010007

doors at train platforms have been shown to reduce suicides by 76% in Japan (Ueda et al., 2015), 89% in South Korea (Chung et al., 2016), and 91% in China (Xing et al., 2019).

Consistent with this evidence, a recent umbrella review (Nevarez-Flores et al., 2025) that integrated 12 international systematic reviews concluded that means restriction strategies are an empirically proven and effective measure for suicide prevention globally. The results indicate that the greatest effectiveness is achieved when interventions are adapted to the most prevalent methods of suicide and the local sociocultural context, minimizing the likelihood of method substitution.

Likewise, significant decreases of 50–61% have been observed through the installation of signage promoting help, and decreases of 47% have followed interventions that increase the likelihood of detection and intervention by third parties (Pirkis et al., 2015).

Furthermore, economic cost-effectiveness assessments of these measures have found them to be profitable investments. Bandara et al. (2022) estimated that installing barriers on bridges in Australia yielded a return of US $2.40 for every US dollar invested over a ten-year period. The evidence was less consistent in the case of cliffs, reinforcing the need for further research in this area.

In Spain, the first Suicide Prevention Action Plan was published in 2025 (Comisionado de Salud Mental, Ministerio de Sanidad, 2025). It considers key preventive strategies to include intensifying measures that limit access to lethal methods, identifying and acting on "critical sites," and improving the design of public spaces to increase safety, along with other measures already initiated years ago, such as strengthening control over the acquisition of toxic substances and the possession of weapons (in collaboration with the Spanish Medicines Ag2015 is changedency and the Ministry of the Interior). However, to date, there are no national publications analyzing the cost-effectiveness of such measures, despite the fact that some locations are socially recognized for their high incidence of suicide. One possible reason may be the scarcity of data on the exact locations of suicide deaths, a relevant factor for social and health policy planning.

In this context, based on the relevance of studying "hotspots" and the lack of available data for the strategic planning of preventive actions, this study was carried out within the framework of a collaboration between the Castilla-La Mancha Health Service and the Institutes of Legal Medicine and Forensic Sciences (IMLCF), as well as several universities in the region and neighboring areas. The primary objective is to analyze suicides recorded between 2020 and 2024 in the provinces of Toledo and Albacete in order to ascertain the geographical distribution of critical sites, whether concentrated in public places (such as elevated infrastructure, natural environments, or transportation areas in Spain) or in private spaces, and to reveal associated sociodemographic characteristics that allow for the adoption of specific prevention strategies. The secondary objective is to identify possible critical sites and propose preventive measures adapted to the local contexts, based on available scientific evidence.

2. Materials and Methods

2.1. Study Design

This observational, descriptive, and retrospective study examines suicides that occurred in two provinces of the Autonomous Community of Castilla-La Mancha, Toledo and Albacete, during the period spanning 2020 to 2024. Data collection was carried out by IMLCF professionals in these provinces through the systematic analysis of records and the study of individual case files, allowing for a comprehensive reconstruction of each event.

https://doi.org/10.3390/bs16010007

2.2. Participants and Scope

The data available in the forensic archives of the IMLCF of Toledo and Albacete, collected during the medico-legal investigations of deaths by suicide between 2020 and 2024, were analyzed. Data from the provinces of Guadalajara, Ciudad Real, and Cuenca were not considered because of diminished accessibility due to differences in registration.

2.3. Study Variables

For each case identified, the following variables were recorded: date of the event (day, month, year); municipality and province; age (in years); sex (male, female, other); place of death; method used; prevention method suggested as likely to be effective (based on the suggestions provided by Too et al., 2025); and other relevant circumstances (qualitative and descriptive information collected to facilitate the identification and classification of locations).

In the case of places of death, data collection used a coded classification based on the situations most frequently reported in the literature, with researchers providing qualitative information that allowed for the identification of high-incidence sites (such as place names). The categories for this variable were: 1. bridge; 2. cliff; 3. tall public building (upper floors or roof); 4. train/subway station or railroad tracks at a location other than a station (differentiated in observations); 5. field; 6. forest; 7. road or path; 8. river/reservoir/lake; 9. public building (interior); 10. other; 11. place not classifiable as a "hotspot" due to being a private space or residence (with observations differentiating between residences, workplaces, and jumps from a residence to a public road). In relation to this last category, to facilitate the researchers´ classification task, several additional criteria were provided for those places that, in contrast, would be "classifiable as critical sites" (Owens et al., 2015; Pirkis et al., 2015; Too et al., 2024), specifically: 1. having public or semi-public access (as opposed to a private residence or workplace); 2. offering access to a highly lethal method (e.g., bridges or other elevated infrastructure, railroad tracks, deep bodies of water, cliffs, or high-speed roads); and 3. being sufficiently isolated to hinder early intervention.

In a second step, after this initial classification, those places "classifiable as critical sites" were considered actual critical sites only if they met the most common definition found in the literature (Bandara et al., 2022), which is those places where more than one suicide had been documented within a 5-year reference period.

Classification of methods chosen followed a standardized typology based on the behaviors most frequently used to die by suicide, namely: 1. jumping from a height; 2. hanging/strangulation/suffocation; 3. firearm; 4. poisoning by drugs or chemicals; 5. inhalation of carbon monoxide or gases; 6. drowning; 7. burns/self-immolation; 8. cutting or sharp weapon; 9. collision with a moving vehicle; 10. electrocution; 11. other.

2.4. Data Analysis

Descriptive analyses were performed to obtain the mean and range of the continuous quantitative variable in the study (age), as well as the absolute and relative frequencies (percentages) of the nominal qualitative variables: sex, province, classification of the location as a critical site, location, and method. The descriptive analysis was both performed for the total sample and stratified by province (Toledo/Albacete) and by type of site (classifiable as critical or not).

For the analysis of association between variables, the age variable was recoded according to age ranges based on the minimum and maximum values observed. The following categories were defined: adolescence (15–17 years), emerging adulthood (18–29 years), young adulthood (30–44 years), middle adulthood (45–59 years), older adulthood (60–74 years), and old age ($\geq$75 years).

https://doi.org/10.3390/bs16010007

3. Results

The analysis included 421 cases of suicide recorded from 2020 through 2024, with a mean age of 56.68 years (SD = 18.34), and a range between 15 and 97 years. Men accounted for 82.4% of cases, and more than half (64.4%) of the cases occurred in the province of Toledo. In both Toledo and Albacete, a higher proportion of men than of women was observed (Toledo: 84.5%; Albacete: 78.7%). The predominant age group was middle adulthood (45–59 years), with 34.7% in Toledo and 38.7% in Albacete.

The most frequent location, chosen in 9% of cases, was the countryside, followed by high places (bridges, cliffs, tall buildings), which accounted for 8.2%, and public buildings, at 4.8%.

As for method, hanging was the most frequent (56.1%), followed by jumping (16.6%) and ingesting drugs or chemicals (9.7%).

The years with the fewest cases were 2020 (76 cases) and 2024 (78 cases), while the highest numbers were recorded in 2022 (93 cases) and 2023 (89 cases). In seasonal terms, 56.1% of cases in Toledo and 61.4% in Albacete occurred during spring and summer.

Overall, 74.3% of the suicides analyzed occurred at public locations, and with regard to locations that could possibly be classified as critical sites, there were only two cases of location coincidence, i.e., of two or more cases occurring at the same location during the five-year period analyzed. Therefore, only one critical site was found during this period, specifically in the province of Toledo.

Table 1 presents the data cross-tabulated between the variables of location and method, using slashes (/) to differentiate between the provinces of Toledo and Albacete.

Table 1. Cross-tabulation by province of the variables *location* and *method* (Toledo = 271; Albacete = 150).

	Method									
Location	**Jumping**	**Hanging**	**Firearm**	**Poisoning**	**Inhalation**	**Drowning**	**Stabbing**	**Vehicle Collision**	**Total Toledo/Albacete**	**Total**
Bridge	5/4	1/0	0/0	0/0	0/0	0/0	0/0	0/0	6/4	10
Cliff	1/3	0/0	0/0	0/0	0/0	0/0	0/0	0/0	1/3	4
High-rise building	12	0/0	0/0	0/0	0/0	0/0	0/0	0/0	12/0	12
Field	1/0	12/14	1/2	1/0	1/0	0/0	0/0	6/0	22/16	38
Forest	0/0	1/1	2/1	0/0	0/0	0/0	0/0	0/0	3/2	5
Highway or road	3/0	5/2	2	1/0	0/0	0/0	1/0	3/1	15/3	18
River, reservoir	0/0	0/0	0/0	0/0	0/0	5/0	0/0	0/0	5/0	5
Public building (interior)	5/1	7/1	1/1	3/0	0/0	0/0	1/0	0/0	17/3	20
Other	0/0	9/3	0/0	1/0	0/0	0/1	1/0	0/0	11/4	15
Not classifiable as critical site	6/29	125/55	15/9	21/14	3/2	0/3	9/3	0/0	179/115	294
Totals	33/37	160/76	21/13	27/14	4/2	5/4	12/4	9/1	271/150	421

Note: The absolute numbers of cases per cell are indicated.

Of the 108 cases that occurred in public places, 10.2% (11 cases) involved women, with the province of Toledo being more highly represented (at 67.6%) than Albacete, where the preponderance of cases occurred in the private sphere.

Figures 1 and 2 show that the predominant age group was middle adulthood (45–59 years) for both men and women. The most commonly used method for men was hanging (46 cases), followed by jumping from a height (21) and firearms (9). For women, it was jumping from a height (4), hanging (4), then poisoning (2) and drowning (1). Thus, the method used varied by sex: women did not use collision with a vehicle, a knife, a firearm, or inhalation of monoxide.

https://doi.org/10.3390/bs16010007

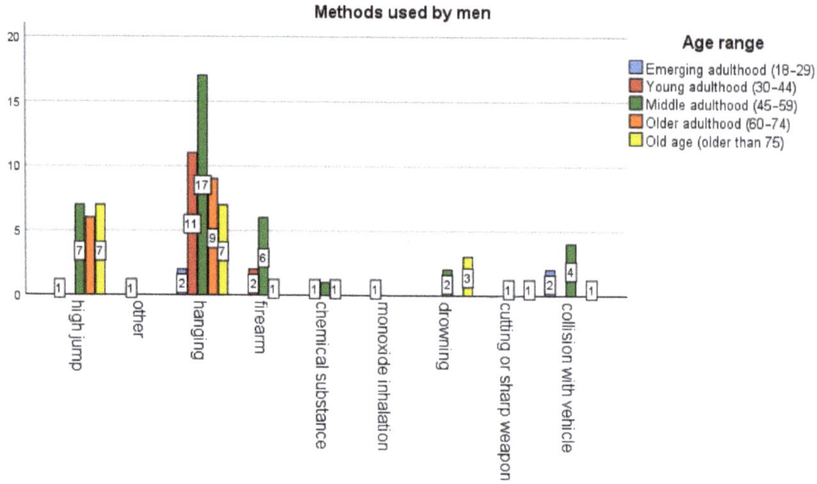

Figure 1. Number of cases involving men (n = 97) at public locations classifiable as critical sites. Analysis by age range and method.

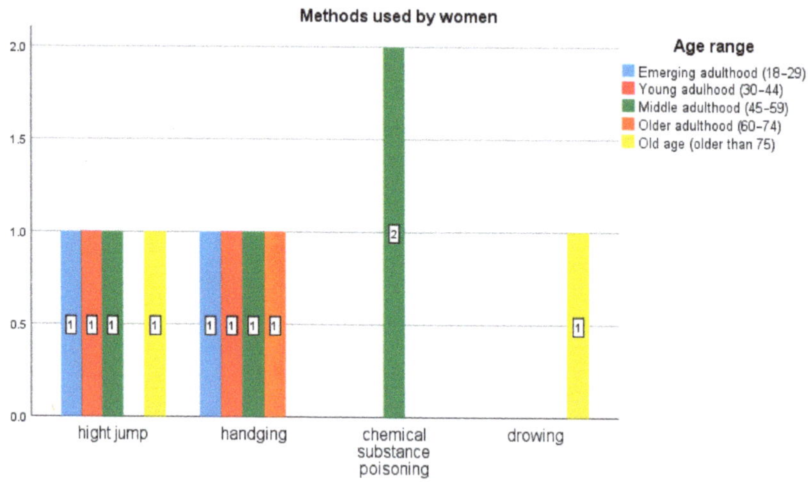

Figure 2. Number of cases involving women (n = 11) at public locations classifiable as critical sites. Analysis by age range and method.

In terms of location (Figures 3 and 4), men died by suicide more frequently in rural or transit areas (fields, highways, roads) and public buildings, while women did not choose locations such as forests or rivers. Specifically, in the case of men, the locations chosen were countryside (29 cases), highway or road (15), public building (18), bridge (9), forest (5), river or lake (5). In contrast, women made a wider variety of choices (while avoiding forests and rivers): countryside (3), road (2), public building (2), bridge (1), cliff (1), tall building (1), and other (1).

 https://doi.org/10.3390/bs16010007

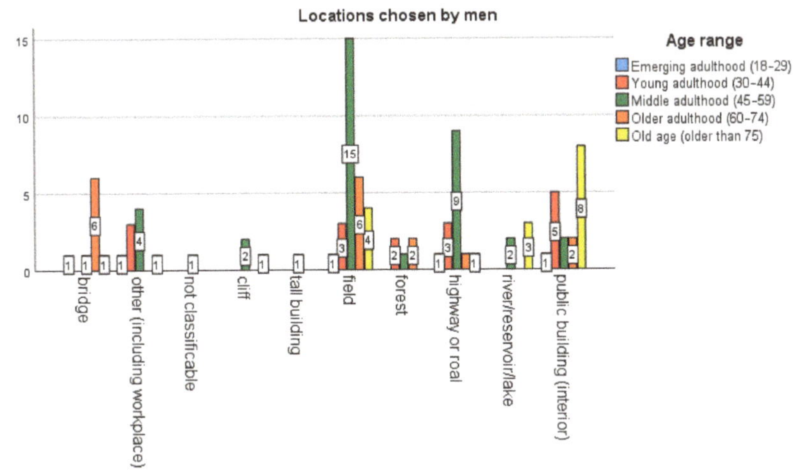

Figure 3. Number of cases involving men (n = 97) at public sites classifiable as critical. Analysis by age range and method.

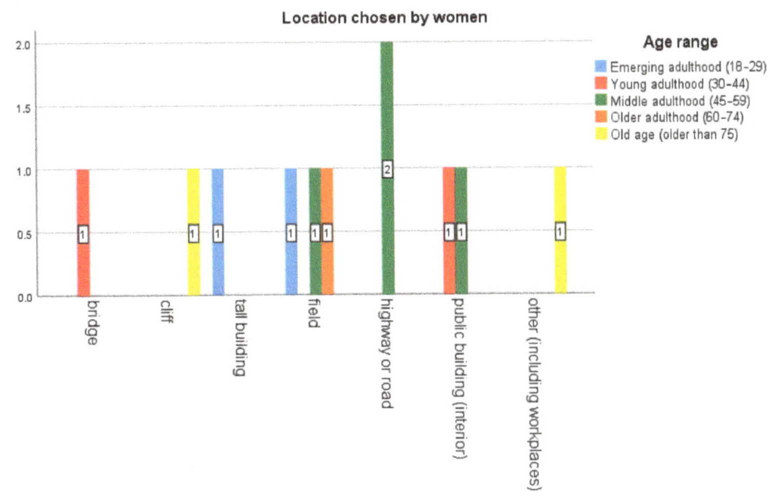

Figure 4. Number of cases involving women (n = 11) at sites classified as critical. Analysis by age range and method.

4. Discussion

The main objective of this study was to identify and characterize suicide locations in the provinces of Toledo and Albacete from 2020 through 2024, with the aim of identifying possible critical sites. Suicides in public places may be more easily preventable than those occurring at home, due to greater potential for observation and intervention. In addition, sociodemographic and contextual characteristics were analyzed, mainly age, sex, date, and method used, in order to generate empirical evidence that contributes to guiding prevention strategies adapted to the regional context of Castilla-La Mancha. Analysis of the sample in this study, with 421 cases, confirmed the existence of differential patterns based on sex, location, method, and seasonality.

In terms of gender, there was a clear male predominance (82%), with a male/female ratio of 5:1, which exceeds the most prevalent ratios of 3:1, not only in Spain, but also in the

https://doi.org/10.3390/bs16010007

European context and in high-income countries in general (GBD 2021 Suicide Collaborators, 2025; World Health Organization, 2025). This finding could be related to specific sociocultural and economic factors in the region, such as greater access to lethal or more violent methods among men, which would make them more vulnerable to dying by suicide, or the persistence of traditional gender roles that make it difficult for men to express emotional vulnerability and seek help (Simion & Jung, 2025).

With regard to age, the average age of deceased persons was 56.6 years, with a wide range from 15 to 97 years. The most highly represented age group, in raw numbers, corresponds to middle adulthood (45–59 years), followed by older adulthood (60–74 years). This pattern coincides with the national trend, where suicide mortality peaks between the ages of 45 and 60, especially among men (National Institute of Statistics [INE], 2024; World Health Organization, 2025). At these ages, vulnerability factors such as unemployment, chronic illness, social isolation, and loss of family and work roles converge (Zalsman et al., 2016). However, when age-adjusted suicide rates are considered instead of crude (absolute) numbers, international studies indicate that the highest rates are found in the population over 70 years of age (GBD 2021 Suicide Collaborators, 2025). Taken together, the results point to the need to design specific prevention strategies for middle-aged and older men in rural or semi-urban contexts, a group with high vulnerability due to a combination of personal and structural risk factors that increase the lethality of suicide attempts (Nevarez-Flores et al., 2025; Shin et al., 2025).

Of the methods used, hanging/strangulation/suffocation was chosen most frequently (56.1%), followed by jumping from a height (16.6%) and poisoning by drugs or chemicals (9.7%), which is consistent with previous studies conducted in similar contexts (GBD 2021 Suicide Collaborators, 2025). Most locations where suicides occurred were homes and private spaces, which cannot be classified as hotspots. As for other locations, a higher concentration of cases was observed in rural and semi-urban areas, especially in Toledo. In Albacete, no cases were recorded on railway tracks. The geographical configuration of Castilla-La Mancha, characterized by large rural expanses and a scarcity of urban infrastructure such as high-rise buildings, favors the occurrence of suicides on bridges and viaducts and in reservoirs and rivers, highlighting the need for adapted preventive measures such as barriers, surveillance in isolated spaces, and signage at critical sites. In any case, the figures highlight the importance of the home and private sphere as the predominant setting for recorded suicides.

The analysis of public places identified a single critical site, located in Toledo, on a high bridge associated with notable symbolism and recognized by the local population, where the main method of suicide is jumping. The interview with the forensic professional overseeing the study indicated that, due to structural and financial constraints and the extensive size of the area, the installation of full barriers may not be feasible. Nonetheless, effective alternatives exist, such as deterrent signage or the provision of helpline phones. Indeed, various authors point out that preventive measures need not completely prevent access to lethal means as partial barriers can also have a deterrent effect (Salgado, 2015).

To the best of our knowledge, this is the first study in Spain to apply a systematic, location-based methodology to identify high-risk suicide locations in public settings, using data from two provinces as a foundation for future nationwide research.

Based on the concentrations of cases in elevated infrastructure and public access spaces, the authors of this study recommend that the installation of physical barriers be considered a priority strategy for suicide prevention that cannot be postponed, as there is strong evidence that restricting access to hazardous sites is associated with a decrease in suicide and is therefore a key strategy that should be integrated into various public policies (Zalsman et al., 2016). The installation of such barriers should be accompanied by

https://doi.org/10.3390/bs16010007

complementary interventions, especially in contexts where complete barrier installation is not feasible. Complementary interventions that can maximize the preventive impact include signage with help resources, crisis hotlines, and/or surveillance systems (Pirkis et al., 2015). Although initial cost and esthetic objections are often presented as obstacles, the benefits in terms of reducing deaths (over 90% in many cases) amply justify their implementation and maintenance as a public health measure.

With regard to recorded data on suicide, various authors highlight the importance of forensic sources in improving the quality of information and reducing the underestimation of cases (Barbería et al., 2018; Giner & Guija, 2014; Santurtún et al., 2016). In Spain, the National Statistics Institute (INE), under a collaboration agreement established for this purpose with the Institutes of Legal Medicine and Forensic Sciences (IMLCF) to directly incorporate causes of death from judicial sources, provides detailed annual information on deaths by suicide, including variables such as sex, age, place of residence, month of death, and the suicide method used. This agreement arose from the need to improve data on judicial deaths which, although representing a small percentage of total deaths, include certain causes that are preventable and affect all age groups, such as completed suicides.

This study has some limitations. First, the data analyzed include only completed suicides, excluding non-fatal attempts recorded by emergency or health services, which limits overall understanding of the problem. It would be advisable to promote the integration of data from the IMLCF records with other relevant sources (emergency services, hospital records, mental health professionals, police forces) in order to obtain a more complete picture that includes both completed suicides and non-fatal attempts. In general, establishing channels for inter-institutional collaboration (involving, e.g., health, justice, social services, or education) would facilitate the implementation of prevention policies based on scientific evidence.

Second, the available information is derived from administrative records whose completeness may vary depending on the quality of reporting and on the coding process, which may introduce biases. For the purpose of conducting more robust interprovincial comparative studies and extrapolations, it would be appropriate to propose that, in the case of records of completed suicides compiled by the Institutes of Legal Medicine and Forensic Sciences and provided to the National Statistics Institute (INE), the variable "place of occurrence" be incorporated in addition to the current variables of sex, age, date, and method of death. This inclusion would be consistent with the data already collected for natural deaths documented by forensic physicians (e.g., public space, residence, workplace, among others), with the aim of identifying critical points or areas of higher incidence (Consejo Médico Forense, 2024).

For future research, it will be essential to extend the analysis to all five provinces of Castilla-La Mancha and to adopt longer observation periods, as this would provide a more complete regional overview and allow meaningful comparisons across territories. The present study was limited to the provinces of Toledo and Albacete due to differences in forensic and healthcare data registration systems, a constraint that underscores the need for greater harmonization of data collection procedures across institutions. Addressing these disparities would reduce selection bias and improve the generalizability of future findings. At the same time, information on non-fatal suicide attempts recorded by emergency and health services should be incorporated into future studies to provide a more comprehensive approach to the phenomenon of suicide. It would also be relevant to incorporate contextual and socioeconomic variables, such as unemployment, education level, rural or urban setting, and accessibility of mental health services, with the aim of exploring possible associations with the critical sites identified, in line with other international studies. Another aspect that has been little researched relates to the impact of the media on the amplification of suicide,

https://doi.org/10.3390/bs16010007

especially at these critical sites, and the potential for managing that impact as a preventive measure (García-Fernández et al., 2024). Also under-researched is the influence of urban design, including the creation of green spaces and facilitators of interpersonal relationships (Barboza-Salerno et al., 2025; Shen et al., 2022). Finally, the development of longitudinal studies will permit analysis of the temporal evolution of these concentrations and a more accurate assessment of the impact of any preventive measures implemented.

Author Contributions: Conceptualization, B.V.-S., V.M. and M.C.; Methodology, B.V.-S., N.S.-P., and A.H.-D.A.; Investigation, V.M., M.C., F.M., and C.A.; Data Curation, B.V.-S.; Formal Analysis, N.S.-P.; Writing—Original Draft Preparation, B.V.-S., N.S.-P., and A.H.-D.A.; Writing—Review & Editing, B.V.-S., N.S.-P., and A.H.-D.A.; Project Administration & Supervision, B.V.-S. All authors have read and agreed to the published version of the manuscript.

Funding: No funding was received for this research.

Institutional Review Board Statement: Ethical review and approval were waived for this study due to its retrospective design based exclusively on the analysis of anonymized forensic and administrative records from deceased individuals, with no involvement of human participants, no collection of identifiable personal data, and no use of biological samples. In accordance with Regulation (EU) 2016/679 (GDPR, Recital 27), Spanish Organic Law 3/2018 on the Protection of Personal Data and Guarantee of Digital Rights, and Spanish Law 14/2007 on Biomedical Research, studies using fully anonymized data from deceased persons for research purposes do not require approval by an Institutional Review Board or Ethics Committee.

Informed Consent Statement: The study involved the analysis of forensic and registry data from deceased individuals who died by suicide. According to Spanish legislation (Organic Law 3/2018 on the Protection of Personal Data and Guarantee of Digital Rights) and European Regulation (EU) 2016/679 (GDPR), informed consent is not required for the use of anonymized data of deceased persons for research purposes. The study adhered to the ethical principles of the Declaration of Helsinki and the national guidelines for biomedical research.

Data Availability Statement: The data that support the findings of this study are available from the corresponding author upon reasonable request, in compliance with ethical guidelines and participant confidentiality.

Acknowledgments: The author acknowledges the support of the Institute of Legal Medicine, Castilla-La Mancha, in the form of access to patient records. During the preparation of this work, the authors used an AI language model developed by OpenAI for writing assistance. After using this service, the authors reviewed and edited the content as needed and take full responsibility for the content of the publication.

Conflicts of Interest: The authors declare no conflicts of interest.

References

Bandara, P., Pirkis, J., Clapperton, A., Shin, S., Too, L. S., Reifels, L., Onie, S., Page, A., Andriessen, K., Krysinska, K., Flego, A., Schlichthorst, M., Spittal, M. J., Mihalopoulos, C., & Le, L. K. (2022). Cost-effectiveness of installing barriers at bridge and cliff sites for suicide prevention in Australia. *JAMA Network Open, 5*(4), e226019. [CrossRef]

Barbería, E., Gispert, R., Gallo, B., Ribas, G., Puigdefàbregas, A., Freitas, A., Segú, E., Torralba, P., García-Sayago, F., & Estarellas, A. (2018). Improving suicide mortality statistics in Tarragona (Catalonia, Spain) between 2004–2012. *Journal of Psychiatry and Mental Health, 11*(4), 227–233. [CrossRef]

Barboza-Salerno, G. E., Watson-Grace, A., Shockley-McCarthy, K., Harrington, T., Warren, K., & Steelesmith, D. (2025). The land cover paradox: Characteristics of blue- and green spaces within and beyond high-risk suicide clusters. *SSM—Population Health, 31*, 101820. [CrossRef]

Chung, Y. W., Kang, S. J., Matsubayashi, T., Sawada, Y., & Ueda, M. (2016). The effectiveness of platform screen doors for the prevention of subway suicides in South Korea. *Journal of Affective Disorders, 194*, 80–83. [CrossRef]

https://doi.org/10.3390/bs16010007

Comisionado de Salud Mental, Ministerio de Sanidad. (2025). *Plan de Acción para la Prevención del Suicidio 2025–2027 [Action plan for suicide prevention 2025–2027]*. Gobierno de España. Available online: https://www.sanidad.gob.es/gabinete/notasPrensa.do?id=6618 (accessed on 15 September 2025).

Consejo Médico Forense. (2024). *Informe sobre mortalidad con intervención judicial. 2022*. Ministerio de la Presidencia, Justicia y Relaciones con las Cortes, Gobierno de España.

Cox, G. R., Owens, C., Robinson, J., Nicholas, A., Lockley, A., Williamson, M., Cheung, Y. T., & Pirkis, J. (2013). Interventions to reduce suicides at suicide hotspots: A systematic review. *BMC Public Health, 13*, 214. [CrossRef]

García-Fernández, D., Marcos del Cano, A. M., & Topa, G. (2024). Suicide and public interest in the Spanish press: Theoretical analysis from the constitutional jurisprudence on freedom of information. *SEECI Communication Journal, 57*, 1–33. [CrossRef]

GBD 2021 Suicide Collaborators. (2025). Global, regional, and national burden of suicide, 1990–2021: A systematic analysis for the Global Burden of Disease Study 2021. *The Lancet Public Health, 10*(3), e189–e202. [CrossRef]

Giner, L., & Guija, J. A. (2014). Número de suicidios en España: Diferencias entre los datos del Instituto Nacional de Estadística y los aportados por los Institutos de Medicina Legal [Number of suicides in Spain: Differences between data from the Spanish Statistical Office and the Institutes of Legal Medicine]. *Revista de Psiquiatría y Salud Mental, 7*(3), 139–146. [CrossRef] [PubMed]

Giupponi, G., Thoma, H., Lamis, D., Forte, A., Pompili, M., & Kapfhammer, H. P. (2019). Posttraumatic stress reactions of underground drivers after suicides by jumping to arriving trains; feasibility of an early stepped care outpatient intervention. *Journal of Trauma & Dissociation, 20*(5), 495–510. [CrossRef] [PubMed]

Hemmer, A., Meier, P., & Reisch, T. (2017). Comparing different suicide prevention measures at bridges and buildings: Lessons we have learned from a national survey in Switzerland. *PLoS ONE, 12*(1), e0169625. [CrossRef] [PubMed]

Jain, N., Wijnen, B., Lohumi, I., Chatterjee, S., & Evers, S. M. A. A. (2024). Economic burden of suicides and suicide attempts in low- and middle-income countries: A systematic review of costing studies. *Expert Review of Pharmacoeconomics & Outcomes Research, 24*(9), 1067–1079. [CrossRef]

Joyner, L., Mackenzie, J. M., Willis, A., Phillips, P., Cliffe, B., Marsh, I., Pettersen, E., Hawton, K., & Marzano, L. (2025). Suicide prevention measures at high-risk locations: A goal-directed motivation perspective. *Behavioral Sciences, 15*(8), 1009. [CrossRef] [PubMed]

LeFevre, M. L. (2014). Screening for suicide risk in adolescents, adults, and older adults in primary care: US Preventive Services Task Force recommendation statement. *Annals of Internal Medicine, 160*(10), 719–726. [CrossRef]

Mackenzie, D. W., Lester, D., Manson, R., & Yeh, C. (2016). Do suicides from the Golden Gate Bridge cluster? *Psychological Reports, 118*(1), 70–73. [CrossRef]

Marzano, L., Spence, R., Marsh, I., Barbin, A., & Kruger, I. (2025). How does news coverage of suicide affect suicidal behavior at a high-frequency location? A 7-year time series analysis. *BMJ Public Health, 3*(1), e002136. [CrossRef] [PubMed]

Merli, R., & Costanza, A. (2024). Effectiveness of physical barriers to prevent suicide by jumping from high-risk bridges: From an integrative review to a northern Italian province's paradigm. *Preventive Medicine Reports, 42*, 102745. [CrossRef]

National Institute for Mental Health in England. (2006). *Guidance on action to be taken at suicide hotspots*. Available online: https://sprc.org/wp-content/uploads/2023/01/SuicideHotspotsGuidance-PDF.pdf (accessed on 15 September 2025).

National Institute of Statistics [INE]. (2024). *Deaths by cause of death. Year 2023*. Available online: https://www.ine.es (accessed on 15 September 2025).

Nevarez-Flores, A. G., Pandey, V., Angelucci, A. P., Neil, A. L., McDermott, B., & Castle, D. (2025). Means restriction for suicide prevention: An umbrella review. *Acta Psychiatrica Scandinavica, 151*(6), 653–667. [CrossRef] [PubMed]

Owens, C., Hardwick, R. J. L., Charles, N., & Watkinson, G. (2015). *Preventing suicides in public places: A practice resource*. Available online: https://assets.publishing.service.gov.uk/media/5c2f6f8b40f0b66cf8298a70/Preventing_suicides_in_public_places.pdf (accessed on 15 September 2025).

Owens, C., Lloyd-Tomlins, S., Emmens, T., & Aitken, P. (2009). Suicides in public places: Findings from one English county. *European Journal of Public Health, 19*(6), 580–582. [CrossRef]

Pirkis, J., Too, L. S., Spittal, M. J., Krysinska, K., Robinson, J., & Cheung, Y. T. (2015). Interventions to reduce suicides at suicide hotspots: A systematic review and meta-analysis. *The Lancet Psychiatry, 2*(11), 994–1001. [CrossRef]

Salgado, P. (2015, August 12). These are some of the places marked by suicide in Spain. *Vice*. Available online: https://www.vice.com/es/article/algunos-de-los-lugares-marcados-por-el-suicidio-en-espana-924/ (accessed on 15 September 2025).

Santurtún, M., Santurtún, A., Agudo, G., & Zarrabeitia, M. T. (2016). Method used in suicide deaths in Spain: Poisoning and non-toxic violent agents. *Cuadernos de Medicina Forense, 22*(3–4), 73–80. Available online: http://scielo.isciii.es/scielo.php?script=sci_arttext&pid=S1135-76062016000200003&lng=es&tlng=es (accessed on 22 October 2025).

Shen, Y. S., Lung, S.-C. C., & Cui, S. (2022). Exploring multiple pathways and mediation effects of urban environmental factors for suicide prevention. *Environmental Pollution, 294*, 118642. [CrossRef]

https://doi.org/10.3390/bs16010007

Shin, S., Spittal, M. J., Clapperton, A., Pirkis, J., & Too, L. S. (2025). Trends in, and risk factors for, suicide in public places: A 17-year case-control study in Australia. *Suicide & Life-threatening Behavior*, *55*(2), e70017. [CrossRef]

Simina-Petra Simion, S.-O., & Jung, H. (2025). Gender disparities in suicide: A deeper look into the complexity of suicidal acts. *Legal Medicine*, *77*, 102679. [CrossRef] [PubMed]

Too, L. S., Shin, S., Mavoa, S., Law, P. C. F., Clapperton, A., Roberts, L., Arensman, E., Spittal, M. J., & Pirkis, J. (2024). High-risk suicide locations in Australia. *JAMA Network Open*, *7*(6), e2417770. [CrossRef] [PubMed]

Too, L. S., Shin, S., Taouk, Y., Pirkis, J., Sinyor, M., Yip, P. S. F., & Hawton, K. (2025). Impact of interventions at frequently used suicide locations on occurrence of suicides at other sites: A systematic review and meta-analysis. *Psychological Medicine*, *55*, E168. [CrossRef] [PubMed]

Ueda, M., Sawada, Y., & Matsubayashi, T. (2015). The effectiveness of installing physical barriers for preventing railway suicides and accidents: Evidence from Japan. *Journal of Affective Disorders*, *178*, 1–4. [CrossRef]

World Health Organization. (2025). *Suicide 2021*. Available online: https://www.who.int/news-room/fact-sheets/detail/suicide (accessed on 20 September 2025).

Xing, Y., Lu, J., & Chen, S. (2019). Evaluating the effectiveness of platform screen doors for preventing metro suicides in China. *Journal of Affective Disorders*, *253*, 63–68. [CrossRef]

Zalsman, G., Hawton, K., Wasserman, D., van Heeringen, K., Arensman, E., Sarchiapone, M., Carli, V., Höschl, C., Barzilay, R., Balazs, J., Purebl, G., Kahn, J. P., Sáiz, P. A., Lipsicas, C. B., Bobes, J., Cozman, D., Hegerl, U., & Zohar, J. (2016). Suicide prevention strategies revisited: 10-year systematic review. *The Lancet Psychiatry*, *3*(7), 646–659. [CrossRef]

 https://doi.org/10.3390/bs16010007

behavioral sciences

MDPI

Article

From Pressure to Peril: Investigating the Drivers of Suicide Planning and Attempts in University Students Struggling with Academic Anxiety

Gulzar H. Shah [1,*], Masha Asad Khan [2], Maham Muzamil [3] and Mahira Ahmed [2]

1 Jiann-Ping Hsu College of Public Health, Georgia Southern University, Statesboro, GA 30460, USA
2 Department of Psychology, Kinnaird College for Women, Lahore 54000, Pakistan; masha.khan@kinnaird.edu.pk (M.A.K.); mahira.ahmed@kinnaird.edu.pk (M.A.)
3 Department of Education, Kinnaird College for Women, Lahore 54000, Pakistan; maham.muzamil@kinnaird.edu.pk
* Correspondence: gshah@georgiasouthern.edu

Abstract

Self-harm is a growing public health concern, particularly among university students facing academic anxiety. This study explored the underlying factors driving suicide planning and attempts in this population. Using a qualitative design, we conducted thematic analysis of interviews with eight counselors and eight students from five public and private universities. Analysis via NVivo Software revealed six core themes: (1) current mental health support and coping strategies, (2) triggers of suicidal ideation linked to family and psychological stressors, (3) perceptions of campus mental health services, (4) cultural and societal misconceptions surrounding suicide, (5) institutional barriers to accessing mental health care, and (6) student-driven recommendations for prevention and support. These findings highlight the complex interplay between academic pressure, emotional distress, and limited institutional support. The study emphasizes the need for universities to enhance access to mental health services, reduce stigma through open dialogue and peer support, and engage families through targeted workshops. Tailored interventions addressing academic, emotional, and familial challenges—such as flexible deadlines and improved counseling access—can significantly reduce suicidal ideation and promote student well-being.

Keywords: suicidal ideation; self-harm; academic anxiety; coping mechanisms; academic pressure; cultural stigma; mental health support; student well-being

1. Introduction

Globally, university students' suicidal tendencies are becoming a serious public health issue. Students are more likely to experience mental health issues, such as suicidal thoughts and behaviors, as a result of the transition from adolescence to adulthood and the academic, social, and personal pressures of university life (Lumivero, 2024; Lipson et al., 2022). The diathesis–stress model provides a valuable framework, suggesting that individual vulnerabilities, such as cognitive biases, impulsivity, or prior mental health issues, interact with environmental stresses like academic demand to increase the risk of suicidal ideation. Suicidal ideation, defined as thoughts of killing or harming oneself, is alarmingly common among the university population and can appear in many forms. These range from brief, passing thoughts to carefully planned intentions (Monroe & Simons, 1991; Landa-Blanco et al., 2024).

Academic pressure is one of the leading causes of mental health difficulties among students. The demanding nature of coursework, frequent examinations, and the pressure to achieve can lead to high levels of stress and anxiety. These factors are closely linked to suicidal ideation (Arria et al., 2021; Eisenberg et al., 2020). Suicidal thoughts and behaviors are prevalent among college students, yet many do not seek help when experiencing a crisis. A survey of over twenty-six thousand undergraduate and graduate students across seventy US colleges found that a substantial proportion reported lifetime or recent suicidal ideation, with academic stress, relationship problems, and emotional distress commonly cited as triggers. Importantly, half of the affected students did not disclose their thoughts or pursue professional support (Drum et al., 2021). This aligns with another research study on student mental health and help-seeking patterns, which found that fifty percent of the students who screened positive for major depressive disorder or anxiety received any mental health services within the past year. Help-seeking behavior was measured as any counseling or psychiatric treatment, and barriers included personal stigma, low perceived need, and limited awareness of services. They found that personal stigma significantly reduced help-seeking, while perceived public stigma showed little impact. Moreover, a substantial treatment gap indicated that many students experiencing mental health issues do not pursue professional help (Hunt & Eisenberg, 2021). A recent 10-year analysis (2007–2017) of 155,026 US college students examined mental health treatment, diagnosis, depressive symptoms, suicidal ideation, and stigma. The study found notable increases in mental health concerns and service utilization alongside a decline in stigma towards seeking help. Despite this improvement, many students with significant symptoms remained untreated. Researchers noted limitations related to self-reported data and survey response bias, highlighting ongoing gaps between mental health needs and service use among students (Jones et al., 2023).

1.1. Academic Stress and Students' Mental Health

Research indicates that students who experience high levels of stress in their academic setting are more susceptible to mental health issues, such as depression and suicidal thoughts (Giancola et al., 2024; Gupta et al., 2024; Gbore & Adebowale, 2023). As they strive for academic success, university students usually struggle with the responsibilities and demands of their educational journey (Gallagher, 2024; T. H. Nguyen et al., 2023; Paredes-Céspedes et al., 2024). On this excursion, some people suffer from extreme academic anxiety, which can set off a domino effect of psychological distress and emotional misery. Given the potential for long-term harm to students' lives in this setting, the threat of suicide becomes a significant concern (Mann, 2003; Muhammad Khir et al., 2024).

The influence of family dynamics and psychological stressors on students' mental health is considered a significant factor. According to Wang and Zhang (2024), having family support significantly reduces the risk of mental health problems, but not having family support can worsen psychological discomfort and have serious consequences, including suicidal thoughts and actions. Psychological discomfort and family problems are frequently associated with psychological triggers, such as panic attacks, self-harm, and hopelessness (M. H. Nguyen et al., 2021; Dobbertin et al., 2024; Mortier et al., 2022). As noted by Drum et al. (2021), the prevalence of suicidal ideation among students reflects profound mental suffering, a deep sense of hopelessness, and the perception that they cannot manage academic demands. Students may feel alone and unsupported due to the stigma associated with mental health concerns and the dearth of candid conversations about emotional health (Corrigan et al., 2024; Urme et al., 2022). Cultural settings can influence students' desire to seek treatment by either helping or impeding the acceptance and support of mental health initiatives (Joiner, 2005).

1.2. Aim of the Current Study

In this study, the authors aim to examine how academic distress contributes to suicidal ideation, planning, and attempts among university students. Specifically, it seeks to explore how psychological, familial, cultural, and institutional factors shape students' experiences with suicidal thoughts and acts. The study also examines how students and university counselors perceive available mental health services, barriers that limit help-seeking, and the kind of support students believe would prevent self-harm. By addressing these questions, the study intends to generate insights that can guide universities in strengthening mental health services.

1.3. From Ideation to Attempt

The occurrence of students thinking about suicidal ideation shows the severity of the mental suffering they go through, indicating a deep sense of hopelessness and a belief that they are unable to handle the demands of academic life (Abualhamael et al., 2024). Given this perspective, individuals usually isolate themselves and plan for suicide, which signifies a significant advancement on the spectrum of suicidal ideation, indicating a final turn towards self-harm and maybe ending one's life (Roberts et al., 2023; Ribeiro et al., 2016; Tang et al., 2024). Suicidal ideation and preparation are essential markers of psychological distress (Diefenbach et al., 2024). Still, the actual act of attempted suicide is a horrific representation of the depths of desperation that college students go through (Heapy et al., 2024; Shaman et al., 2024).

1.4. Prevalence and Severity of Suicide Attempts Among University Students

Among full-time college students aged 18–22, about 0.9% reported suicide attempts in the past year compared with approximately 1.9% among adults of the same groups not enrolled in college (Substance Abuse and Mental Health Services Administration, 2024). Among the broader adult population (all ages), the past-year attempt rate is approximately 0.6% (Centers for Disease Control and Prevention, 2025; Corrigan et al., 2024). The act of causing bodily harm to end life, known as an injurious suicide attempt, embodies the severe outcomes of failing to address academic anxiety and untreated mental health issues (da Conceição et al., 2024). The prevalence of harmful suicide attempts among university students needs immediate interventions to reduce the risk factors that lead to such concerning results (Fadipe et al., 2025; Fauk et al., 2023).

1.5. Barriers to Accessing Mental Health Services

A crucial concern is that mental health services in academic settings are insufficient or unavailable after the initial session (Guenthner et al., 2023). Students frequently report that counseling services are scarce (Li et al., 2025). Therefore, the majority of students suffer a lot due to this lack of mental health care at the university level (Li et al., 2025). Matar et al. (2024) emphasized that students face several obstacles in receiving mental health treatment, such as the scarcity of counselors, ignorance of available services, and the stigma attached to asking for assistance (Steare et al., 2023). These barriers prevent students from receiving the necessary support, which raises the risk of untreated mental health issues, suicidal thoughts, and actions (Walker et al., 2023).

1.6. Limitations of Existing Research

There is an increasing amount of research on suicide ideation and actions among university students. However, there are still many gaps in the precise causes and socio-environmental influences of these problems. Critical characteristics that have been linked to suicidal thoughts in students include sleep quality, social media consumption, self-esteem, and perceived barriers to getting psychiatric treatment (Matar et al., 2024; Mortier et al., 2022). However, rather than delving into students' complex experiences and perspectives, these studies often focus on broad generalizations. In addition, a significant void in the current body of literature is the dearth of qualitative studies that document the actual experiences of students grappling with suicidal ideation and actions. Gaining insight into the individual experiences and unique stressors that students encounter, especially those associated with academic anxiety, can provide a more comprehensive picture of the issue.

1.7. Rationale of Current Study

This study intends to shed light on the underlying causes that drive vulnerable college students from feeling under pressure to the risky verge of planning and attempting suicide by examining the intricate connection between academic distress and suicidal actions. By concentrating on the precise ways that academic demands influence suicidal thoughts and attempts, this study seeks to close this knowledge gap and offer recommendations for improved mental health practices in educational settings. By focusing on how academic pressures influence suicidal ideation and attempts, this research will bridge these gaps to inform customized interventions. The long-term impact will be improved awareness and a lower prevalence of suicidal behaviors in this susceptible group.

2. Materials and Methods

2.1. Research Paradigm

The present study was guided by a constructivist paradigm, which emphasizes that people create meaning through their individual experiences and social interactions. According to this paradigm, individuals' interpretations of their lived experiences shape reality, which is seen as subjective and context-dependent (Creswell, 2008). This paradigm supports the study's goal of examining how people interpret their social and psychological reality in relation to their particular surroundings. To ensure that participants' viewpoints were understood within their individual and cultural settings. The constructivist orientation guided the study's design, data collection, and analysis.

2.2. Research Design and Sampling

The study employed a qualitative research design to analyze data collected from university students and college counselors through open-ended interview guides. The study focuses on university students and counselors from public and private institutions, and draws a purposive sample of 16 participants, comprising eight counselors and eight students from 3 public and private universities. We limited the sample size to eight because of the nature of the study. Since the study was about the sensitive issue of suicidal thoughts and attempts, it initially posed difficulties in participant recruitment. Several students opted out of interviews, citing concerns about sharing their personal experiences due to worries related to research publication and potential stigma. To address this challenge, we requested that the college campus counselors concerned help connect us with willing participants, ensuring they felt supported and at ease throughout the process. Invitations were sent to students recommended by the counselors. Counselors who provided referrals for students also participated as interviewees. To reduce potential selection bias, we ensured that referrals represented a diverse range of student experiences across disciplines, academic years, and levels of distress.

After completing eight thorough interviews, we reached data saturation. The responses began to reveal common themes, and no new significant information emerged. Acknowledging this repetition, we decided to conclude data collection after eight interviews, as qualitative research aims to gain comprehensive insights and depth rather than focus on a large sample size.

2.3. Research Instrument

One research instrument was developed based on open-ended qualitative interview guides. We used two instruments: one for students and one for counselors (Appendix A). The research instrument for students consists of two sections. The first section included questions about students' demographics, including their gender, age, and discipline. The second section included seven questions about the drivers that influence suicide planning and attempts in university students struggling with academic anxiety. The research tool for counselors consists of seven questions on causes of suicidal planning, its trends and frequency among students, with coping interventions, and recommendations. Diathesis Model (Mann, 2003) and Joiner's Interpersonal Theory of Suicide (Joiner, 2005) guided the formulation of inquiries regarding perceived burdensomeness, obstructed belongingness, and coping strategies. The tools were pilot tested with two students and two counselors to assess clarity and contextual relevance. This phase proposed minor alterations in phrasing and sequencing to enhance emotional sensitivity and narrative coherence. Each interview lasted approximately 30 min, enabling participants to convey their experiences and insights. Ethical approval for this study was obtained from the Institutional Review Board (IRB) of Kinnaird University, with the protocol ID KC/ORIC/ERC/2025/004.

2.4. Data Collection Procedure

Given that suicide attempts and planning are sensitive topics, we collected all of the data using Zoom and WhatsApp calls rather than face-to-face interviews. Participants were informed that their responses would be recorded for transparency and accuracy. For privacy's sake, participants were instructed to turn off their cameras. All the data were collected from February to March 2025. We conducted a total of 16 interviews, consisting of eight with students and eight with counselors. After that, the responses began to reveal common themes, and no new significant information emerged. Acknowledging this repetition, we decided to conclude data collection after 16 interviews, as qualitative research aims to gain comprehensive insights and depth rather than focus on a large sample size. Informed consent was obtained from all participants in the study, including parental/guardian consent from participants under 18. The checklist of Consolidated Criteria for Reporting Qualitative Research (COREQ) is included in Appendix B.

2.5. Data Analysis

We used NVivo software version 15 (Lumivero, 2024) for the thematic analysis of the qualitative data employed to synthesize students' perspectives of the drivers influencing their academic anxiety and suicide plans and attempts. NVivo facilitated organizing the data, systematic coding, visualization of thematic connections, and identification of cross-group themes and trends, thereby enhancing analytic rigor and transparency. We used three coding passes: open, coaxial, and selective. Open codes were allocated to all potential themes. Using axial coding, specific thematic codes were selected as subthemes to create a word cloud structure for each more comprehensive subject. Preliminary codes were generated from unprocessed transcripts to facilitate the natural development of themes from participants' narratives. The transcripts were read multiple times before coding to ensure immersion and familiarity. All transcripts were systematically coded and categorized into themes according to the interview guide. Discrepancies were addressed through consensus, leading to the refinement of the codebook. A separate ID was assigned to each participant to maintain confidentiality and anonymity throughout the study. Non-relevant themes and sub-themes were removed using selective coding to reduce the amount of data.

3. Results

Table 1 shows the demographic information of study participants. The study consisted of 16 participants, equally split between students (n = 8) and counselors (n = 8). The students ranged in age from 18 to 27 (three male, five female); they studied a variety of fields, including psychology, education, law, and the social sciences. The counselors ranged in age from 30 to 55 years and were all female; their professional careers included clinical psychology, educational counseling, and student affairs.

Table 1. Participants' Demographics information.

Group	Number (n)	Age Range	Gender	Academic/Professional Background
Students	8	18–27 years	3 Males, 5 females	Psychology, Education, Law, Social Sciences
Counselors	8	30–55 years	All female	Clinical Psychology, Educational Guidance, Student Affairs

The word cloud (Figure 1) depicts the key terms aligning with the constructs from the thematic analysis. For instance, it shows that "support" is a critical factor in preventing or addressing suicidal ideation, as individuals who lack adequate support systems are more likely to experience persistent suicidal impulses.

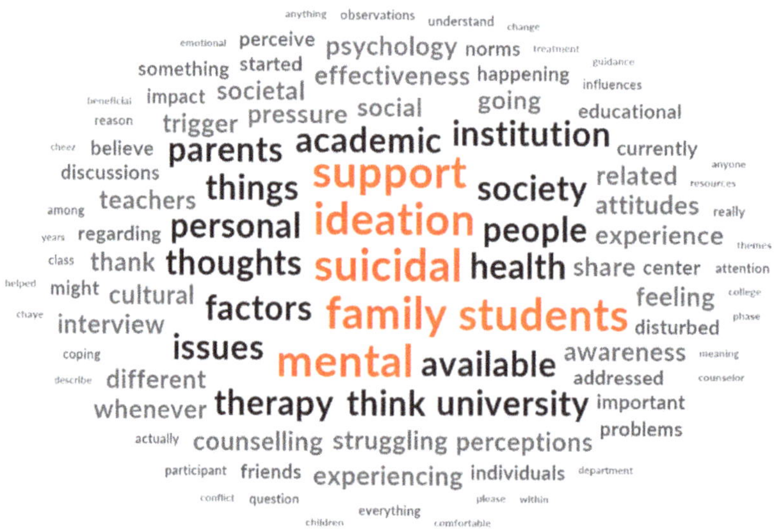

Figure 1. Word cloud representing students' concerns regarding the drivers of suicide planning and attempts.

Our thematic analysis, discussed later, also revealed that both social support networks and accessible mental health services provide emotional stability, mental health support, and prompt intervention, which serve as protective factors. The term "Family" is also prominent in the word cloud. It is supported by the importance of family influences in suicidal ideation, as suicidal tendencies can be significantly influenced by family dynamics, as specific relationships or parental attitudes can either alleviate or intensify emotional distress, as supported by our thematic analysis. Suicidal thoughts can develop or escalate as a result of family environments that are either unsupportive or strained. "Parents," "people," and "mental" are among the most prominent words in our word cloud and thematic analysis.

The themes and subthemes of our analysis are given in the tables below regarding the students' concerns of suicidal ideation. These themes emphasize the pressing necessity for multi-level support systems and the intricate interplay of personal, social, institutional, and cultural factors that affect students' mental health. The themes indicate that the students stressed the need for therapy, self-improvement, and awareness programs. The thematic analysis also highlighted that family troubles, stress, lack of support, stigmatizing cultural misconceptions, and pessimism were psychological and emotional triggers for suicidal ideation. The participating students reported confusion, lack of assistance, and cultural stereotypes concerning mental health in academic settings as challenges. Students also indicated that family relationships, societal expectations, and mental health stigma extenuated suicidal ideation. The thematic analysis showed that academic institutions of higher learning, especially private ones, often had inadequate or inaccessible mental health treatments beyond initial sessions. The students suggested the role of workshops, inclusive environments, empathic counselors, and motivating support to prevent suicide and enhance mental health. The subsequent section presents the main themes along with selected quotes.

Theme 1: Current Mental Health Support

Sub-theme: Coping Mechanisms/Effective Coping Strategies

Table 2 represents the subtheme related to coping mechanisms/effective coping strategies. The majority of students shared that they had experienced suicidal ideation a range of times, from a few months to many years. Most students indicated that seeking diverse therapeutic outlets and participating in various activities were essential coping mechanisms.

Theme 2: Triggers of Suicidal Ideation

Sub-theme: Family and Psychological Triggers

Table 3 provides an overview of the subthemes identified in this theme. The majority of students noted that a range of emotional and psychological factors triggered their suicidal thoughts and actions. They expressed emotional suffering, resulting from isolation, withdrawal, and having unsettled mental health issues that were often worsened by institutional and societal expectations. These severe internal conflicts made students feel worthless, and for some, recurring ideation of self-harm.

Theme 3: Perceptions of Campus Mental Health Services

Sub-theme: Campus Mental Health Services/perceptions/influences

Table 4 presents the core subthemes related to campus mental health services. Several students emphasized their failure to understand the complexity of suicidal situations in the absence of the necessary health education and empathetic attitudes, perceptions, and actions of peers and society. This unfamiliarity may lead to misinterpretation and stigmatization, further isolating individuals who require assistance. Cultural norms and societal beliefs greatly influence attitudes toward mental health, yet these factors are usually disregarded. To promote a more knowledgeable and caring society where people feel empowered to seek support and assistance for mental health issues, this awareness gap must be closed.

Table 2. Description of the themes and subthemes used for the interviews conducted with undergraduate students regarding Current Mental Health Support.

Major Themes	Subthemes	Descriptions	Selected Quotes
Current Mental Health Support	Coping Mechanisms/Effective Coping Strategies	**Coping Mechanisms/Effective Coping Strategies:** Techniques and methods individuals use to manage and reduce suicidal ideation. **Personal Improvement:** Personal growth and changes that help mitigate suicidal thoughts. **Therapy is Important:** The role of therapeutic interventions in preventing and managing suicidal ideation. **Awareness Programs:** The impact of programs aimed at raising awareness about suicidal ideation and prevention.	Here is what different students said: • I've experimented with various therapeutic techniques and kept myself occupied with calligraphy and photography. Depending on how severe the problem is, different exercises are performed. Academic webinars and seminars help people understand the value of different treatments. One book altered my perspective, and I gained a deeper understanding of life's purpose through a class assignment. I used to think that killing myself would make me happy, but then I saw that I had to accomplish something positive for both my life and the lives of others. • In my experience, discovering joy in minor accomplishments can be a potent barrier against hopelessness. • I use constructive coping mechanisms daily that help me turn my gloomy moments into learning experiences. • I prefer to seek assistance from others is a brave first step on the road to recovery and fortitude. Other respondents said: • Participating in joyful activities helps me stay anchored during stressful moments. Creating a network of dependable people is a lifesaver when things go tough. Self-care and mindfulness exercises build a wall against overpowering ideas. Making a safety plan with people you can trust gives you hope and security. Concentrating on future goals and aspirations facilitates redirecting my negative thoughts toward positive outcomes.

Table 3. Description of the themes and subthemes used for the interviews conducted with undergraduate students regarding Triggers of Suicidal Ideation.

Major Themes	Subthemes	Descriptions	Selected Quotes
Triggers of Suicidal Ideation	Family and Psychological Triggers	**Family-related Factor Triggers:** How family dynamics and issues can initiate or exacerbate suicidal thoughts and behaviors. **Academic Stressors:** The influence of academic pressures and stress on suicidal ideation. **Lack of Support System:** The effect of not having a supportive network on individuals experiencing suicidal thoughts. **Pessimistic Attitude/Negative Attitude Towards Life:** How negative thinking patterns contribute to suicidal behaviors. **Hopelessness:** The role of feelings of hopelessness in suicidal ideation. **Pressures:** Various pressures that contribute to suicidal thoughts. **Panic Attacks During Suicidal Ideation:** The occurrence of panic attacks alongside suicidal thoughts.	Some representative quotes are listed below: • I experienced a constant sense of deprivation and criticism for my beliefs. Psychologists stated I was fine except for being agitated. Teachers' disregard for their students resulted in poor self-worth and worthlessness. My in-laws' thoughts caused panic attacks, which led to self-harm. I felt alone because of my introverted personality and my inability to handle constant pressure; devoid of enthusiasm for studying and despondent about finishing my degree or thesis. • Emotional distress frequently drives me to the verge of hopelessness, where psychological factors trigger me to set off a tempest of suicidal ideas, leaving me as a victim who feels helpless. • I feel an ongoing struggle with inner demons that set me on a hazardous route toward self-destruction due to unresolved emotional suffering. • I feel incessant attacks of the mind might cause me to contemplate the impossibly extreme, resulting in detrimental manifestations of psychological discomfort and thoughts of suicide.

Table 4. Description of the themes and subthemes used for the interviews conducted with undergraduate students regarding Perceptions of Campus Mental Health Services.

Major Themes	Subthemes	Descriptions	Selected Quotes
Perceptions of Campus Mental Health Services	Campus Mental Health Services/perceptions/influences	Campus Mental Health Services How campus Mental Health Services impacts the recognition and management of suicidal ideation. Lack of Awareness: There is a general lack of understanding about suicidal issues within the community. Lack of Adequate Support/Support System: Insufficient support systems for individuals experiencing suicidal thoughts. External Factors: Outside influences that affect suicidal ideation. Ignore Internal Factors: Neglecting personal, internal factors that contribute to suicidal thoughts.	Here is what different students said: • I am accused of my behavior. • The teacher in our department made fun of my problems. • I face criticism for my deeds, but nobody acknowledges the suffering they caused. • People treat suicidal thoughts as attention-seeking, dismissing their actuality. • Society frequently dismisses those who exhibit suicidal thoughts and behaviors as mentally ill, neglecting their underlying issues. • People make fun of such suicidal ideation concepts. • Society started giving the excuse that if a person shows certain behaviors related to suicide, it might be because of a mental illness. • Whenever I showed suicidal behaviors or whenever I got panic attacks, everyone made fun of me as if I was pretending or something. • I was ridiculed when I showed my distress, as if my suffering was a show. • People did not hear my pleas for assistance; they thought my panic attacks were dramatic.

Theme 4: Cultural and Societal Impact

Sub-theme: Influences of cultural and Societal factors on Suicidal Ideation

Table 5 shows how participant narratives clustered into cultural and Societal factors on Suicidal Ideation. Many students experience suicidal thoughts for a variety of reasons, including social, family, and educational issues. Overwhelming feelings of hopelessness may result from academic difficulties, such as financial burdens and high performance expectations. Parental attitudes, toxic relationships, and conflicts within the family all have a significant impact on mental health. In addition, shame and isolation among those who are struggling are exacerbated by society and cultural beliefs toward mental health and suicide.

Reflecting on their adverse childhood experiences, some students discussed the subtleties of poor parent–child relationships, unresolved parental disputes, and the nuances of joint family systems that can negatively impact children's mental health, feeding into suicidal thoughts and necessitating effective therapy options.

A few students shared their struggles with academic pressure, which were complicated by financial difficulties and family pressures. They believed that feeling trapped by these negative influences necessitated social support, and that a lack of it could lead to losing sight of one's purpose.

Theme 5: Institutional Support and Response to Suicide Ideation

Sub-theme: Mental health support availability in the university/institution

Table 6 presents a summary of themes and subthemes related to the mental health support available in educational institutions. Inadequate mental health care provided by educational institutions is a significant problem in our culture. Many students encounter obstacles in their quest for efficient mental health care, such as stigma, insufficient funding, and ignorance. These difficulties may cause them to feel isolated, anxious, or depressed, which can harm their overall well-being and academic performance. Even while specific programs are offered, their quality and accessibility are often lacking, depriving many students of the support they need. It is essential to close these gaps to create a nurturing atmosphere where children can flourish intellectually and personally. It is time for our educational systems to prioritize mental health.

Table 5. Description of the themes and subthemes used for the interviews conducted with undergraduate students regarding Perceptions of Cultural and Societal Impact.

Major Themes	Subthemes	Descriptions	Selected Quotes
Cultural and Societal Impact	Influences of cultural and Societal factors on Suicidal Ideation	**Academic Stressors:** The pressure and stress from academic responsibilities that lead to suicidal thoughts. **Family Relationships/Parental Attitude:** The impact of family dynamics and parental attitudes on suicidal ideation. **Family-related Issues:** Specific issues within the family that contribute to suicidal thoughts. **Society and Culture Attitude:** The broader societal and cultural attitudes towards suicide and mental health. **Social Support/Support System:** The importance of having a strong support network in mitigating suicidal thoughts. **Treatment Suggestions:** Recommendations for treatments to manage and reduce suicidal ideation. **Personal Improvement/Realization:** How personal growth and self-awareness can help control suicidal thoughts.	Here are the responses from different students: • I am demoralized by my parents' ongoing arguments. I genuinely know people who had suicidal thoughts because of their parents. Parent workshops are also necessary. Suicidal thoughts, in my opinion, stem from familial problems. I believe that masculine dominance permeates both my family and our society. I find societal conventions disturbing, particularly the notion that girls should be married by the time they are 20 or 22. I feel better when I talk to someone about my issues. Treatment, in my opinion, ought to be based on how serious suicidal thoughts are. After discussing, if my problems are fixed, I feel at ease. To console myself, I have to work hard. • I know it is due to family matters; others also know it. I have known individuals who have suicidal thoughts because of their parents. Others said: • Suicidal thoughts, in my opinion, are a result of unresolved parental disputes and arguments. Suicidal thoughts may arise from a bad parent–child connection. The mental health of their children is greatly influenced by the way parents live together and how they parent. Disturbances might also result from family disputes. Joint family systems, in my opinion, involve a variety of elements that can impact kids' mental health. In a shared family arrangement, elders are unable to provide each child with the individual attention they need because there are many of them. Therapy conducted in person is prohibited in joint family systems. I believe it is essential to have a range of therapy options. The ineffectiveness of online therapy can be attributed to improper interactions between psychologists. Individuals going through difficult times or those who have suicidal thoughts need to know that they are not alone. A few students shared that: • I had to retake the entire semester because I was unable to administer my final exams. I believe there are not many people who could offer you guidance. Supportive people surround me. My buddies helped to create a network of social support. I think that listening to someone can be therapeutic. During the intermediate, my relatives put pressure on me. My background was middle-class, and the academy was expensive. My relatives used to rage at me and accuse me of not getting the grades they wanted. For me, the combination of these elements created a loop. I believe that when something is removed from its intended purpose, people can become lost.

Table 6. Description of the themes and subthemes used for the interviews conducted with undergraduate students regarding Institutional Support and Response to Suicide Ideation.

Major Themes	Subthemes	Descriptions	Selected Quotes
Institutional Support and Response to Suicide Ideation	Mental health support availability in the university/institution	Mental Health Support Availability in University/Institution: The availability and effectiveness of mental health services within educational institutions. Mental Health Support Availability in Private Universities/Institutions: Access to mental health services in private universities and institutions. Lack of Effective Counseling Services: The insufficiency of counseling services to address suicidal ideation effectively.	Most of the students shared that: • Despite being an excellent student, I was unable to attend lectures on mental health awareness at my university due to the absence of a counseling committee. Organizations ought to create these committees to promote the psychological health of their students. Teachers frequently do not consider the personal or family difficulties that students may encounter. While some older educators may offer empathy, it is often ineffective to raise issues related to missed deadlines; in fact, some educators may make light of them. • Not many counselors are available, and the ones who are may not remain so after the initial session. Although webinars and seminars aim to raise awareness, receiving assistance from friends and teachers depends on emotional expression. Despite its high cost, my academy did not address the mental health concerns of its students. I do not think any educator has ever asked why something was occurring. Although there is still a long way to go, private colleges are beginning to take their students' mental health and well-being into account.

Theme 6: Recommendations for Support and Prevention

Sub-theme: Student-Driven Suggestions and Solutions

Table 7 provides participant quotes on suggestions and solutions. Many students reported that there are insufficient awareness programs and support systems on campus. To prevent suicidal ideation, educational institutions should provide a supportive environment and a sufficient resource system to prevent suicidal commitments.

Table 7. Description of the themes and subthemes used for the interviews conducted with undergraduate students regarding "Recommendations for Support and Prevention".

Major Themes	Subthemes	Descriptions	Selected Quotes
Recommendations for Support and Prevention	Student-Driven Suggestions and Solutions	Conduct seminars/workshops: Conducting seminars/workshops for those who do not want to share their feelings with anyone. Supporting/Inclusive environment in educational institutions Provision of a supportive/Inclusive environment in educational institutions. Motivational talk on general topics during class. Teacher motivational talk, constructive feedback, and one-on-one meetings with those who find studying difficult. Cooperative behavior of the campus counselor Campus counselor positive behavior that allows the patient to discuss/share thoughts without judgment.	Most students stated that: • Awareness programs, support systems, and family counseling should be made available to address these issues. They further elaborated, saying that a counselor who is more empathetic towards you, listens to you, and can offer you comfort and solace in a particular environment. It will provide a supportive environment for counselees to express their concerns regarding why they want to commit suicide. A few students reported that: • They tried reading motivational books that have changed their perspective. They further said that people sometimes get lost because their lives lack meaning, and they find it difficult to solve the problems they face. Additionally, doing some exercise also helped them to divert their attention from the suicidal planning and attempts.

Services: The following tables (Tables 8–14) present the themes and sub-themes, with selected quotes emanating from counselors' perceptions. Their interviews provided insights into student suicide ideation prevalence, causes, and institutional reactions. They observed persistent discomfort stemming from academic, familial, and cultural demands, as well as inadequacies in the major support infrastructure. The following themes capture a sophisticated understanding of these difficulties and evidence-based strategies to improve school mental health support systems.

Table 8. Description of the themes and subthemes used for the interviews conducted with counsellors regarding Prevalence and Patterns of Suicidal Ideation.

Major Themes	Sub-Themes	Description	Selected Quotes
Prevalence and Patterns of Suicidal Ideation	Frequency of Encounter and Observed Trends	Investigates the frequency with which experts come across pupils who are planning suicide and focuses on recurring trends among impacted students who make suicidal attempts, or triggers.	The majority of counselors stated that: • They frequently meet students with suicidal ideation, especially during exam periods, after the exam results are announced, and relationship breakups. "Forced study" by the parents, i.e., the student wanted to study medicine but was sent by the parents to an engineering university. The number of such cases is not so many, but in every semester, 3–4 students come with this type of thought. Especially students from the 7th semester come with suicidal ideation because they have spent a long time at university with poor grades and even never tell their parents, especially residents of hostels, as they are away from home. Still, when the last year is finished, parents will ask, "When will you start your job to help us?" This fear pushes them to think about suicide. A few counselors highlighted that: • The typical patterns/trends of social ideation include family issues, neglected child, history of sexual abuse, absence of parents, unpleasant home environment, academic stress, bullying, pressure from parents, peer pressure, low self-esteem, social media pressure, and underlying mental health disorders.

Table 9. Description of the themes and subthemes used for the interviews conducted with counsellors regarding Contributing Factors to Suicidal Ideation.

Major Themes	Sub-Themes	Description	Selected Quotes
Contributing Factors to Suicidal Ideation	Social and Family Factors and Academic Stressors	Examines how parental pressure, family conflict, and academic failure trigger suicidal ideation.	Most of the counselors shared that: • Most of the social factors include loneliness, homesickness, hostility, and peer pressure. Strict parenting, Lack of emotional support, domestic violence, Lack of trust, Low self-esteem, Peer pressure, Substance abuse, Identity crisis, bullying, Body-shaming, Sexual abuse, and Emotional abuse are common issues that lead to severe mental health issues and result in suicide. • Family-related issues are mainly linked with the comparisons within or between families, financial problems, and relationship issues that include parental quarrels and cross-gender friendships. • Others reported that the most frequent academic challenges include fear of failure, heavy course loads, poor time management, and extreme competition, which are common among engineering students. A few stated that: • Some students feel shame when they cannot meet their own set goals, start to blame themselves, overthink about unprecedented outcomes, and commit suicide.

Table 10. Description of the themes and subthemes used for the interviews conducted with counsellors regarding the Institutional Support and Mental Health Services.

Major Themes	Sub-Themes	Description	Selected Quotes
Institutional Support and Mental Health Services	Availability of Resources and Effectiveness of Support Services	Evaluates the availability and use of on-campus counseling and mental health services. Moreover, assess the quality and effectiveness of the available psychological support services.	Many of the counseling staff reported that: • Relevant resources are available, and faculty members are also provided with basic training. They said they have expert doctors and psychologists in their educational institution who deal with students suffering from mental health issues. Others reported that: • Various relevant interventions and strategies are employed, including Cognitive Behavioral Therapy (CBT) for emotional regulation. Reported cases are given proper treatment until they recover fully; alternatively, severe cases are hospitalized for proper medication and treatment.

Table 11. Description of the themes and subthemes used for the interviews conducted with counsellors regarding Cultural and Societal Influences on Help-Seeking.

Major Themes	Sub-Themes	Description	Selected Quotes
Cultural and Societal Influences on Help-Seeking	Cultural Norms and Stigma	Explains how students' desire to ask for aid is impacted by cultural ideas, stigma, or fear of being judged.	Many of the counselors stated that: • In Pakistani society, we do not address the problem at its initial level but instead wait for it to worsen. Some parents discourage female students from seeing a counselor who is struggling with finding a life partner, believing it affects their social image. This shame-based thinking keeps many students from reaching out until a crisis has deteriorated. Others said that: • If mental health is stigmatized or seen as a sign of weakness, students may feel ashamed or fearful of being judged, which discourages them from reaching out. Conversely, in environments that promote openness, empathy, and emotional well-being, students are more likely to seek support early.

Table 12. Description of the themes and subthemes used for the interviews conducted with counsellors regarding Institutional Challenges in Providing Support.

Major Themes	Sub-Themes	Description	Selected Quotes
Institutional Challenges in Providing Support	Internal Barriers	Identify institutional limitations, including shortages of qualified personnel, financial constraints, and policy inconsistencies.	Many counselors said that: • The most significant obstacle is Low funding: we lack sufficient funds for awareness campaigns, workshops, and online resources related to mental health services. A few reported that: • There is insufficient staff in one counseling center. Only one or two counselors cannot serve thousands of students. Additionally, 24/7 Availability is necessary on campus for Hostilities students who frequently experience emergencies on weekends or at night when services are unavailable. Others said we need properly trained hostel Resident Tutors (RTs) who provide services when the counselor is off duty.

Table 13. Description of the themes and subthemes used for the interviews conducted with counsellors regarding Effective Interventions and Strategies.

Major Themes	Sub-Themes	Description	Selected Quotes
Effective Interventions and Strategies	Successful Approaches	Offer pupils professional advice on interventions that have yielded favorable results.	Most of the counselors said: • It is difficult to specify one intervention or support strategy because each case is different when addressing suicidal ideation. They said it is essential first to identify the trigger and urge behind the suicidal ideation systematically by providing emotional support and creating an atmosphere of love and care around the counselee. • Others suggested that various interventions can be applied, including psychoeducation, active listening, Cognitive Behavioral Therapy (CBT), Rational Emotive Behavior Therapy (REBT), Acceptance and Commitment Therapy (ACT), Non-judgmental presence, and Peer support programs. A few stated that: • Incorporating Mindfulness and self-regulation, as well as religious coping techniques, is also very useful, depending on the nature of the case. During this process, collaborating with psychiatrists is crucial for cases that require medication or intensive therapy.

Table 14. Description of the themes and subthemes used for the interviews conducted with counsellors regarding Recommendations for Improvement.

Major Themes	Sub-Themes	Description	Selected Quotes
Recommendations for Improvement	Service Enhancement	Provide suggestions for enhancing or growing the university's outreach and mental health services.	Most of the counselors recommended that: • Different suicide prevention campaigns, awareness campaigns, and Emergency contacts for support should be conducted. These awareness campaigns should be conducted for all faculty members, students, parents, and the community, including college staff members, by highlighting the signs and severe outcomes of mentally disturbed individuals. A few reported that: • There should be an increase in the budget for mental health services. Hiring sufficient staff, such as counselors and psychiatrists, is crucial in educational institutions to meet the growing demands of an increasing number of students enrolled.

4. Discussion

4.1. Summary of Findings

This qualitative study investigated perspectives of university students and counselors about the drivers of students' suicidal ideation and attempts, especially those resulting from academic distress. Interviews were conducted with eight students and eight counselors from five public and private universities. This study's primary objective was to investigate how academic pressures contribute to suicidal ideation and attempts among university students. Several themes emerged from qualitative data from students and counselors. Both groups emphasized the critical role of academic pressure, family expectations, and lack of emotional support in triggering suicidal ideation. Furthermore, participants agreed on the value of reducing mental health stigma and enhancing the availability of timely and compassionate institutional support services. Both students and counselors emphasized the interplay between intense academic demands, limited emotional, and insufficient institutional resources as critical pathways leading to suicidal ideation. The findings highlight the urgent need for culturally sensitive mental health interventions that address both individual vulnerabilities and environmental stressors.

4.2. Thematic Discussion

4.2.1. Current Mental Health Support and Coping Strategies

The results show that students face severe emotional distress and frequently feel overwhelmed to the point of contemplating withdrawal because of the demanding academic schedule. Family dynamics, societal views, and the accessibility of mental health resources significantly shape students' mental health status. These findings highlight the necessity of all-encompassing mental health interventions in school settings to address the complex factors contributing to suicidal behaviors among students. Students' experiences of severe emotional distress, including suicidal thoughts and behaviors, align with previous studies highlighting the prevalence of mental health problems among young adults. For instance, Landa-Blanco et al. (2024) found that university students are particularly vulnerable to suicidal thoughts and actions because of the significant academic and social pressures they encounter. This is in line with our study findings, indicating that students frequently struggle with intense internal distress that pushes them to emotional collapse, particularly if they lack effective coping mechanisms. Furthermore, their emotional immaturity and lack of life experience may make their mental health issues worse.

Our findings add to previous research, providing a culturally sensitive viewpoint on the elements influencing students' mental health issues. Hetrick and Sharma (2025) noted that counselors often come across students contemplating suicide during stressful academic times, especially final-year students who are feeling overburdened by expectations from their families and educational failure. In contrast, counselors in our study emphasized culturally specific triggers, such as forced career paths, authoritarian parenting, and social pressures related to honor and reputation. These issues are less stressed in Western research but are highly relevant in South Asian contexts (Alshareef & Alfuqaha, 2024). Additionally, while other research has shown financial stress as a significant contributing factor (Yao et al., 2023), the counselors participating in our study underscored relational trauma and emotional neglect as more pressing concerns.

4.2.2. Triggers of Suicidal Ideation Linked to Family and Psychological Stressors

The influence of family dynamics and psychological stressors on the mental health of students is significant. Our findings suggest that psychological distress and family problems are linked with panic episodes, self-harm, and hopelessness. Research from Makhubela (2021) demonstrates that family support is the main factor against mental health difficulties in university students. On the other hand, a lack of family support can make psychological anguish worse, which can have severe consequences like suicidal thoughts and actions. One additional important feature in your findings is the general lack of understanding regarding suicide issues among students and the community at large. Numerous students have never participated in mental health lectures or workshops, indicating inadequate mental health education. Another study by Mortier et al. (2022) highlights the need for greater mental health awareness and education to avoid suicidal attempts. The lack of these programs can make kids more susceptible to suicidal planning since they are ill-prepared to deal with their mental health issues.

Most study participants reported that societal and cultural expectations have a significant impact on their mental health. Students often experience feelings of loneliness and lack of support due to the stigma related to mental health concerns and the absence of candid conversations about emotional well-being. This is consistent with findings from Corrigan et al. (2024), who contend that societal stigma is a significant obstacle to getting mental health treatment. The acceptance and support of mental health efforts can be influenced by cultural context, which can either positively or negatively affect students' desire to seek help. Students who are under academic pressure, have personal and familial difficulties, and lack emotional support are among the many variables that lead to suicidal planning. Our results are consistent with previous research, like that of Lipson et al. (2022), who found that personal problems and academic stress are significant predictors of suicidal thoughts in college students. These problems are exacerbated by limited access to mental health resources and effective counseling (Andrew et al., 2011; Yorgason et al., 2024).

4.2.3. Perception of Campus Mental Health Services

A critical theme that emerged in our findings was institutional deficiencies in addressing the issue of suicidal ideation, in addition to individual and cultural influences. Fadipe et al. (2025) and Fauk et al. (2023) highlighted a persistent gap between institutional best practices and the mental health treatments currently offered in educational institutions. While some colleges provide basic counseling services, their effectiveness is compromised by a shortage of qualified personnel, outdated evaluation methods, inadequate privacy, and limited infrastructure. The counselors noted that weak institutional support and fragmented referral networks were issues that mirrored global trends but were exacerbated by regional limitations. On the other hand, some components, such as the use of cognitive behavioral therapy and spiritual counseling, were considered culturally congruent. However, long-term progress is still impeded by uneven training and administrative carelessness. Compared to Western institutions with formalized mental health frameworks, Pakistani universities continue to fall short of properly prioritizing psychological care, reinforcing systemic neglect (Asad & Dawood, 2025).

4.2.4. Cultural and Societal Misconceptions Surrounding Suicide

A pervasive cultural stigma surrounding mental health is considered a significant contributory factor to suicidal ideation, where social judgment and victim-shaming prevent students from seeking mental health counseling and care (Rahman et al., 2025; Shah & Alamian, 2023). Although awareness and openness have improved over the past decade, students still tend to worry about social stigma and adverse reactions (Karnwal & Sharmila, 2024; Zhai et al., 2025).

4.2.5. Institutional Barriers to Accessing Mental Health Care

One crucial concern raised by our findings is the accessibility of mental health services in academic settings. Numerous students complain about the shortage of counseling services, and those that are offered are sometimes inadequate or inaccessible beyond the first few sessions. Studies such as Gallagher (2024) support this finding, showing that, although many colleges provide counseling services, they are often underfunded and unable to meet demand. Students may not have the tools they need to properly manage their mental health because of this gap in mental health care. Furthermore, accessibility issues with mental health services are another critical element of our research. Students encounter numerous challenges, including the scarcity of counselors, limited awareness of available services, and the stigma associated with seeking help. This aligns with research in the literature, where studies such as Zhou et al. (2023) highlight comparable obstacles that prevent students from accessing mental health services. These obstacles raise the possibility of suicidal planning and attempts by contributing to untreated mental health problems.

4.2.6. Student-Driven Recommendation for Prevention and Support

Our study findings are consistent with existing literature on student suicidal planning and attempts. Several important variables that affect students' mental health include themes of emotional turmoil, family dynamics, societal attitudes, and institutional support. Educational institutions must address these factors to ensure students have access to appropriate mental health resources and support. Institutions can promote general well-being and prevent suicidal tendencies among students by recognizing and addressing these variables. This entails raising family support levels, decreasing the stigma associated with mental illness, raising mental health awareness, and expanding the availability and accessibility of mental health treatments in university settings.

4.3. Limitations of the Study

Our study used a qualitative research design to explore university students' and counselors' perceptions about suicidal ideation, resulting in study limitations with implications for the generalizability of our findings. First, the study included only 16 individuals from five universities, which may not fully represent Pakistan's diverse experiences and opinions across regions, disciplines, and institutions. Secondly, suicidal ideation and mental health are sensitive; therefore, students and counselors may have suppressed information or altered their opinions to fit societal norms. Third, the study only captured individuals' experiences and perceptions at one point in time, making it difficult to determine how suicidal ideation or support mechanisms change. Fourth, the findings rely exclusively on interviews, without including institutional data (e.g., the number of reported mental health cases and resource allocation), which could have strengthened the analysis and validation of observed trends. Fifth, the study did not use any standardized clinical assessments of depression or personality traits to select participants. While participants were included based on prior behavioral health service use, the lack of standardized screening for personality or behavioral disorders limits the ability to contextualize their experiences within established diagnostic frameworks. Finally, the qualitative interviews yield context-specific results. They are not statistically applicable to Pakistani or international students.

4.4. Future Directions and Implications

This qualitative study provides avenues for developing theory in suicidal ideation, while contributing to the development of culturally relevant interventions. The qualitative nature of the study has highlighted the complexity of an individual regarding the major mental health issue of suicidal ideation. By revealing culturally ingrained interpretations of distress and suicide, qualitative research contributes to the formulation of interventions that align with individuals' lived experiences (Richardson et al., 2025; Amiri et al., 2025). Such alignment ensures that interventions and strategies tackle not only psychological risk factors but also sociocultural dynamics that affect help-seeking and coping mechanisms. Gangemi et al. (2019, 2021) explain how reasoning strategies and emotional reasoning processes worsen cognitive misrepresentations such as despair and entrapment, which are pivotal to suicidal ideation. These insights suggest that future interventions should incorporate cognitive–behavioral elements to help individuals restructure their maladaptive reasoning patterns. Qualitative studies can provide further insight into how an individual forms their perception of the world around them through relationships and cultural norms. Future qualitative research aimed to provide research evidence to inform suicide prevention efforts could also use tested theoretical frameworks, such as Rasmussen et al.'s (2025) integrated Motivational/Volitional model of suicide prevention and treatment, and suggest that, in addition to addressing the motivational states associated with self-stifling and humiliation, in order to prevent progression to suicidal behaviors. In sum, future research may build on these findings and generate additional research evidence to integrate qualitative narratives into clinical practice, enabling therapists to respond to the subjective meanings individuals assign to their distress.

The following recommendations, based on the study findings, can inform programs aimed at addressing the issue of suicidal behaviors among university students: To begin with, the educational institutions can introduce structured teacher training programs and capacity-building workshops aimed at enhancing teachers' ability to recognize early indicators of psychological distress among students, such as sudden mood changes, withdrawal from peers, or academic decline. In addition, teachers should be guided on the referral mechanism to connect at-risk students with school counsellors or psychological support units. Furthermore, schools can integrate brief, structured mental well-being activities into daily routines or before high-stress events, such as examinations. These may include mindfulness and breathing exercises, simplified cognitive behavioral techniques (CBT), and Emotion regulation exercises. To extend these efforts beyond the school setting and to reinforce school-based efforts, a community-based awareness campaign can be organized in collaboration with local NGOs and psychologists. These initiatives can train peer facilitators to support your mental health, encourage open discussions on emotional well-being, and provide information on accessible counselling resources in both urban and rural settings.

5. Conclusions

The results of this study revealed the influence of different drivers, such as academic pressure, family distress, and emotional misery, on suicidal planning and suicidal thoughts among university students, as well as the intense mental distress they go through. Without healthy coping strategies, students frequently experience inner demons that push them to the verge of despair, which can result in self-destructive behavior and suicidal thoughts. Families are a significant source of stress for many people with mental health disorders, and mental health interventions must take family dynamics into account. The problem is worsened due to a noticeable ignorance about suicide issues and students' inability to identify the warning signs of mental health issues, which delays seeking assistance and intervention.

Societal and cultural beliefs also greatly influence students' mental health. Students often experience feelings of loneliness and lack of support due to the stigma associated with mental health concerns and the absence of candid conversations about emotional well-being. This social stigma may discourage students from getting the necessary support, worsening their mental health issues. To provide a setting where students feel comfortable and encouraged to talk about their mental health concerns, these societal and cultural barriers must be addressed. Students may experience significant levels of stress and anxiety as a result of the demanding academic requirements, and these conditions are intimately linked to suicidal ideation. These problems are worsened by the lack of adequate mental health resources and counseling in educational institutions, which deprives students of the assistance they need to manage their mental health properly. A comprehensive, multi-level strategy is necessary to address the issues highlighted by our findings. By increasing services, lowering stigma, and creating supportive environments, educational institutions must put mental health first. Universities can foster a culture of care that supports student well-being and reduces the incidence of suicidal behaviors by incorporating mental health education, involving families, and enhancing institutional infrastructure.

Author Contributions: Conceptualization, G.H.S., M.A.K. and M.M.; methodology, G.H.S., M.A.K., and M.M.; formal analysis, G.H.S. and M.M.; data collection, M.A.K., M.M. and M.A.; writing—original draft preparation, G.H.S. and M.M.; writing—review and editing, G.H.S., M.M. and M.A.K.; supervision, G.H.S. and M.A.K. All authors have read and agreed to the published version of the manuscript.

Funding: This research received no external funding.

Institutional Review Board Statement: The study was conducted in accordance with the Declaration of Helsinki, and approved by the Institutional Review Board of Kinnaird University (protocol code: ID KC/ORIC/ERC/2025/004, date of approval: 11 February 2025).

Informed Consent Statement: Informed consent was obtained from all subjects involved in the study.

Data Availability Statement: The institutional data protection policies of Kinnaird College for Women restrict public access to individual-level qualitative data due to the sensitive nature of the topic, behavioral health issues, and the risk of participant re-identification. De-identified transcripts and materials supporting the findings of this study may be made available upon reasonable request under a data use agreement subject to approval by the Kinnaird College Institutional Review Board and Data Access Committee. Data requests can be emailed to masha.khan@kinnaird.edu.pk with a statement of research purpose, assurance of confidentiality and ethical use, and institutional ethics committee approval.

Acknowledgments: The authors gratefully acknowledge the administrative support provided by the Office of Research, Innovation, and Commercialization (ORIC) at Kinnaird College. During the preparation of this manuscript, the authors used Microsoft Office and NVivo (version 15) for data analysis. The authors have reviewed and edited the output and take full responsibility for the content of this publication.

Conflicts of Interest: The authors declare no conflicts of interest. The funders had no role in the design of the study; in the collection, analyses, or interpretation of data; in the writing of the manuscript; or in the decision to publish the results.

Appendix A

Research Tools:

From Pressure to Peril: Investigating the Drivers of Suicidal Ideation and Attempts in University Students

Questions Guide for Counselors

Instructions:

Thank you for your participation. This study aims to understand the social, family-related, and academic factors contributing to suicidal ideation and attempts in university students. The interview will take approximately 30 min. Your responses are confidential and anonymous. You may skip any question or stop at any time.

1. How often do you encounter students experiencing suicidal ideation, and are there any common patterns or trends you've observed?
2. What factors do you believe are most significant in triggering suicidal thoughts among students? *Possible probes: Social factors, family-related issues, and academic pressures.

3. How do you evaluate the effectiveness of the mental health resources currently available to students with suicidal ideation at the Guidance and Counseling Center?
4. In your opinion, how do societal norms and cultural attitudes impact students' willingness to seek help for mental health concerns?
5. What barriers within the institution limit your ability to provide adequate support for students struggling with suicidal ideation?
6. Based on your professional expertise, what interventions or support strategies have you found to be most successful in addressing suicidal ideation?
7. What improvements or changes do you suggest for enhancing mental health services for students experiencing suicidal thoughts?

From Pressure to Peril: Investigating the Drivers of Suicidal Ideation and Attempts in University Students

Questions Guide for Students

Instructions:

Thank you for your participation. This study aims to understand the social, family-related, and academic factors contributing to suicidal ideation and attempts in university students. The interview will take approximately 30 min. Your responses are confidential and anonymous. You may skip any question or stop at any time.

1. For how long have you been experiencing suicidal ideation?
2. Are you currently receiving any therapy or support? If yes, please specify.
3. Please share your thoughts on what type of social, family-related, or academic factors trigger your suicide ideation.
    a. *Probe: If a student fails to mention any of the social, family-related, or academic factors triggers, ask for the follow-up example (1-A). So you have talked about the social factors, but what are academic factors, such as homework workload, class environment, etc., that contribute to suicide ideation?
4. How do you perceive the availability and effectiveness of mental health resources available at Guidance and Counseling Center for students experiencing suicidal thoughts?
5. In what ways do you think cultural attitudes and societal norms in our society impact discussions and perceptions of suicide and mental health?
6. Could you describe any personal experiences or observations regarding how suicide ideation is addressed within our educational institution?
7. What kind of support or treatment do you believe would be most beneficial for individuals struggling with thoughts of suicide?

Appendix B

COREQ checklist

From Pressure to Peril: Investigating the Drivers of Suicidal Ideation and Attempts in University Students

Domain 1: Research Team and Reflexivity

Item	Description
Interviewer/facilitator	Prof. Dr. Gulzar Shah, Prof. Dr. Masha Asad Khan, Ms. Maham Muzamil, and Ms. Mahira Ahmed
Credentials	Department Chair & Professor, Academic Dean & Professor, Lecturer, Assistant Professor.
Experience and training	Experienced qualitative researchers and educators
Relationship established	No prior relationship with participants
Participant's knowledge of the interviewer	Participants were informed of the researchers' institutional affiliation and study purpose
Interviewer characteristics	Researchers maintained neutrality and followed IRB-approved ethical protocols

Domain 2: Study Design

Item	Description
Methodological approach	Thematic analysis
Theoretical framework	Interpersonal Theory of Suicide (Joiner, 2005); Stress-Diathesis Model (Mann, 2003)
Participant selection	Purposive sampling
How participants were approached	Via institutional channels and direct invitation
Sample size	16 total (8 students, 8 counselors)
Non-participation	3 reported
Setting of data collection	Remote interviews via Zoom and WhatsApp
Description of sample	University students and counselors from different Universities in Lahore City, Punjab, Pakistan.
Interview guide	Developed from literature; pilot tested and refined
Repeat interviews	No
Audio/visual recording	Yes
Field notes	Reflexivity journals and analytic memos are maintained
Duration	Average interview duration: 30 min
Data saturation	Yes, discussed and achieved
Transcripts returned	Yes, transcripts and findings were shared with participants for validation

Domain 3: Analysis and Findings

Item	Description
Number of data coders	Two independent coders for reliability checks
Description of coding tree	Codes derived inductively and clustered into themes
Derivation of themes	Themes emerged from data; not pre-identified
Software used	NVivo 14 for coding and thematic analysis
Participant checking	Yes, findings reviewed by participants
Quotations presented	Yes, anonymized quotations are used to support themes
Data and findings are consistent	Yes, findings grounded in participant narratives
Clarity of major/minor themes	Major and minor themes are clearly distinguished and discussed

References

Abualhamael, S. A., Baig, M., Alghamdi, W., Gazzaz, Z. J., Al-Hayani, M., & Bazi, A. (2024). Quality of life, stress, anxiety and depression and associated factors among people with type 2 diabetes mellitus in western region Saudi Arabia. *Frontiers in Psychiatry, 14*, 1282249. [CrossRef]

Alshareef, B. E., & Alfuqaha, O. A. (2024). The effect of a spiritual intelligence-based counselling programme on suicidal ideation and self-concept among retirement. *Counselling and Psychotherapy Research, 24*(4), 1337–1344. [CrossRef]

Amiri, I., Knettel, B. A., Tarimo, C. S., Stewart, K. A., Palmquist, A. E. L., Mwobobia, J. M., Katiti, V., Knippler, E., Minja, L., Madundo, K., Msoka, E. F., Martinez, A., Boshe, J., Relf, M. V., Mmbaga, B. T., & Goldston, D. B. (2025). "Everyone is fighting their own battles": A qualitative study to explore the context of suicidal ideation among people with HIV in Tanzania. *PLoS Mental Health, 2*(1), e0000318. [CrossRef]

Andrew, D. P., Pedersen, P. M., & McEvoy, C. D. (2011). *Research methods and design in sport management*. Human Kinetics.

Arria, A. M., O'Grady, K. E., Caldeira, K. M., Vincent, K. B., Wilcox, H. C., & Wish, E. D. (2021). Suicide ideation among college students: A multivariate analysis. *Archives of Suicide Research, 13*(3), 230–246. [CrossRef]

Asad, S., & Dawood, S. (2025). Factors predicting intentions to seek psychological counseling among undergraduate university students of Lahore, Pakistan. *International Journal for the Advancement of Counselling, 47*(1), 171–198. [CrossRef]

Centers for Disease Control and Prevention. (2025). *Suicide data and statistics*. U.S. Department of Health and Human Services. Available online: https://www.cdc.gov/suicide/facts/data.html (accessed on 20 April 2025).

Corrigan, P. W., Druss, B. G., & Perlick, D. A. (2024). The impact of mental illness stigma on seeking and participating in mental health care. *Psychological Science in the Public Interest, 15*(2), 37–70. [CrossRef]

Creswell, J. W. (2008). *Educational research: Planning, conducting, and evaluating quantitative and qualitative research* (3rd ed.). Pearson Education, Inc.

da Conceição, V., Mesquita, E., & Gusmão, R. (2024). Effects of a stigma reduction intervention on help-seeking behaviors in university students: A 2019–2021 randomized controlled trial. *Psychiatry Research, 331*, 115673. [CrossRef]

Diefenbach, G. J., Stubbing, J., Rice, T. B., Lord, K. A., Rudd, M. D., & Tolin, D. F. (2024). Uncovering the role of substance use in suicide attempts using a mixed-methods approach. *Suicide and Life-Threatening Behavior, 54*(1), 70–82. [CrossRef] [PubMed]

Dobbertin, M., Blair, K. S., Aloi, J., Bajaj, S., Bashford-Largo, J., Mathur, A., Zhang, R., Carollo, E., Schwartz, A., Elowsky, J., Ringle, J. L., Tyler, P., & Blair, R. J. (2024). Neural correlates of automatic emotion regulation and their association with suicidal ideation in adolescents during the first 90-days of residential care. *Translational Psychiatry, 14*(1), 54. [CrossRef]

Drum, D. J., Brownson, C., Denmark, A. B., & Smith, S. E. (2021). New data on the nature of suicidal crises in college students: Shifting the paradigm. *Professional Psychology: Research and Practice, 40*(3), 213–222. [CrossRef]

Eisenberg, D., Gollust, S. E., Golberstein, E., & Hefner, J. L. (2020). Prevalence and correlates of depression, anxiety, and suicidality among university students. *American Journal of Orthopsychiatry, 77*(4), 534–542. [CrossRef] [PubMed]

Fadipe, R. A., Adefila, O. J., Oladosu, T. D., & Adetoyese, E. O. (2025). Relationship between substance abuse and suicidal ideation among undergraduates in Kwara state, Nigeria: Implications for school counselling. *Journal of Guidance and Counselling Studies, 9*(1), 29–43.

Fauk, N. K., Asa, G. A., McLean, C., & Ward, P. R. (2023). "I was very shocked, I wanted it to be over": A qualitative exploration of suicidal ideation and attempts among women living with HIV in Indonesia. *International Journal of Environmental Research and Public Health, 21*(1), 9. [CrossRef]

Gallagher, R. P. (2024). *National survey of college counseling centers 2024*. The International Association of Counseling Services.

Gangemi, A., Dahò, M., & Mancini, F. (2021). Emotional reasoning and psychopathology. *Brain Sciences, 11*(4), 471. [CrossRef]

Gangemi, A., Tenore, K., & Mancini, F. (2019). Two reasoning strategies in patients with psychological illnesses. *Frontiers in Psychology, 10*, 2335. [CrossRef]

Gbore, M. A., & Adebowale, O. F. (2023). Effectiveness of three counselling modes on suicidal ideation among undergraduates in a Nigerian university. *Turkish International Journal of Special Education and Guidance & Counselling, 12*(2), 94–105.

Giancola, N., Bentley, K. H., & Torous, J. (2024). Social media and suicidal behavior in youth: Slippery slope or simply overstressed? *Current Treatment Options in Psychiatry, 11*(3), 141–144. [CrossRef]

Guenthner, L., Baldofski, S., Kohls, E., Schuhr, J., Brock, T., & Rummel-Kluge, C. (2023). Differences in help-seeking behavior among university students during the COVID-19 pandemic depending on mental health status: Results from a cross-sectional survey. *Behavioral Sciences, 13*(11), 885. [CrossRef] [PubMed]

Gupta, S., Fischer, J., Roy, S., & Bhattacharyya, A. (2024). Emotional regulation and suicidal ideation—Mediating roles of perceived social support and avoidant coping. *Frontiers in Psychology, 15*, 1377355. [CrossRef]

Heapy, C., Haddock, G., & Pratt, D. (2024). The relationship between social problem-solving and suicidal ideation and behavior in adults: A systematic review and meta-analysis. *Clinical Psychology: Science and Practice, 31*, 419–432. [CrossRef]

Hetrick, S., & Sharma, V. (2025). Debate: Where to next for universal school-based mental health interventions? Can research led by young people shape universal solutions for mental health and suicide prevention in school settings? *Child and Adolescent Mental Health, 30*, 92–95. [CrossRef] [PubMed]

Hunt, J., & Eisenberg, D. (2021). Mental health problems and help-seeking behavior among college students. *Journal of Adolescent Health, 46*(1), 3–10. [CrossRef] [PubMed]

Joiner, T. E. (2005). *Why people die by suicide*. Harvard University Press.

Jones, A. A., Hard, G., Gray, J., Apsley, H. B., & Santos-Lozada, A. R. (2023). The role of substance use disorders on suicidal ideation, planning, and attempts: A nationally representative study of adolescents and adults in the United States. *Substance Abuse: Research and Treatment, 17*, 11782218231216233. [CrossRef]

Karnwal, R., & Sharmila, K. (2024). Perspective view of stress, anxiety, and depression among pregnant women: A review. *Journal of Ecophysiology and Occupational Health, 24*(1), 1–13. [CrossRef]

Landa-Blanco, M., Romero, K., Caballero, I., Gálvez-Pineda, E., Fúnes-Henríquez, M. J., & Romero, R. (2024). Exploring suicide ideation in university students: Sleep quality, social media, self-esteem, and barriers to seeking psychological help. *Frontiers in Psychiatry, 15*, 1352889. [CrossRef]

Li, Q., Li, J., & Fan, Y. (2025). Addressing mental health in university students: A call for action. *Frontiers in Public Health, 13*, 1614999. [CrossRef]

Lipson, S. K., Lattie, E. G., & Eisenberg, D. (2022). Increased rates of mental health services utilization by US college students: 10-year population-level trends (2007–2017). *Psychiatric Services, 70*(1), 60–63. [CrossRef]

Lumivero. (2024). *NVivo (version 15)* [computer software]. Available online: https://www.lumivero.com (accessed on 27 January 2025).

Makhubela, M. (2021). Suicide and depression in university students: A possible epidemic. *South African Journal of Psychology, 51*(1), 3–5. [CrossRef]

Mann, J. J. (2003). Neurobiology of suicidal behaviour. *Nature Reviews Neuroscience, 4*(10), 819–828. [CrossRef]

Matar, J. L., Laletas, S., & Lubman, D. I. (2024). Mental health concerns and help-seeking behaviors among adolescents in high socioeconomic status groups: A scoping review. *Adolescent Research Review, 9*(1), 93–134. [CrossRef]

Monroe, S. M., & Simons, A. D. (1991). Diathesis–stress theories in the context of life stress research: Implications for the depressive disorders. *Psychological Bulletin, 110*(3), 406–425. [CrossRef]

Mortier, P., Demyttenaere, K., Auerbach, R. P., Green, J. G., Kessler, R. C., Kiekens, G., Nock, M. K., & Bruffaerts, R. (2022). The impact of lifetime suicidality on academic performance in college freshmen. *Journal of Affective Disorders, 225*, 97–103. [CrossRef]

Muhammad Khir, S., Wan Mohd Yunus, W. M. A., Mahmud, N., Wang, R., Panatik, S. A., Mohd Sukor, M. S., & Nordin, N. A. (2024). Efficacy of progressive muscle relaxation in adults for stress, anxiety, and depression: A systematic review. *Psychology Research and Behavior Management, 17*, 345–365. [CrossRef]

Nguyen, M. H., Le, T. T., Nguyen, H. K. T., Ho, M. T., Nguyen, H. T. T., & Vuong, Q. H. (2021). Alice in suicideland: Exploring the suicidal ideation mechanism through the sense of connectedness and help-seeking behaviors. *International Journal of Environmental Research and Public Health, 18*(7), 3681. [CrossRef]

Nguyen, T. H., Shah, G., Muzamil, M., Ikhile, O., Ayangunna, E., & Kaur, R. (2023). Association of in-school and electronic bullying with suicidality and feelings of hopelessness among adolescents in the United States. *Children, 10*(4), 755. [CrossRef] [PubMed]

Paredes-Céspedes, D. M., Vélez, N., Parada-López, A., Toloza-Pérez, Y. G., Téllez, E. M., Portilla, C., González, C., Blandón, L., Santacruz, J. C., & Malagón-Rojas, J. (2024). The effects of nature exposure therapies on stress, depression, and anxiety levels: A systematic review. *European Journal of Investigation in Health, Psychology and Education, 14*(3), 609–622. [CrossRef] [PubMed]

Rahman, M., Kabir, M. I., Sultana, S., Abdullah, I., & Shimu, A. T. (2025). Suicidal behaviours and associated factors among Bangladeshi medical students: A systematic review and meta-analysis (2000–2024). *BMJ Open, 15*(3), e095573. [CrossRef] [PubMed]

Rasmussen, S., Martin, B., & Cramer, R. J. (2025). Multidimensional impulsivity and suicidal behaviour: A partial test of the integrated motivational-volitional (IMV) model of suicide. *Archives of Suicide Research: Official Journal of the International Academy for Suicide Research, 29*(1), 26–44. [CrossRef]

Ribeiro, J. D., Franklin, J. C., Fox, K. R., Bentley, K. H., Kleiman, E. M., Chang, B. P., & Nock, M. K. (2016). Self-injurious thoughts and behaviors as risk factors for future suicide ideation, attempts, and death: A meta-analysis of longitudinal studies. *Psychological Medicine, 46*(2), 225–236. [CrossRef]

Richardson, S. C., Phipps-Bennett, M., Gryglewicz, K., Vance, M., Williams, J. A., Bey, I., Herbert, R., Dennis, S., & Karver, M. S. (2025). Making deep-structure adaptations: A community-engaged qualitative study for culturally adapting suicide prevention interventions for Black youth. *Cultural Diversity & Ethnic Minority Psychology. advanced online publication*. [CrossRef]

Roberts, M. E., Bell, E. A., & Meyer, J. L. (2023). Mental health and academic experiences among U.S. college students during the COVID-19 pandemic. *Frontiers in Psychology, 14*, 1166960. [CrossRef]

Shah, G. H., & Alamian, A. (2023). COVID-19, health inequities, and behavioral health issues facing children. *International Journal of School Health, 10*(1), 1–2. [CrossRef]

Shaman, J., Kandula, S., Pei, S., Galanti, M., Olfson, M., & Gould, M. (2024). Quantifying suicide contagion at population scale. *Science Advances, 10*, eadq4074. [CrossRef]

Steare, T., Muñoz, C. G., Sullivan, A., & Lewis, G. (2023). The association between academic pressure and adolescent mental health problems: A systematic review. *Journal of Affective Disorders, 339*, 302–317. [CrossRef] [PubMed]

Substance Abuse and Mental Health Services Administration. (2024). *Key substance use and mental health indicators in the United States: Results from the 2023 national survey on drug use and health*. U.S. Department of Health and Human Services. Available online: https://www.samhsa.gov/data/data-we-collect/nsduh-national-survey-drug-use-and-health/national-releases (accessed on 9 February 2025).

Tang, S., Chen, R., Ma, Z., Li, X., Chen, J., & Zhao, J. (2024). Associations of problematic smartphone use with depressive symptoms and suicidal ideation in university students before and after the COVID-19 outbreak: A meta-analysis. *Addictive Behaviors, 152*, 107969. [CrossRef] [PubMed]

Urme, S. A., Islam, M. S., Begum, H., & Chowdhury, N. R. A. (2022). Risk factors of suicide among public university students of Bangladesh: A qualitative exploration. *Heliyon, 8*(6), e09659. [CrossRef]

Walker, A., Tait-McCutcheon, S. L., & Gilbert, A. (2023). Tutors' responses to student disclosures: From suicidal ideation to feeling a little stressed. *Journal of University Teaching and Learning Practice, 20*(7), 1–22.

Wang, Q., & Zhang, Y. (2024). The impact of academic stress on suicidal ideation among college students: A longitudinal study. *Journal of Affective Disorders, 315*, 45–52. [CrossRef]

Yao, Y., Dong, F., & Qiao, Z. (2023). Perceived abusive supervision and graduate students' suicidal ideation: From the perspective of interpersonal psychological theory of suicide. *BMC Psychology, 11*(1), 80. [CrossRef]

Yorgason, J. B., Linville, D., & Zitzman, B. (2024). Mental health among college students: Do those who need services know about and use them? *Journal of American College Health, 57*(2), 173–182. [CrossRef] [PubMed]

Zhai, Y., Boitet, L. M., Soldner, J., Lockman, J. D., & Du, X. (2025). Trends in clinically significant anxiety, depression, suicidal ideation and services utilisation among US medical students, 2018–2023. *BMJ Mental Health, 28*(1), e301528. [CrossRef]

Zhou, H. Y., Luo, Y. H., Shi, L. J., & Gong, J. (2023). Exploring psychological and psychosocial correlates of non-suicidal self-injury and suicide in college students using network analysis. *Journal of Affective Disorders, 336*, 120–125. [CrossRef] [PubMed]

behavioral sciences

MDPI

Article

The Relation Between Violence and Suicidality in Mexico: The Impact of Different Types of Violence in Suicidal Behaviour Detected by a Massive Mental Health Screening App (MeMind)

Cristian Antonio Molina-Pizarro [1,†], Olatz Lopez-Fernandez [2,*,†], Paula Villasante-Soriano [3], Ismael Martinez-Nicolas [4,5], Fuensanta Aroca-Bisquert [6], Pablo Méndez-Bustos [7], Lucas Giner [8] and Enrique Baca-García [3,9,10,11,12,13,*]

1 Instituto de Salud Mental del Gobierno de Yucatán (Institute of Mental Health of the Government of Yucatan), Merida 97000, Mexico; molina_cripiz@gva.es
2 Department of Behavioural Sciences Methodology, Faculty of Psychology, Universidad Nacional de Educación a Distancia (UNED), Moncloa-Aravaca, 28040 Madrid, Spain
3 Department of Psychiatry, University Hospital Jimenez Diaz Foundation, 28040 Madrid, Spain; pvillasante@uoc.edu
4 Faculty of Life Sciences, Universidad Católica San Antonio de Murcia (UCAM), 30107 Guadalupe, Spain; ismael.martinez2@carm.es
5 Sistema Español de Notificación en Seguridad en Anestesia y Reanimación (SENSAR), IDEhA Simulatio Centre, Fundación Alcorcon University Hospital, 28922 Alcorcon, Spain
6 Instituto de Matemáticas, Universidad Nacional Autónoma de México (UNAM), Mexico City 14610, Mexico; fuen@im.unam.mx
7 Department of Psychology, Universidad Católica del Maule, Talca 3460000, Maule, Chile; pmendez@ucm.cl
8 Department of Psychiatry, Universidad de Sevilla, 41009 Seville, Spain; lginer@us.es
9 Department of Psychiatry, Universidad Autónoma de Madrid, 28029 Madrid, Spain
10 Department of Psychiatry, Hospital Rey Juan Carlos, 28933 Móstoles, Spain
11 Department of Psychiatry, Central Hospital de Villalba, 28400 Villalba, Spain
12 Department of Psychiatry, University Hospital Infanta Elena, 28034 Valdemoro, Spain
13 CIBERSAM, Research Group CB/07/09/0025, 28007 Madrid, Spain
* Correspondence: olatz.lopez@psi.uned.es (O.L.-F.); ebacgar2@yahoo.es or research.fjd@gmail.com (E.B.-G.)
† These authors contributed equally to this work.

Abstract

The construct of violence has scarcely been researched in relation to suicidality in Mexico. The aim of the present study was to explore the role of different types of violence (e.g., violence at home, non-suicidal self-injury) in suicidal behaviour (e.g., suicidal ideation, suicidal acts) of the citizens of the Yucatan State using a massive online screening approach through a smartphone application. A prospective cohort study design was undertaken during 2022 including 32,531 Mexican participants aged between 15 and 80 years old, which constituted the second wave of the SmartScreen project, through the TEDUCA survey. We selected as the main variables violence at home, non-suicidal self-injuries, and suicidal behaviour (Columbia—Suicide Severity Rating Scale; C-SSRS). A set of univariate regression analyses was performed for the entire sample connecting the variables with the C-SSRS. Subsequently, a multiple linear regression model was used. The model explained a significant portion of the variance in C-SSRS scores (R^2adj = 0.3227) indicating the following as predictors affecting suicidality: perceived violence at home, followed by a history of NSSI, and previous mental health service attendance, among other associations between the sociodemographic predictors and suicidal behaviour. Significant interactions between perceived violence and NSSI history were also found. In conclusion, our study highlights the significant role of perceived violence at home and NSSI history in shaping suicide risk understood as the ideation and intention of suicidality among Yucatan citizens. The

 https://doi.org/10.3390/bs15081117

interaction between these factors and sociodemographic variables such as gender and age underscore the complex nature of suicide risk.

Keywords: violence at home; self-injury; suicide ideation; suicide attempt; smartphone screening; Mexico

1. Introduction

The construct of violence has been explicitly identified as a significant public health issue, as it can harm the physical and mental well-being of individuals (Rutherford et al., 2007). At present, the framework of the United Nations' 2030 Agenda for Sustainable Developments has recognized violence as a critical topic, and different proposals have targeted goals related to violence prevention to work on global public health actions worldwide (Lee et al., 2016b).

According to the World Report on Violence and Health (WRVH) (World Health Organization [WHO], 2004), violence is defined as the intentional use of force or power, threatened or actual, against oneself, another person, or against a group or community, whilst suicide refers to the deliberate act of ending one's own life, and suicidal behaviour pertains to non-fatal suicidal thoughts and actions, such as suicide ideation, planning, and attempts, following the terminology established by Posner et al. (2007) and Silverman et al. (2007a, 2007b). Violence can occur in four modes (i.e., physical, sexual, psychological, and deprivation), and three sub-types have been described based on the victim–perpetrator relationship: (i) self-directed violence (i.e., self-injury, self-abuse, and suicide); (ii) interpersonal violence at the family level (e.g., child maltreatment, intimate partner violence (IPV), or elder abuse); and (iii) the non-family level (e.g., community violence perpetrated by an acquaintance or stranger). Studies show that suicidal behaviour is usually associated with violence types (Centers for Disease Control and Prevention [CDC], 2016; Decker et al., 2018), such as violence at home (Brown & Seals, 2019) or self-injury (Liu et al., 2022). Angelakis et al. (2020) quantified the association between the core types of childhood maltreatment and suicide behaviour in children and young adults, all of which induced 2.5-fold greater odds of suicide ideation, except for child sexual abuse (CSA), which caused a 4.0-fold increase in suicide plans.

Conceptual models of suicidal behaviour have identified a history of violence as a critical risk factor. A systematic and narrative review conducted by Díaz-Oliván et al. (2021) has outlined, from theoretical models of suicidal behaviour, a set of variables associated with various types of violence: (i) self-directed violence (e.g., feelings of defeat, entrapment, aggression, and self-injury); (ii) family-related violence (e.g., neglect, CSA and physical abuse); and (iii) non-family violence (e.g., social exclusion or traumatic life events). Although self-injuries is a classic risk factor, CSA emerged as the most prevalent factor linked to suicidality according to the theoretical models.

In the American continent, violence is one of the leading sources of morbidity and mortality (Decker et al., 2018). It is noteworthy that empirical studies in the United States of America (USA) have reinforced the relationship between violence and suicide in which the interplay exists in both directions, with self-directed and other-directed violence serving as underlying factors causing, at least, suicidal ideation. For instance, North American cross-sectional studies indicate that exposure to violence acts as a risk factor for future suicidal behaviour, with self-directed and interpersonal violence frequently occurring in conjunction. Research in the USA has demonstrated that the impact of exposure to violence on suicidal ideation is fully mediated and stronger in females and adolescents (Farrell & Zimmerman, 2018). Similarly, in longitudinal studies, a reciprocal relationship between violence and suicidality has been observed from adolescence into adulthood, especially in males during early adulthood (Van Dulmen et al., 2013).

Nevertheless, most of the global violence occurs in regions such as Latin American countries (Lee et al., 2016a). Indeed, a surge in the incidence of violent deaths among young individuals, particularly males, has been noted in Mexico (González-Pérez et al., 2017) where both violence and suicidal behaviour are more prevalent compared to other regions (World Health Organization [WHO], 2021). However, the relationship between different types of violence and suicidal behaviour has been scarcely investigated in Mexico, although previous research has studied the prevalence and associated psychological factors of attempted suicide in a sample of Mexican adolescents (Valdez-Santiago et al., 2018a). Exposure to interpersonal and community violence is strongly linked to adverse mental health outcomes among Mexican adolescents, including heightened risks of anxiety, depression, and suicidal behaviour. Experiences such as domestic violence, school bullying, and exposure to organized crime contribute to a recurring cycle of trauma that frequently goes unaddressed due to systemic deficiencies in institutional support for youth (Valdez-Santiago et al., 2020). Y. Cruz-Manrique et al. (2021) found that school-based victimization, compounded by a lack of family support, was a strong predictor of suicidal ideation among adolescents in Yucatán.

Comprehending the magnitude of the connection between violence types and suicidal behaviour is crucial for understanding the relationship between both to develop effective interventions and policies to address the problem contextualized to specific population groups. Consequently, the main aim of the present study is to explore the role of different types of violence, such as violence at home, non-suicidal self-injury, and a lack of well-being, in the suicidal behaviour (i.e., suicidal ideation and suicidal acts) of the Yucatan State (Mexico) general population using massive online screening approach.

2. Methods

2.1. Design

This investigation was conducted under a quantitative, positivist paradigm using a cross-sectional survey design. Data were collected in a single wave in 2023 via the SmartScreen project's platform (MeMind app), targeting residents of the State of Yucatán, Mexico.

2.2. Participants

This study included 32,531 Mexican participants from the general population in the State of Yucatan, from which 16,267 (50.0%) were women. In total, 192 (0.6%) participants identified their gender as non-binary or as not falling within the categories of woman or man. The age range was 15 to 80 years old.

Our inclusion criteria were as follows: (1) age 15 years or above with enrolment at a participating institution (e.g., education centres, organizations); (2) the ability to use their smartphones; (3) the ability to understand the nature, purpose, and methodology of the study; and (4) participation following express informed consent granted in the app. The exclusion criteria were as follows: (1) students protected by law (e.g., conservatorship) and (2) individuals deprived of liberty (e.g., prisoners).

2.3. Instruments

Our main variables were violence at home (VH), non-suicidal self-injuries (NNSI), and suicidal behaviour (SB). These were derived from reported theoretical models' systematic review and empirical studies, which are described as follows:

The variable violence at home (VH) was assessed using a 5-point Likert scale ranging from "unusual" to "very frequent." This ordinal measure captured the participant's perception of the frequency of violence currently occurring within their home environment, specifically focusing on intrafamilial violence (e.g., "Do you think violence at home or in the family is...").

NNSI was an item about NSSI adapted from DMS 5-2: Have you ever intentionally injured yourself without the intent to take your own life (e.g., cut yourself, hit yourself, stuck yourself with needles, burned yourself, scratched your skin with force, etc.)?

SB was measured through the Columbia—Suicide Severity Rating Scale (C-SSRS) (Mundt et al., 2013; Posner et al., 2011). It includes seven yes/no items regarding the participant's risk of suicidality. The Spanish version used (Al-Halabí et al., 2016) showed good internal consistency (Cronbach's $\alpha = 0.81$) and has also been used in a previous study with another cohort of participants (Martínez-Nicolás et al., 2022b).

These mental health tests have demonstrated adequate validity as a screening tool in several countries including Mexico. Additionally, we employed the following variables: previous mental health service attendance, NSSI history, gender, age, occupation, number of household members, and marital status as secondary variables.

For more information regarding the selection of the tests and items for the SmartScreen Project in Mexico, please see Arenas-Castañeda et al. (2020).

2.4. Procedure

The data were retrieved in 2023 from the second wave of the SmartScreen project, through the TEDUCA survey (Martínez-Nicolás et al., 2022b), through a large suicide risk and NSSI behaviour assessment. The TEDUCA is an ongoing online survey through a mHealth smartphone app named MeMind (Berrouiguet et al., 2015) and, according to SmartScreen's protocol (Martínez-Nicolás et al., 2022a), its primary purpose is to identify the correlates of potential unhealthy populations concerning suicide. For all the details about the SmartScreen protocol survey, please see Arenas-Castañeda et al. (2020). Ethical approval (002/2019) was granted by the Ethics Review Board of the 'Hospital Psiquiátrico Yucatán', Yucatan (Mexico). This protocol has been registered in ClinicalTrials.gov. as the SmartScreen Project (Arenas-Castañeda et al., 2020).

Answers to MeMind questions compiled within the app were uploaded to a secure web server. Usernames and personal data were pseudonymized with a code. Data were encrypted using AES-256 algorithms and 256-bit keys protected by a professional key management infrastructure externally audited.

2.5. Analysis

Descriptive and exploratory analyses were performed to describe participant characteristics. After that, univariate regressions were conducted to determine if the selected variables (violence at home, NSSI history, gender, age, occupation, number of household members, and marital status) were significant in the total score of the C-SSRS test following the purposeful selection process, whereby any variable with a statistically significant result in the univariate analysis was selected as a candidate for the multivariate analysis (Bursac et al., 2008).

Upon confirming that all variables were significant in the univariate regression analyses, including the interaction between violence at home and NSSI, a multiple linear regression model was constructed to analyse the relationship between the predictor variables, the interaction and the total score of the C-SSRS test.

Statistical analyses were conducted using R statistical software. R is available as an open access software under the terms of the GNU General Public License (Lafaye de Micheaux et al., 2013).

3. Results

The descriptive statistics are reported in Table 1. Significant differences across genders were observed across all variables analysed ($p < 0.001$). Gender was balanced (50% women), and among the age groups studied, those situated between the late adolescence and middle-aged adulthood categories were more prevalent than in the elderly age group (1%). The majority of the participants (90%) used to live in homes with a small number of cohabitants (from two to six persons), in which almost half of the sample was single and did not have a child under their care. Regarding current labour activity, more than half of the sample was active as a third were high school and undergraduate students. Concerning the aggressive variables, only a tenth (10%) committed NSSI behaviours, almost a fifth (17%) had some type of suicide risk, and more than a half of the sample (61%) reported to have experienced violence at home.

Table 1. Descriptive statistics and sociodemographics.

		Overall	Man	Woman	Other	*p*-Value
Age	<18	5083 (15.6)	2188 (13.6)	2802 (17.2)	93 (48.4)	<0.001
	18–25	6791 (20.9)	3512 (21.9)	3228 (19.8)	51 (26.6)	
	25–35	6862 (21.1)	3281 (20.4)	3556 (21.9)	25 (13.0)	
	35–50	9875 (30.4)	5021 (31.2)	4837 (29.7)	17 (8.9)	
	50–65	3623 (11.1)	1873 (11.7)	1745 (10.7)	5 (2.6)	
	>65	297 (0.9)	197 (1.2)	99 (0.6)	1 (0.5)	
Marital status	Single	13,788 (52.1)	6376 (49.0)	7300 (54.8)	112 (78.9)	<0.001
	Common-law partner	2279 (8.6)	1079 (8.3)	1188 (8.9)	12 (8.5)	
	Married	8738 (33.0)	4942 (38.0)	3782 (28.4)	14 (9.9)	
	Separated/divorced	1448 (5.5)	545 (4.2)	899 (6.7)	4 (2.8)	
	Widowed	215 (0.8)	64 (0.5)	151 (1.1)	0 (0.0)	
Current activity	Retired	86 (0.3)	48 (0.3)	37 (0.3)	1 (0.6)	<0.001
	Active	18,906 (65.1)	9654 (67.5)	9210 (63.2)	42 (27.3)	
	Homemaker	560 (1.9)	110 (0.8)	445 (3.1)	5 (3.2)	
	Student	8462 (29.2)	4057 (28.4)	4309 (29.6)	96 (62.3)	
	Unemployed	144 (0.5)	62 (0.4)	77 (0.5)	5 (3.2)	
	Underemployed	870 (3.0)	379 (2.6)	486 (3.3)	5 (3.2)	
Number of cohabitants	Alone	1127 (4.3)	614 (4.7)	504 (3.8)	9 (6.2)	<0.001
	1–3	12,581 (47.5)	6045 (46.5)	6477 (48.6)	59 (41.0)	
	4–6	11,133 (42.1)	5571 (42.8)	5500 (41.3)	62 (43.1)	
	More than 6	1625 (6.1)	777 (6.0)	834 (6.3)	14 (9.7)	
Violence at home	Non-existent	10,645 (37.1)	5673 (40.1)	4941 (34.2)	31 (20.9)	<0.001
	Very frequent	3319 (11.6)	1075 (7.6)	2229 (15.4)	15 (10.1)	
	Frequent	5571 (19.4)	2449 (17.3)	3076 (21.3)	46 (31.1)	
	Not very frequent	7870 (27.4)	4258 (30.1)	3571 (24.7)	41 (27.7)	
	Do not know	1318 (4.6)	690 (4.9)	613 (4.2)	15 (10.1)	
NSSI	No	26,390 (89.6)	13,667 (94.3)	12,652 (85.4)	71 (46.1)	<0.001
	Yes	3066 (10.4)	827 (5.7)	2156 (14.6)	83 (53.9)	
CSSRS		5.86 (2.20)	5.71 (2.07)	5.99 (2.27)	6.97 (4.17)	<0.001
	TOTAL	32,531	16,072 (49.4)	16,267 (50.0)	192 (0.6)	

Table 2 presents the outcomes of multiple linear regression (MLR) applied to the training data. Significance was found in all model parameters concerning the effectiveness of treatment ($p < 0.0001$).

The model demonstrated good fit, explaining a significant portion of variance in C-SSRS scores.

Perceived violence at home was a significant predictor, with individuals perceiving very frequent ($b = 0.103$, $p < 0.001$), frequent ($b = 0.096$, $p < 0.001$), and somewhat frequent violence ($b = 0.087$, $p < 0.001$) compared to those who did not perceive violence at home (Table 2).

Table 2. Multiple linear regression (MLR).

Predictor	β	95% CI	*p*-Value
Intercept	6.57 **	[6.26, 6.88]	<0.01
Had sought any mental health services (ref: no)			
Yes	0.30 **	[0.27, 0.33]	<0.01
Violence at home (ref: inexistent violence)			
Very frequent	0.10 **	[0.05, 0.15]	<0.01
Frequent	0.10 **	[0.06, 0.14]	<0.01
Not frequent	0.09 **	[0.05, 0.12]	<0.01
Does not know how often violence occurs at home	0.07	[−0.00, 0.14]	0.06
Had intentionally inflicted NSSI before (ref: no)			
Yes	1.57 **	[1.49, 1.66]	<0.01
Gender (ref: Man)			
Woman	0.04 *	[0.01, 0.06]	0.01
Other	1.09 **	[0.91, 1.28]	<0.01
Current activity (ref: retired)			
Active	−0.13	[−0.43, 0.16]	0.38
Homemaker	0.27	[−0.05, 0.58]	0.09
Student	0.00	[−0.30, 0.30]	0.99
Unemployed	0.81 **	[0.46, 1.16]	<0.01
Underemployed (temporary)	−0.03	[−0.34, 0.27]	0.83
Household members (ref: 0)			
1–3	−0.16 **	[−0.23, −0.09]	<0.01
4–6	−0.17 **	[−0.24, −0.10]	<0.01
More than 6	−0.15 **	[−0.24, −0.06]	<0.01
Family status			<0.01
Domestic partner	0.10 **	[0.05, 0.15]	<0.01
Married	0.00	[−0.04, 0.04]	0.87
Divorced/separated	0.06	[−0.00, 0.13]	0.06
Widowed	0.05	[−0.10, 0.20]	0.53
Age group (ref: <18)			
18–25	−0.14 **	[−0.18, −0.09]	<0.01
25–35	−0.29 **	[−0.35, −0.22]	<0.01
35–50	−0.34 **	[−0.41, −0.28]	<0.01
50–65	−0.34 **	[−0.42, −0.27]	<0.01
>65	−0.45 **	[−0.63, −0.28]	<0.01
Violence at home: had intentionally inflicted NSSI before (ref: Inexistent violence: No)			<0.01
Very frequent: Yes	0.57 **	[0.43, 0.71]	<0.01
Frequent: Yes	0.33 **	[0.21, 0.45]	<0.01
Not frequent: Yes	0.44 **	[0.32, 0.55]	<0.01
Does not know: Yes	0.20 *	[0.00, 0.39]	0.05

* $p < 0.1$; ** $p < 0.01$.

A history of NSSI was strongly associated with higher C-SSRS scores ($b = 1.573$, $p < 0.001$). Gender also played a role, with women having slightly higher scores compared to men ($b = 0.035$, $p = 0.013$) and individuals identifying as non-binary having significantly higher scores ($b = 1.094$, $p < 0.001$).

Previous mental health service attendance was another significant predictor, with individuals who had previously accessed mental health services having higher C-SSRS scores ($b = 0.301$, $p < 0.001$).

Regarding occupation, those who were unemployed had higher C-SSRS scores compared to retired individuals ($b = 0.812$, $p < 0.001$). Homemakers showed a marginal increase in scores ($b = 0.268$, $p = 0.094$), while other occupations did not show significant differences.

The number of household members was inversely related to C-SSRS scores, with individuals living with 1–3 ($b = -0.161$, $p < 0.001$), 4–6 ($b = -0.169$, $p < 0.001$) or more than 6 members ($b = -0.150$, $p < 0.001$) having lower scores compared to those living by their own. Marital status was significant, with individuals in a couple ($b = 0.096$, $p < 0.001$) showing higher scores.

Age showed a significant negative relationship with C-SSRS scores. Younger individuals (18–25 years) had lower scores ($b = -0.139$, $p < 0.001$) compared to individuals between 15 and 18 years old, and the scores continued to decrease significantly across the older age groups (25–35, 35–50, 50–65, and 65+).

Significant interactions between perceived violence and NSSI history were found, indicating that the relationship between violence perception and C-SSRS scores is moderated by NSSI history. Individuals perceiving very frequent violence combined with a history of NSSI ($b = 0.569$, $p < 0.001$), frequent violence combined with NSSI ($b = 0.329$, $p < 0.001$), somewhat frequent violence combined with NSSI ($b = 0.435$, $p < 0.001$), and an uncertain frequency of violence combined with NSSI ($b = 0.198$, $p = 0.048$) had significantly higher C-SSRS scores compared to non-perceived violence at home combined with no NSSI history.

4. Discussion

Our study investigated the associations between perceived violence at home, NSSI history, and suicide risk among individuals assessed using the Columbia—Suicide Severity Rating Scale. The main findings underscore the significance of perceived violence at home and NSSI history as pivotal factors influencing suicide risk scores. However, gender and sociodemographic characteristics such as age, and occupation were found also as meaningful predictors. Each of these factors contributes uniquely to the overall risk. Hence, our results contribute to a better understanding of the multifaceted nature of suicide risk in relation to violence types, necessitating a comprehensive approach in both assessment and intervention strategies.

Specifically, the multivariate analysis revealed that the perception of frequent violence at home significantly increased C-SSRS scores, with a gradient effect observed across categories from frequent to very frequent violence. This trend remained significant after adjusting for sociodemographic variables such as gender and age. Furthermore, a history of NSSI was strongly associated with elevated C-SSRS scores, particularly when interacting with the perception of violence at home, as also shown in females in previous studies.

The impact of interpersonal violence on suicide risk has been well documented. MacIsaac et al. (2017) systematically reviewed the association between exposure to interpersonal violence and completed suicide among women, either as victims or perpetrators, finding a connection with no clear association among mental health factors. Similarly, Angelakis et al. (2020) conducted a systematic review and meta-analysis, quantifying the association between various forms of childhood maltreatment and suicide behaviour in young individuals. They found a 2.5-fold greater risk for suicide ideation, with child sexual abuse leading to a 4.0-fold increase in suicide plans. Moreover, a global study on intimate partner violence and mental health outcomes in women revealed increased odds for suicidality (OR = 2.17–5.52), further demonstrating the serious mental health consequences of violence exposure (R. G. White et al., 2024). A. Clarke et al. (2019) also highlighted the broader context of NSSI, encompassing various forms of violence and their connections to suicidality.

Hence, our findings in the present study applied to Mexico are consistent with previous research highlighting the link between violence and suicide risk. Studies have repeatedly demonstrated that individuals exposed to domestic violence are at a heightened risk for developing suicidal ideation and behaviours, particularly when compounded by a history of NSSI. Moreover, the gender differences in suicide risk observed in our study align with global patterns that suggest women may experience more severe mental health impacts from domestic violence.

Indeed, gender seems to play a notable role in suicide risk. Valdez-Santiago et al. (2018b) explored attempted suicide among Mexican adolescents, finding a 2.7% prevalence, with women being significantly more at risk than men. Women and non-binary individuals had significantly higher C-SSRS scores compared to men when controlling for the perception of violence and NSSI history (Mendoza-Pérez et al., 2021; Valdez-Santiago et al., 2018a). Interestingly, the interactions between gender and perceived violence suggest that women and non-binary individuals may experience an amplified suicide risk in environments of domestic violence compared to men.

Additionally, adolescents who had experienced violence-related health damage in the previous year had over four times the risk of engaging in suicide attempts. Indeed, younger age groups and individuals who had previously sought mental health services demonstrated higher suicide risk scores, emphasizing the importance of early mental health intervention in this population (Liu et al., 2022). Social factors should be considered in future locally adapted population-based interventions. For instance, A. L. Cruz-Manrique et al. (2021) found that school victimization and a lack of family support were important predictors of suicidal ideation among adolescents in the State of Yucatan. These findings reflect the need for considering younger, female and minorities populations (e.g., Mexican homosexual and bisexual men). They also add to the broader literature on the cumulative effects of adverse childhood experiences on long-term mental health outcomes (Anda et al., 2006), which require in turn a dedicated, priority effort to be addressed.

4.1. Clinical and Policy Implications

The findings from this study have important clinical implications, particularly in the context of screening and intervention for suicide risk. Given the strong association between perceived violence and NSSI, clinicians should prioritize comprehensive assessments that include questions about domestic violence and NSSI behaviours when evaluating suicide risk.

The gendered disparities found in this study reflect broader social and structural inequalities that disproportionately affect women and sexual and gender minorities in Mexico (Mendoza-Pérez et al., 2021; Valdez-Santiago et al., 2018b). These groups often face compounded forms of violence, including gender-based discrimination, limited access to healthcare, and social stigmatization (A. L. Cruz-Manrique et al., 2021; S. J. White et al., 2024), all of which may exacerbate suicide risk. Previous studies have shown that non-binary and LGBTQ+ individuals in Mexico experience higher levels of psychological distress and suicidal ideation due to these intersecting vulnerabilities (Angelakis et al., 2020; Anda et al., 2006). As such, interventions must go beyond clinical assessment to incorporate gender-sensitive and culturally responsive approaches—ensuring that prevention and care strategies address the specific needs, vulnerabilities, and strengths of diverse gender populations (S. Clarke et al., 2019; MacIsaac et al., 2017).

This is particularly crucial for younger individuals and those with a history of mental health service use (Dube et al., 2001). Furthermore, interventions should be gender-sensitive, as women and non-binary individuals appear to be disproportionately affected by violence in relation to suicide risk.

From a policy perspective, our results support the need for robust domestic violence prevention programmes and the integration of mental health services for individuals exposed to violence. Public health initiatives aimed at reducing domestic violence and providing timely mental health support may significantly mitigate the suicide risk among vulnerable populations (Krug et al., 2002).

4.2. Limitations

One of the main limitations of our study is its reliance on self-reported measures of violence and suicide risk, which may be subject to social desirability bias. Additionally, the cross-sectional design limits our ability to infer causal relationships between perceived violence and suicide risk. Future longitudinal studies are needed to establish the temporal sequence between these variables. However, the large sample size and comprehensive statistical analysis employed in this study are notable strengths that enhance the reliability of our findings (Friedman & Sudak, 2019).

5. Conclusions

In conclusion, our study highlights the significant role of perceived violence at home and NSSI history in shaping suicide risk as measured by the C-SSRS. The interaction between these factors and sociodemographic variables such as gender and age underscore the complex nature of suicide risk. Future research should focus on longitudinal analyses to better understand the causal pathways involved. Clinicians and policymakers should prioritize the early identification of risks and intervention for individuals exposed to violence and those with a history of NSSI to reduce the burden of suicide in these populations.

Author Contributions: Conceptualization, C.A.M.-P., F.A.-B. and E.B.-G.; Formal Analysis, C.A.M.-P., O.L.-F., P.V.-S. and I.M.-N.; Funding Acquisition, C.A.M.-P. and E.B.-G.; Investigation, C.A.M.-P., O.L.-F., P.V.-S. and I.M.-N.; Methodology, C.A.M.-P., I.M.-N., F.A.-B. and E.B.-G.; Resources, C.A.M.-P.; Supervision, E.B.-G.; Writing—Original Draft, O.L.-F., P.V.-S. and I.M.-N.; Writing—Review and Editing, C.A.M.-P., O.L.-F., P.V.-S., I.M.-N., F.A.-B., P.M.-B., L.G. and E.B.-G. All authors have read and agreed to the published version of the manuscript.

Funding: This research was supported by CIBER-Consorcio Centro de Investigación Biomédica en Red (código CIBER), Instituto de Salud Carlos III, Ministerio de Ciencia e Innovación and Unión Europea—European Regional Development Fund (ISCIII PI20/01555), by Ministerio de Ciencia e Innovación/a Agencia Estatal de Investigación MCIN/AEI/10.13039/501100011033 and "NextGenerationEU"/PRTR (TED2021-131120B-I00) by the Madrid Regional Government (S2022/BMD-7216, AGES 3-CM), and by Fundació La Marató de TV3 (202226-31).

Institutional Review Board Statement: The study was conducted in accordance with the Declaration of Helsinki, and approved by the NAME OF INSTITUTE Ethics Review Board of the 'Hospital Psiquiátrico Yucatán' (approval code 002/2019, date of approval 27 August 2019). This protocol has been registered in ClinicalTrials.gov. (NCT04067063) as the SmartScreen Project (Arenas-Castañeda et al., 2020).

Informed Consent Statement: Informed consent was obtained via the express informed consent given during the application process.

Data Availability Statement: The datasets used and/or during the current study are available from the corresponding author on reasonable request.

Conflicts of Interest: E.B.-G. has been a consultant to or has received honoraria or grants from Janssen Cilag, Lundbeck, Otsuka, Pziffer, Servier and Sanoffi. E.B.-G. designed the MEmind application. The other authors confirm they have no conflicts of interest.

References

Al-Halabí, S., Sáiz, P. A., Burón, P., Garrido, M., Benabarre, A., Jiménez, E., Cervilla, J., Navarrete, M. I., Díaz-Mesa, E. M., García-Álvarez, L., Muñiz, J., Posner, K., Oquendo, M. A., García-Portilla, M. P., & Bobes, J. (2016). Validation of a Spanish version of the Columbia-suicide severity rating scale (C-SSRS) [Validación de la versión en Español de la Columbia-suicide severity rating scale (escala columbia para evaluar el riesgo de suicidio)]. *Revista de Psiquiatria y Salud Mental, 9*(3), 134–142. [CrossRef] [PubMed]

Anda, R. F., Felitti, V. J., Bremner, J. D., Walker, J. D., Whitfield, C., Perry, B. D., Dube, S. R., & Giles, W. H. (2006). The enduring effects of abuse and related adverse experiences in childhood. *European Archives of Psychiatry and Clinical Neuroscience, 256*(3), 174–186. [CrossRef]

Angelakis, I., Austin, J. L., & Gooding, P. (2020). Association of childhood maltreatment with suicide behaviors among young people: A systematic review and meta-analysis. *JAMA Network Open, 3*(8), e2012563. [CrossRef]

Arenas-Castañeda, P. E., Aroca Bisquert, F., Martinez-Nicolas, I., Castillo Espíndola, L. A., Barahona, I., Maya-Hernández, C., Lavana Hernández, M. M., Manrique Mirón, P. C., Alvarado Barrera, D. G., Treviño Aguilar, E., Barrios Núñez, A., De Jesus Carlos, G., Vildosola Garcés, A., Flores Mercado, J., Barrigon, M. L., Artes, A., de Leon, S., Molina-Pizarro, C. A., Rosado Franco, A., ... Baca-Garcia, E. (2020). Universal mental health screening with a focus on suicidal behaviour using smartphones in a Mexican rural community: Protocol for the SMART-SCREEN population-based survey. *BMJ Open, 10*(7), e035041. [CrossRef]

Berrouiguet, S., Courtet, P., Perez-Rodriguez, M., Oquendo, M., & Baca-Garcia, E. (2015). The Memind project: A new web-based mental health tracker designed for clinical management and research. *European Psychiatry, 30*(Suppl. S1), 974. [CrossRef]

Brown, S., & Seals, J. (2019). Intimate partner problems and suicide: Are we missing the violence? *Journal of Injury & Violence Research, 11*(1), 53–64. [CrossRef]

Bursac, Z., Gauss, C. H., Williams, D. K., & Hosmer, D. W. (2008). Purposeful selection of variables in logistic regression. *Source Code for Biology and Medicine, 3*, 17. [CrossRef] [PubMed]

Centers for Disease Control and Prevention (CDC). (2016). *Preventing multiple forms of violence: A strategic vision for connecting the dots*. Division of Violence Prevention, National Center for Injury Prevention and Control, CDC. Available online: https://www.cdc.gov/suicide/pdf/strategic_vision.pdf (accessed on 7 July 2025).

Clarke, A., Patalay, P., Allen, E., Knight, L., Naker, D., & Devries, K. (2019). Patterns and predictors of self-harm in poor urban young adolescents in sub-Saharan Africa: A prospective cohort study. *BMC Public Health, 19*, 1209.

Clarke, S., Allerhand, L. A., & Berk, M. S. (2019). Recent advances in understanding and managing self-harm in adolescents. *F1000Research, 8*, 1794. [CrossRef]

Cruz-Manrique, A. L., Martínez-Valle, A., & Medina-Mora, M. E. (2021). Prevalencia e impacto de la victimización escolar en la ideación suicida de adolescentes en Yucatán. *Salud Mental, 44*(5), 221–228. [CrossRef]

Cruz-Manrique, Y., Olaizola, J. H., Cortés-Ayala, L., & Malvaceda-Espinoza, E. (2021). Effect of violence and school victimization on suicidal ideation in Mexican adolescents. *International Journal of Psychological Research, 14*(2), 30–36. [CrossRef]

Decker, M. R., Wilcox, H. C., Holliday, C. N., & Webster, D. W. (2018). An integrated public health approach to interpersonal violence and suicide prevention and response. *Public Health Reports (Washington, D.C.: 1974), 133*(Suppl. S1), 65S–79S. [CrossRef]

Díaz-Oliván, I., Porras-Segovia, A., Barrigón, M. L., Jiménez-Muñoz, L., & Baca-García, E. (2021). Theoretical models of suicidal behaviour: A systematic review and narrative synthesis. *The European Journal of Psychiatry, 35*(3), 181–192. [CrossRef]

Dube, S. R., Anda, R. F., Felitti, V. J., Chapman, D. P., Williamson, D. F., & Giles, W. H. (2001). Childhood abuse, household dysfunction, and the risk of attempted suicide throughout the life span: Findings from the adverse childhood experiences study. *JAMA, 286*(24), 3089–3096. [CrossRef]

Farrell, C., & Zimmerman, G. M. (2018). Violent lives: Pathways linking exposure to violence to suicidal behavior in a national sample. *Archives of Suicide Research: Official Journal of the International Academy for Suicide Research, 23*(1), 100–121. [CrossRef]

Friedman, R. A., & Sudak, D. M. (2019). Suicide prevention: A public health imperative. *Journal of the American Medical Association, 322*(16), 1561–1562.

González-Pérez, G. J., Vega-López, M. G., Souza, E. R., & Pinto, L. W. (2017). Violence deaths and its impact on life expectancy: A comparison between Mexico and Brazil [Mortalidad por violencias y su impacto en la esperanza de vida: Una comparación entre México y Brasil]. *Ciencia & Saude Coletiva, 22*(9), 2797–2809. [CrossRef]

Krug, E. G., Dahlberg, L. L., Mercy, J. A., Zwi, A. B., & Lozano, R. (Eds.). (2002). *World report on violence and health*. World Health Organization.

Lafaye de Micheaux, P., Drouilhet, R., & Liquet, B. (2013). *The R software*. Springer.

Lee, B. X., Gilligan, J., Kaaya, S. F., & Schuder, K. K. (2016a). Violence and health: Implications of the 2030 agenda for South-North collaboration. *International Journal of Public Health, 61*(8), 861–862. [CrossRef]

Lee, B. X., Kjaerulf, F., Turner, S., Cohen, L., Donnelly, P. D., Muggah, R., Davis, R., Realini, A., Kieselbach, B., MacGregor, L. S., Waller, I., Gordon, R., Moloney-Kitts, M., Lee, G., & Gilligan, J. (2016b). Transforming our world: Implementing the 2030 agenda through sustainable development goal indicators. *Journal of Public Health Policy, 37*(Suppl. 1), 13–31. [CrossRef] [PubMed]

Liu, R. T., Walsh, R. F. L., Sheehan, A. E., Cheek, S. M., & Sanzari, C. M. (2022). Prevalence and correlates of suicide and nonsuicidal self-injury in children: A systematic review and meta-analysis. *JAMA Psychiatry, 79*(7), 718–726. [CrossRef] [PubMed]

MacIsaac, M. B., Bugeja, L. C., & Jelinek, G. A. (2017). The association between exposure to interpersonal violence and suicide among women: A systematic review. *Australian and New Zealand Journal of Public Health, 41*(1), 61–69. [CrossRef]

Martínez-Nicolás, I., Arenas Castañeda, P. E., Molina-Pizarro, C. A., Rosado Franco, A., Maya-Hernández, C., Barahona, I., Martínez-Alés, G., Aroca Bisquert, F., Baca-García, E., & Barrigón, M. L. (2022a). Impact of depression on anxiety, well-being, and suicidality in Mexican adolescent and young adult students from Mexico city: A mental health screening using smartphones. *The Journal of Clinical Psychiatry, 83*(3), 20m13806. [CrossRef]

Martínez-Nicolás, I., Molina-Pizarro, C. A., Franco, A. R., Arenas Castañeda, P. E., Maya, C., Barahona, I., Martínez-Alés, G., Bisquert, F. A., Delgado-Gomez, D., Dervic, K., Lopez-Fernandez, O., Baca-García, E., & Barrigón, M. L. (2022b). What seems to explain suicidality in yucatan mexican young adults? Findings from an app-based mental health screening test using the smart-screen protocol. *Current Psychology: A Journal for Diverse Perspectives on Diverse Psychological Issues, 42*, 30767–30779. [CrossRef]

Mendoza-Pérez, J. C., González-Forteza, C., Borges, G., & Benjet, C. (2021). Suicide risk and associated factors in Mexican LGBTQ+ youth. *Revista Latinoamericana de Psicología, 53*, 29–37. [CrossRef]

Mundt, J. C., Greist, J. H., Jefferson, J. W., Federico, M., Mann, J. J., & Posner, K. (2013). Prediction of suicidal behavior in clinical research by lifetime suicidal ideation and behavior ascertained by the electronic Columbia-suicide severity rating scale. *The Journal of Clinical Psychiatry, 74*(9), 887–893. [CrossRef] [PubMed]

Posner, K., Brown, G. K., Stanley, B., Brent, D. A., Yershova, K. V., Oquendo, M. A., Currier, G. W., Melvin, G. A., Greenhill, L., Shen, S., & Mann, J. J. (2011). The Columbia-suicide severity rating scale: Initial validity and internal consistency findings from three multisite studies with adolescents and adults. *The American Journal of Psychiatry, 168*(12), 1266–1277. [CrossRef]

Posner, K., Oquendo, M. A., Gould, M., Stanley, B., & Davies, M. (2007). Columbia classification algorithm of suicide assessment (C-CASA): Classification of suicidal events in the FDA's pediatric suicidal risk analysis of antidepressants. *The American Journal of Psychiatry, 164*(7), 1035–1043. [CrossRef]

Rutherford, A., Zwi, A. B., Grove, N. J., & Butchart, A. (2007). Violence: A glossary. *Journal of Epidemiology and Community Health, 61*(8), 676–680. [CrossRef]

Silverman, M. M., Berman, A. L., Sanddal, N. D., O'carroll, P. W., & Joiner, T. E. (2007a). Rebuilding the tower of babel: A revised nomenclature for the study of suicide and suicidal behaviors. Part 1: Background, rationale, and methodology. *Suicide & Life-Threatening Behavior, 37*(3), 248–263. [CrossRef]

Silverman, M. M., Berman, A. L., Sanddal, N. D., O'carroll, P. W., & Joiner, T. E. (2007b). Rebuilding the tower of babel: A revised nomenclature for the study of suicide and suicidal behaviors. Part 2: Suicide-related ideations, communications, and behaviors. *Suicide & Life-Threatening Behavior, 37*(3), 264–277. [CrossRef]

Valdez-Santiago, R., Gonzalez-Forteza, C., Juarez, F., & Borges, G. (2018a). Suicide attempts among Mexican adolescents: Prevalence and associated factors. *Salud Pública de México, 60*(4), 397–405.

Valdez-Santiago, R., Híjar, M., Rojas-Martínez, R., & Heredia-Pi, I. (2020). Violencia en adolescentes mexicanos: Prevalencia y factores asociados. *Salud Pública de México, 62*(1), 33–40. [CrossRef]

Valdez-Santiago, R., Solórzano, E. H., Iñiguez, M. M., Burgos, L. Á., Gómez Hernández, H., & Martínez González, Á. (2018b). Attempted suicide among adolescents in Mexico: Prevalence and associated factors at the national level. *Injury Prevention: Journal of the International Society for Child and Adolescent Injury Prevention, 24*(4), 256–261. [CrossRef] [PubMed]

Van Dulmen, M., Mata, A., Claxton, S., Klipfel, K., Schinka, K., Swahn, M., & Bossarte, R. (2013). Longitudinal associations between violence and suicidality from adolescence into adulthood. *Suicide & Life-Threatening Behavior, 43*(5), 523–531. [CrossRef]

White, R. G., Liu, A., Gong, E., & Heise, L. (2024). Intimate partner violence and mental health outcomes in women: A global systematic review and meta-analysis. *The Lancet Psychiatry, 11*(2), 123–134. [CrossRef]

White, S. J., Sin, J., Sweeney, A., Salisbury, T., Wahlich, C., Montesinos Guevara, C. M., Gillard, S., Brett, E., Allwright, L., Iqbal, N., Khan, A., Perot, C., Marks, J., & Mantovani, N. (2024). Global prevalence and mental health outcomes of intimate partner violence among women: A systematic review and meta-analysis. *Trauma, Violence & Abuse*, *25*(1), 494–511. [CrossRef]

World Health Organisation [WHO]. (2004). *Violence prevention alliance (VPA): World report on violence and health*. Available online: https://www.who.int/groups/violence-prevention-alliance/approach (accessed on 21 May 2024).

World Health Organization [WHO]. (2021). *Suicide worldwide in 2019: Global health estimates*. WHO. Available online: https://iris.who.int/bitstream/handle/10665/341728/9789240026643-eng.pdf?sequence=1 (accessed on 7 July 2025).

behavioral sciences

MDPI

Article

Network Analysis of Psychopathological Dimensions in Patients with and Without Suicidal Ideation

Elena Huguet [1,*], Teresa Paniagua-Granados [1], Miriam Romero [1], Ignacio Fernández-Arias [2] and Cristina Larroy [2]

1 Psychology Department, European University of Madrid, 28670 Madrid, Spain; teresa.paniagua@universidadeuropea.es (T.P.-G.)
2 Personality, Assessment and Clinical Psychology, Complutense University of Madrid, 28223 Madrid, Spain; igfernan@ucm.es (I.F.-A.); clarroyg@ucm.es (C.L.)
* Correspondence: elena.huguet@universidadeuropea.es

Abstract

Knowing the configuration of psychopathological dimensions in patients according to suicidal ideation in an applied context is fundamental in clinical approaches. A cross-sectional and retrospective single-measurement study was carried out in 625 patients of the University Psychology Clinic of the Complutense University of Madrid (CUP-UCM) divided into two groups: with and without suicidal ideation. Network analysis was used as the main methodology. Anxiety and interpersonal variables appeared as core symptoms of the group with suicidal ideation, reinforcing theoretical models where the social component is a key part of present suicidal ideation. Even though the configuration of networks was not significantly different between the two groups, the severity of symptoms in the group with suicidal ideation was higher. In the predictive analyses, depressive symptoms, hostility, somatization, paranoid ideation, and psychoticism were independently associated with suicidal ideation. This result highlights the complex and multidimensional nature of suicide risk, which cannot be fully explained by depressive symptoms alone. Anxiety and interpersonal variables stand out as core symptoms with influence on others, which may guide clinicians in prioritization in therapeutic goals.

Keywords: suicidal ideation; network analysis; psychopathological dimensions; anxiety; interpersonal variables; hostility

1. Introduction

Suicide, understood as death caused by self-directed harmful behaviour with the intention to die (Crosby et al., 2011), has become one of the major public health problems at national and international level. Already in 2014, the WHO raised the alarm on this issue and urged institutions to take specific measures and not to underestimate the risk (World Health Organization, 2014). According to the most updated figures from the National Institute of Statistics, in 2023 in Spain there were 4116 completed suicides, 5.6% more than in 2021, 1.6% more than in 2020, and 7.4% more than in 2019 (Instituto Nacional de Estadística, 2024).

Considering the entire suicide continuum, which also includes suicidal ideation and attempts of varying degrees of intensity and planning (Posner et al., 2011), the presence of suicidal ideation is a proven risk for suicide (De Leo et al., 2013; Hubers et al., 2018; Klonsky et al., 2016; Large et al., 2020). Across the board, the prevalence of suicidal ideation is higher than that of attempts (Castillejos et al., 2021) and 10 times higher than that of completed suicides (Nock et al., 2008).

In relation to the above-mentioned rising figures, and with the intention of focusing on suicide prevention, attempts have been made to identify the elements that are associated with suicidal behaviour. Although suicide is a complex phenomenon influenced by multiple factors—including demographic and sociosituational variables (Kim et al., 2016; Lorant et al., 2018; Nock et al., 2008; Sadock et al., 2015; Shah, 2011; Westefeld et al., 2015)—this study focuses specifically on the psychopathological dimensions (Nock et al., 2009; Nock et al., 2010) associated with suicidal ideation, as they are often the most proximal indicators of risk in clinical outpatient settings. Hopelessness (Franklin et al., 2017), despair (Glenn et al., 2022), psychological pain (Klonsky & May, 2015), impulsivity (Moore et al., 2022), and suicidality (Joiner, 2005; O'Connor & Kirtley, 2018) are some of the factors that clinicians should be aware of, as they are mechanisms related to the development and increased risk of suicidal behaviour.

Risk factors are known to transcend purely individual components, as they are also related to sociosituational factors such as periods of economic crisis, job instability, marital status or the absence of sociofamilial support networks (Blakely et al., 2003; Dehara et al., 2021; Milner et al., 2013a, 2013b). Therefore, the complexity of the phenomenon means that it should be approached from a global rather than an individualistic perspective (Al-Halabí & Fonseca-Pedrero, 2023).

Once it is known which factors are related to suicidal behaviour, it seems undeniable to ask the questions: is it sufficient to know these factors to address the current suicide crisis, and why are deaths still not preventable?

Klonsky et al. (2016) argued that the failure to predict completed suicide is due to a lack of knowledge about the processes underlying ideation and action, so theoretical explanatory models and related research should focus along these lines. Methodological approaches such as network analysis could overcome the tautological conceptualizations and reification of the common latent disorder model applied to psychology (Borsboom & Cramer, 2013). Psychopathological symptoms are conceived as networks of symptoms that evolve over time and are causally interrelated (Borsboom, 2017; Borsboom & Cramer, 2013; Fonseca-Pedrero, 2018; Fried et al., 2016), which is why this analytical approach has been applied to suicidal behavior in recent years (D. P. De Beurs et al., 2017; D. De Beurs et al., 2019; Fonseca-Pedrero et al., 2020b, 2022; Rath et al., 2019).

Most epidemiological studies have focused either on the general population or on specific psychiatric populations (psychotic patients, BPD or adolescents) (Ducasse et al., 2020; Fonseca-Pedrero et al., 2020a; Taylor et al., 2010; Yates et al., 2019). In fact, the Clinical Practice Guideline on the prevention and treatment of suicidal behaviour in Spain (2012) refers only to healthcare settings (primary care, mental health centers, and hospital emergency departments) for detection and intervention within the National Health System, without including the outpatient context outside the public health system. However, this context, a priori of a less urgent and/or serious nature than the hospital, may be the ideal setting for the detection of suicidal ideation at the beginning of its development, prior to its intensification or entry into the hospital circuit after attempts.

Thus, the main objective of this study is to explore the configuration and interrelationships of psychopathological symptoms in patients attending an outpatient clinical setting, according to the presence or absence of suicidal ideation. As a second objective, another aim is to analyze whether the relationships between dimensions are different in comparison with those for the group without suicidal ideation. For this purpose, we used a methodology based on psychopathological network analysis (Borsboom, 2017; Epskamp et al., 2018) and a predictive model that considers these dimensions.

It was hypothesized that symptom intensity would be higher in the group with suicidal ideation, with depressive and anxious symptomatology being the most central factors in the network. Furthermore, it was expected that there would be significant differences between the networks of both groups: depression would be more central in the network of people with ideation and there would be a positive relationship between depressive and anxious symptoms and suicidal ideation.

2. Materials and Methods

2.1. Participants

The sample was incidental composed of patients attending the University Psychology Clinic of the Complutense University of Madrid (CUP-UCM), which has been shown to have similar characteristics to other outpatient settings (Labrador et al., 2010). The participants in this study were all over 18 years of age, requested general psychological care, and signed the corresponding informed consent form.

The sample finally selected was 625 people, aged between 18 and 79 years, whose sociodemographic and clinical characteristics are summarized in Table 1.

Table 1. Sociodemographic and clinical characteristics of the sample (625).

Variables	n (%)/M (DT)
Age	27.76 (11.323)
Sex	
Female	435 (66.0%)
Male	190 (30.4%)
Nationality	
Spanish	565 (90.4%)
Other	60 (9.6%)
Occupational Status	
Student	386 (66.3%)
Employed	104 (17.9%)
Student and employed	60 (10.3%)
Unemployed	7 (1.2%)
Data not available	68 (4.3%)
Educational level	
Incomplete basic education	5 (0.9%)
Completed basic education	28 (4.8%)
Secondary education	309 (53.1%)
Professional education	34 (5.8%)
Bachelor's degree	109 (18.7%)
Postgraduate degree	62 (10.7%)
Doctorate	7 (1.2%)
Data not available	71 (4.3%)
Marital Status	
Single	473 (81.3%)
Married/In a Stable Relationship	78 (13.4%)
Separated/Divorced	5 (0.9%)
Data not available	69 (4.3%)
Previous Psychological Treatment	
Yes	242 (41.6%)
No	308 (52.9%)
Data not available	75 (5.5%)

Table 1. *Cont.*

Variables	n (%)/M (DT)
Depressive Symptoms (BDI-II)	21.59 (11.47)
Suicidal Ideation (Item 9 BDI-II)	394 (66.1%)
Absence of Suicidal Ideation	184 (30.8%)
Mild Suicidal Ideation	12 (2%)
Severe Suicidal Ideation	7 (1.2%)
Very Severe Suicidal Ideation	28 (4.5%)

Note. n = number of persons, % = percentage, M = mean, SD = standard deviation.

Inclusion criteria required participants to be patients at the onset of the assessment process whose full clinical records were available in the archive of CUP-UCM. Participants had to be of legal age at the time of data collection and have completed the full assessment process. In addition, quantitative data from the required psychometric instruments had to be available, and all variables considered in the analysis had to be fully completed

Patients were excluded if the assessment responded to specific demands requiring alternative protocols, if therapy was conducted in a joint format that made it impossible to match individual patients to their corresponding questionnaires, or if the required psychometric data were incomplete or missing.

2.2. *Instruments*

- The Symptom Checklist-90-R (SCL-90-R) (Derogatis, 2001; González de Rivera et al., 2002). This self-administered instrument consists of 90 items that assess the presence of various psychopathological characteristics over the past seven days, specifically evaluating nine symptomatic dimensions and three global distress indices expressed in percentiles and T-scores. The items are structured on a Likert-type scale with five response options (0 to 4), where a higher score indicates greater symptom severity. Internal consistency for the instrument could not be assessed in our study, as item-level responses were not available—only the dimension scores were accessible. However, previous studies have reported adequate reliability for this version of the instrument. In similar clinical samples (Carrasco et al., 2003), the test has shown high internal consistency, both for the total scale (0.97) and for each of its subscales, which correspond to the nine pathological dimensions assessed: Somatization (0.87), Obsessive-Compulsive (0.87), Interpersonal Sensitivity (0.83), Depression (0.89), Anxiety (0.84), Hostility (0.84), Phobic Anxiety (0.88), Paranoid Ideation (0.80), and Psychoticism (0.76). In this study, T-scores of the nine psychopathological dimensions and the PSDI (Positive Symptom Total) were collected. For a detailed interpretation of each dimension, refer to the work of González de Rivera et al. (2002).
- To assess suicidal ideation, item 9 of the Beck Depression Inventory-II (BDI-II; Beck et al., 1996) was used, as has been done in previous research (Arria et al., 2009; Hom et al., 2018; Joiner et al., 2005; Pelizza et al., 2020). This particular item evaluates the presence of suicidal thoughts over the past two weeks using the following response format: 0 = I do not have any thoughts of killing myself; 1 = I have thoughts of killing myself, but I would not do it; 2 = I would like to kill myself; 3 = I would kill myself if I had the chance to do so. Following Taylor et al. (2015) and with the aim of dividing the sample into two groups, this item was dichotomized as follows: absence of suicidal ideation (level 0) and presence of suicidal ideation (levels 1, 2, and 3). In the present study, the full BDI-II scale showed excellent internal consistency ($\alpha = 0.91$; $\omega = 0.91$).

2.3. Procedure

The project was reviewed and approved by the Research Ethics Committee of CUP-UCM and complied with the requirements of the updated version of the Declaration of Helsinki (World Medical Association, 2013). All patients were informed and signed the informed consent, which outlined the general and specific objectives of the research and data collection process. The data were extracted from the clinical records filed at CUP-UCM. These records included, in addition to the patient's clinical record, the initial data collection protocol and the psychometric tests administered.

Once it was verified that the subjects had given their consent to participate in the data collection, the elements relevant to this study were incorporated into the database. This database was subsequently stored in the general archive.

2.4. Data Analysis

A stability and accuracy analysis of the global network was conducted using the total sample (n = 625) as a reference. To avoid potential content overlap and enable a clearer conceptual and statistical distinction between depressive symptoms and suicidal ideation, we recalculated the Depression score using item-level data from the Beck Depression Inventory–II (BDI-II), excluding Item 9 (suicidal ideation). Specific undirected weighted psychometric networks were estimated for groups without suicidal ideation (n = 394) and with suicidal ideation (n = 203) using the bootnet (Epskamp et al., 2018) and qgraph (Epskamp et al., 2012) packages, following the standard guidelines suggested by Burger et al. (2022), Epskamp et al. (2018), and Epskamp and Fried (2018).

Using the bootnet package, a Gaussian graphical model (GGM) was estimated through the EBIC-glasso function, which applies the graphical least absolute shrinkage and selection operator (Graphical-LASSO or G-LASSO) for parameter regularization (Jones et al., 2018). For each network configuration, centrality measures, including strength centrality and expected influence, were computed. Strength centrality identifies the node with the highest number of connections (Borsboom & Cramer, 2013; Epskamp & Fried, 2018; Fonseca-Pedrero, 2018), while expected influence—defined as the sum of all edges connected to a node—determines which nodes exert the greatest influence within the network (Fonseca-Pedrero, 2022; Robinaugh et al., 2016). For each estimated network model, edge weights, standard errors, and p values were calculated to assess the strength and significance of the connections. These estimates are reported in supplementary tables in Appendix A (Tables A3–A5), allowing for a detailed evaluation of the model parameters. Additionally, predictability and stability analyses were performed (Fonseca-Pedrero, 2017).

Finally, a comparative analysis between the two networks was conducted using the averageLayout function from the qgraph package (Epskamp et al., 2012), and the network comparison test (NCT) (Van Borkulo et al., 2022) was applied to assess differences between them. This permutation-based test evaluates network similarity across three dimensions: network structure (M), global network strength (S), and edge weight equality. The estimated edge weights, along with their standard errors and p values, are presented in supplementary tables in the Appendix A. These tables provide a detailed overview of the strength and statistical significance of the connections in the network models.

Finally, to identify psychopathological characteristics with predictive capacity for suicidal ideation, a binary logistic regression was performed. For the logistic regression analysis, the Depression variable was calculated using the total score from the BDI-II, excluding Item 9 (suicidal ideation), to avoid content overlap with the suicidal ideation predictor. Although the SCL-90-R also includes a Depression subscale, item-level data were not available for this measure, preventing the removal of its suicidal ideation item.

Therefore, the BDI-II was used to ensure a cleaner separation between the constructs of depression and suicidal ideation in the analysis. Additionally, multicollinearity between the variables was assessed using the tolerance and variance inflation factor (VIF) indices, which help determine the extent of collinearity present, as high multicollinearity can lead to inflated variance in regression estimates.

3. Results

3.1. Descriptive and Comparative Statistics

The sample of patients with suicidal ideation (Table 2) consisted of 68.0% women (n = 138), with a mean age of 27.16 (SD = 10.366). The sample of the group without suicidal ideation was composed of 70.6% women (n = 278), with a mean age of 28.21 (SD = 11.91). There were no significant differences in sex ($\chi^2(1) = 0.421$, $p = 0.516$) or age (t(595) = 1.063, $p = 0.288$) between the two groups.

Table 2. Means, standard deviations, average ranks, and Mann–Whitney U tests of the sample with suicidal ideation (n = 203) and without suicidal ideation (n = 394).

Variables	Clinical Population with Suicidal Ideation (n = 203) M (SD)/Average Rank	Clinical Population Without Suicidal Ideation (n = 394) M (SD)/Average Rank	Mann–Whitney U	Z	Sig.(bil)
Somatization	1.29 (0.80)/355.74	0.90 (0.71)/269.77	28,473.5	−5.77	<0.01 ***
Obsessive-Compulsive	1.93 (0.78)/381.74	1.32 (0.79)/256.61	23,290.0	−8.37	<0.01 ***
Interpersonal Sensitivity	1.70 (0.79)/384.89	1.08 (0.83)/254.75	22,556.0	−8.74	<0.01 ***
Depression	2.26 (0.70)/416.58	1.40 (0.73)/238.89	16,123.0	−11.96	<0.01 ***
Anxiety	1.53 (0.82)/371.56	1.02 (0.72)/261.61	25,261.0	−7.38	<0.01 ***
Hostility	1.32 (0.96)/382.77	0.68 (0.67)/255.84	22,985.5	−8.55	<0.01 ***
Phobic Anxiety	0.79 (0.75)/356.82	0.47 (0.61)/269.21	28,254.5	−5.93	<0.01 ***
Paranoid Ideation	1.24 (0.81)/367.21	0.78 (0.71)/263.85	26,143.5	−6.95	<0.01 ***
Psychoticism	1.14 (0.65)/392.29	0.62 (0.55)/250.94	21,053.5	−9.50	<0.01 ***

Note. M = mean, SD = standard deviation; *** $p < 0.001$, Z = Z score, Sig.(bil) = Asymptotic two-tailed significance.

Statistically significant differences were found in each of the psychopathological dimensions of the SCL-90-R between the groups. The group with suicidal ideation exhibited more pronounced symptoms in each of the subscales of the SCL-90-R than the group without suicidal ideation.

3.2. Network Analysis of the Global Network of Patients (n = 625)

Figure 1 shows the network of regularized partial correlations. Most of the edges represented positive correlations. The strongest relationships were found between "Somatization" and "Anxiety" (0.44), "Interpersonal Sensitivity" and "Paranoid Ideation" (0.38), and "Anxiety" and "Phobic Anxiety" (0.35). Additionally, relationships were observed between "Depression" and "Suicide" (0.32) and between "Hostility" and "Paranoid Ideation" (0.22).

Figure 2 shows graphs of the standardized centrality measures. The elements that showed the greatest expected influence were "Anxiety" (1.6), "Psychoticism" (1.03), and "Interpersonal Sensitivity" (0.26), with similar functioning in both the main sample and that derived from bootstrapping.

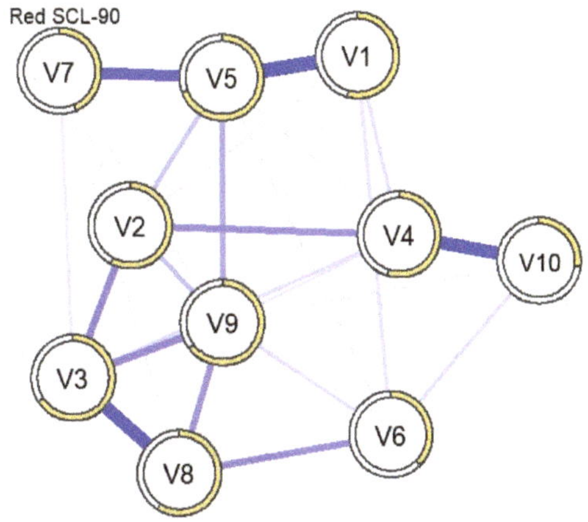

Figure 1. Network structure of the total sample using a Gaussian graphical model (n = 625). Note: V1 = Somatization, V2 = Obsessive-Compulsive, V3 = Interpersonal Sensitivity, V4 = Depression, V5 = Anxiety, V6 = Hostility, V7 = Phobic Anxiety, V8 = Paranoid Ideation, V9 = Psychoticism, V10 = Suicide.

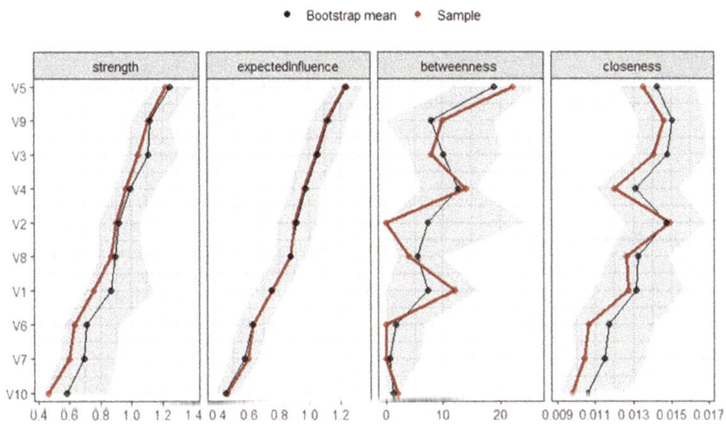

Figure 2. Graph of standardized centrality measures (n = 625). Note: V1 = Somatization, V2 = Obsessive-Compulsive, V3 = Interpersonal Sensitivity, V4 = Depression, V5 = Anxiety, V6 = Hostility, V7 = Phobic Anxiety, V8 = Paranoid Ideation, V9 = Psychoticism, V10 = Suicide.

Figure 3 presents the accuracy of the connections between all nodes using bootstrapping-based techniques (CI = 95%). The confidence intervals are wide, but we observed specific connections between nodes, and the estimated connections from the original sample were within the confidence interval, with an average predictability of 99.2%, ranging from 19.4% (V7 = Phobic Anxiety) to 66.9% (V4 = Depression).

The network stability analysis (Figure 4) indicated that the strength centrality was moderate (CSstrength = 0.75), being above the cutoff point of 0.25 required for interpretation, considering the corresponding limitations (Burger et al., 2022), and above 0.50, ensuring that the centrality index has adequate stability (Epskamp, 2017; Hevey, 2018).

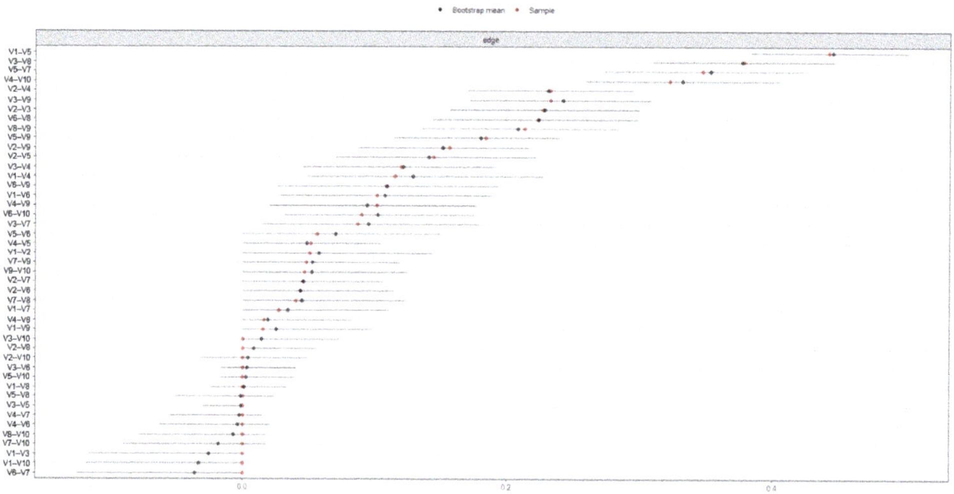

Figure 3. Bootstrap analysis of connections between nodes (n = 625). Note: V1 = Somatization, V2 = Obsessive-Compulsive, V3 = Interpersonal Sensitivity, V4 = Depression, V5 = Anxiety, V6 = Hostility, V7 = Phobic Anxiety, V8 = Paranoid Ideation, V9 = Psychoticism, V10 = Suicide.

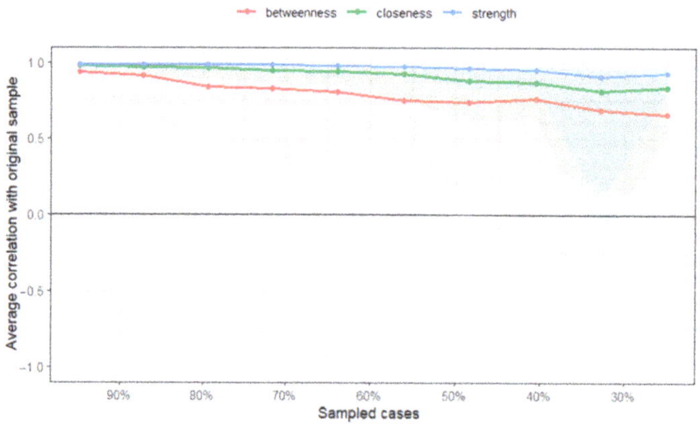

Figure 4. Stability of centrality indices (n = 625).

3.2.1. Network Analysis of the Sample with Suicidal Ideation (n = 203)

The majority of edges represented positive correlations (Figure 5). The strongest relationships were found between "Interpersonal Sensitivity" and "Paranoid Ideation" (0.36), "Somatization" and "Anxiety" (0.39), "Anxiety" and "Phobic Anxiety" (0.35), "Hostility" and "Paranoid Ideation" (0.25), and "Depression" and "Obsessive-Compulsive" (0.26). There were also small negative correlations between "Interpersonal Sensitivity" and "Somatization" (−0.08) and between "Hostility" and "Phobic Anxiety" (−0.04).

Figure 6 shows the plots of the standardised centrality measures. The dimensions with the greatest expected influence were "Anxiety" (1.50), "Psychoticism" (0.8), "Interpersonal Sensitivity" (0.83), and "Obsessive-Compulsive" (0.14). The elements with lower expected influence were "Phobic Anxiety" (−1.63), "Hostility" (−1.12), and "Paranoid Ideation" (−0.52).

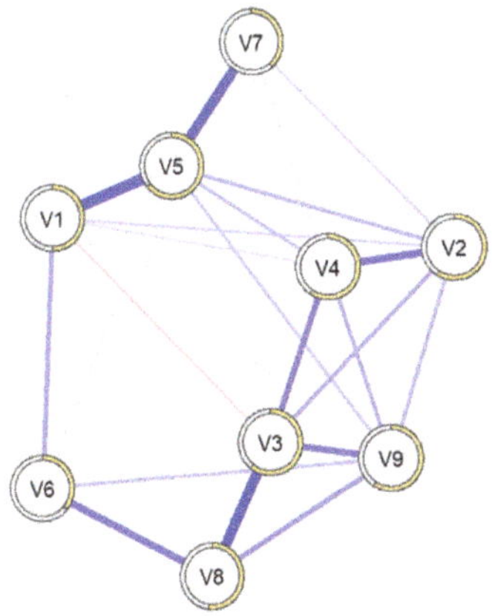

Figure 5. Structure of network configurations for patients with suicidal ideation (n = 203). Note: V1 = Somatization, V2 = Obsessive-Compulsive, V3 = Interpersonal Sensitivity, V4 = Depression, V5 = Anxiety, V6 = Hostility, V7 = Phobic Anxiety, V8 = Paranoid Ideation, V9 = Psychoticism.

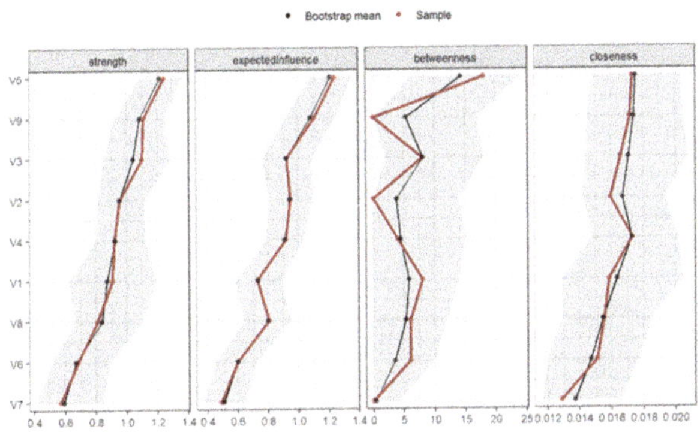

Figure 6. Graph of standardized centrality measures of networks of patients with suicidal ideation (n = 203). Note: V1 = Somatization, V2 = Obsessive-Compulsive, V3 = Interpersonal Sensitivity, V4 = Depression, V5 = Anxiety, V6 = Hostility, V7 = Phobic Anxiety, V8 = Paranoid Ideation, V9 = Psychoticism.

The dimensions with the highest betweenness centrality (i.e., the greatest power of connection between nodes) were "Anxiety" (2.17), "Interpersonal Sensitivity" (0.42), and "Somatization" (0.42). Those with the lowest betweenness centrality were "Psychoticism" (−0.97), "Obsessive-Compulsive" (−0.97), and "Phobic Anxiety" (−0.97). In this case, the functioning was not as similar in the main sample and the bootstrap-derived sample.

Finally, the dimensions with the highest closeness centrality, indicating the greatest global power or access to the other nodes, were "Anxiety" (1.01), "Depression" (1.01), "Psychoticism" (0.91), and "Interpersonal Sensitivity" (0.06). The dimensions with the lowest closeness centrality were "Phobic Anxiety" (−2.16), "Hostility" (−0.57), and "Paranoid Ideation" (−0.25).

The precision of the connections for all nodes was calculated using bootstrapping-based techniques (CI = 95%) as shown in Figure 7. The confidence intervals were wide, but there were specific connections between the nodes, and the estimated connections from the original sample fell within the confidence interval, with an average predictability of 53.5%, ranging from 36.4% (V6 = Hostility) to 64.5% (V5 = Anxiety).

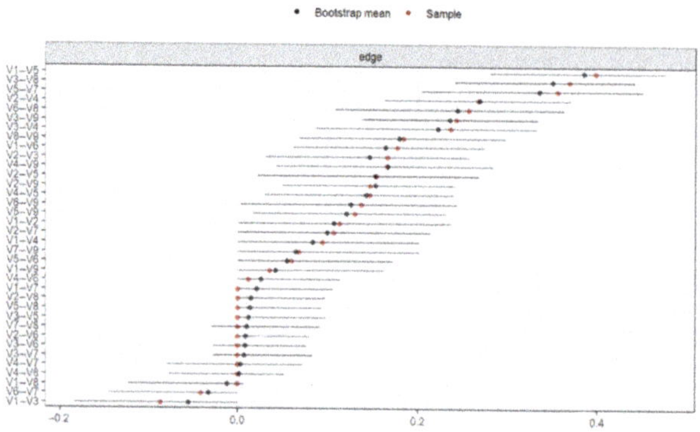

Figure 7. Bootstrap analysis of the connections between nodes (n = 203). Note: V1 = Somatization, V2 = Obsessive-Compulsive, V3 = Interpersonal Sensitivity, V4 = Depression, V5 = Anxiety, V6 = Hostility, V7 = Phobic Anxiety, V8 = Paranoid Ideation, V9 = Psychoticism.

The network stability analysis indicated that the centrality of strength is moderate (CSstrenght = 0.59), being above the threshold of 0.25, required for interpretation with the corresponding limitations, and above 0.50, ensuring that the centrality index has adequate stability.

3.2.2. Network Analysis of the Sample Without Suicidal Ideation (n = 394)

At a topographic level, as shown in Figure 8, the symptom grouping was similar to that of the group with suicidal ideation. In this case, all the edges represented positive correlations. The strongest relationships were found between "Interpersonal Susceptibility" and "Paranoid Ideation" (0.36), "Somatization" and "Anxiety" (0.44), "Anxiety" and "Phobic Anxiety" (0.33), "Hostility" and "Paranoid Ideation" (0.20), and "Depression" and "Obsessive-Compulsive" (0.29).

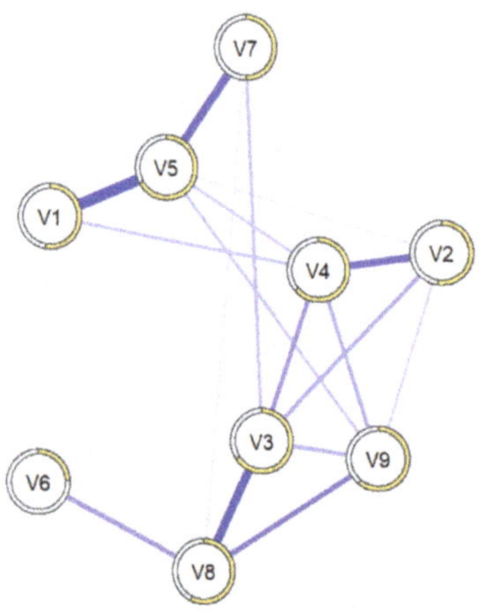

Figure 8. Structure of the network of the group without suicidal ideation using a Gaussian graphical model (n = 394). Note: V1 = Somatization, V2 = Obsessive-Compulsive, V3 = Interpersonal Sensitivity, V4 = Depression, V5 = Anxiety, V6 = Hostility, V7 = Phobic Anxiety, V8 = Paranoid Ideation, V9 = Psychoticism.

Figure 9 shows the standardized centrality measures, with similar performance in both the main sample and the bootstrapped sample. The elements that showed the greatest expected influence were "Anxiety" (1.37), "Interpersonal Susceptibility" (0.92), and "Depression" (0.72). The dimensions with the highest strength centrality were "Anxiety" (1.37), "Interpersonal Susceptibility" (0.92), and "Depression" (0.72).

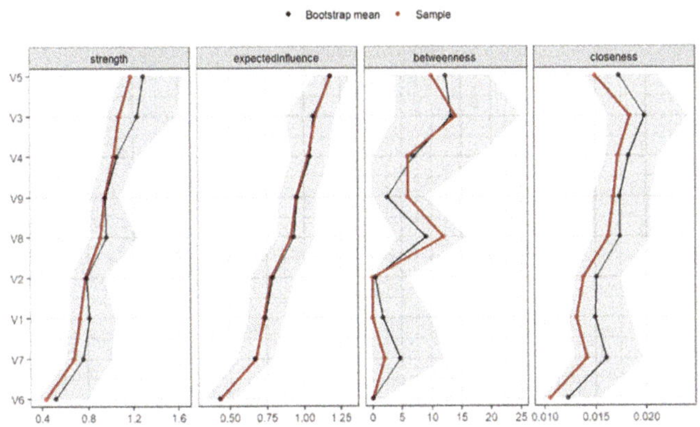

Figure 9. Centrality measure graphs of the networks of patients without suicidal ideation (n = 394). Note: V1 = Somatization, V2 = Obsessive-Compulsive, V3 = Interpersonal Sensitivity, V4 = Depression, V5 = Anxiety, V6 = Hostility, V7 = Phobic Anxiety, V8 = Paranoid Ideation, V9 = Psychoticism.

The dimensions with the greatest strength centrality, as expected, were "Anxiety" (1.37), "Interpersonal Susceptibility" (0.92), "Depression" (0.72), "Psychoticism" (0.37), and "Paranoid Ideation" (0.21). The dimensions with the lowest centrality indices were "Hostility" (−1.85), "Phobic Anxiety" (−0.80), and "Somatization" (−0.58).

The dimensions with the highest betweenness centrality were "Interpersonal Susceptibility" (1.57), "Anxiety" (0.80), "Paranoid Ideation" (1.18), and "Depression" (0.08). The dimensions with the lowest betweenness centrality were "Somatization" (−1.01), "Obsessive-Compulsive" (−1.01), and "Hostility" (−1.01). In this case, and as happened in the group with suicidal ideation, the performance was not as similar in the main sample as in the bootstrapped sample.

Finally, the dimensions with the highest closeness centrality, those with the greatest global power or access to the rest of the nodes, were "Interpersonal Susceptibility" (1.42), "Depression" (0.79), "Paranoid Ideation" (0.52), and "Psychoticism" (0.74). The dimensions with the lowest closeness centrality were "Hostility" (−1.87), "Somatization" (−0.77), "Obsessive-Compulsive" (−0.49), and "Phobic Anxiety" (−0.34).

For a detailed comparison of centrality indices (expected influence, strength, closeness, and betweenness) across the three networks, see Appendix A, Table A2.

In Figure 10, the precision of the connections between all the nodes is shown. There were specific connections between the nodes, and these were within the confidence interval. This indicates the precision with which we can assert that the connections between the nodes in our network were significantly different from zero, although with lower precision. The average predictability of the network was 54.7%, ranging from 36.4% (V6 = Hostility) to 64.5% (V5 = Anxiety).

The network stability analysis for patients without suicidal ideation reveals greater stability in the network (CSstrenght = 0.75), so the network can be interpreted with the same caution mentioned earlier, as it is above the reference value.

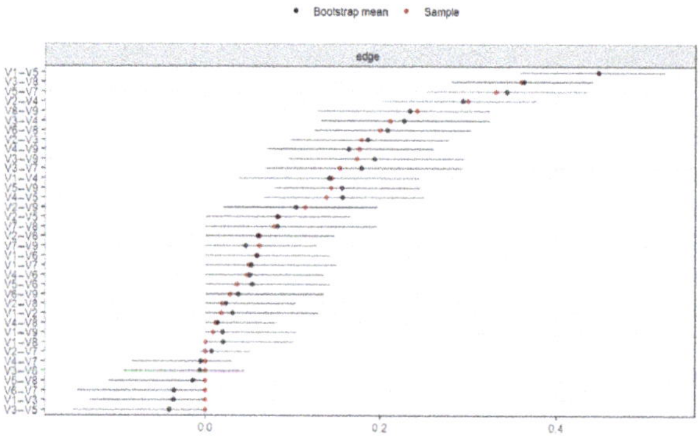

Figure 10. Bootstrap analysis of the connections between nodes (n = 394). Note: V1 = Somatization, V2 = Obsessive-Compulsive, V3 = Interpersonal Sensitivity, V4 = Depression, V5 = Anxiety, V6 = Hostility, V7 = Phobic Anxiety, V8 = Paranoid Ideation, V9 = Psychoticism.

3.2.3. Comparison of Networks Between Groups with and Without Suicidal Ideation

Figure 11 displays both psychometric networks side by side to illustrate their overall configuration. In addition, bivariate comparisons of edge weights between the networks with and without suicidal ideation were also conducted and are presented in Appendix A, Table A1. In parallel, differences between the two network configurations regarding structure, strength, and equality were calculated (Table 3). The results first reflected that there was no difference in the structure of the networks, meaning both networks had the same number of connections between dimensions. There were also no differences in the strength of both networks, meaning the values between the nodes of both networks were similar.

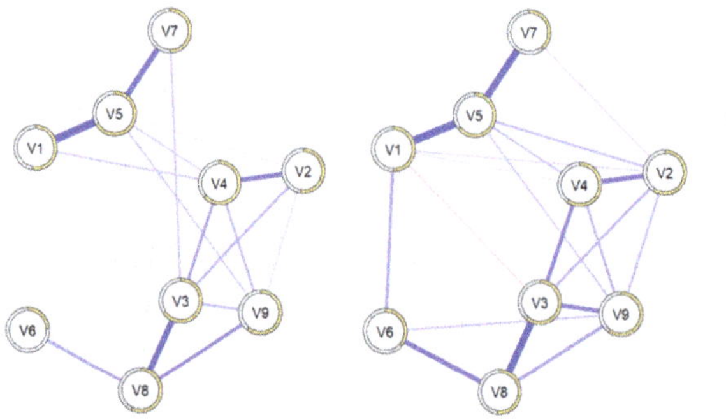

Figure 11. Network configuration structures of patients without suicidal ideation (left) and with suicidal ideation (right). Note: V1 = Somatization, V2 = Obsessive-Compulsive, V3 = Interpersonal Sensitivity, V4 = Depression, V5 = Anxiety, V6 = Hostility, V7 = Phobic Anxiety, V8 = Paranoid Ideation, V9 = Psychoticism.

Table 3. Results of the network comparison test between groups.

Contrasts	Statistic	Significance
Network Structure	M = 0.15	0.43
Network Strength	S = 0.26	0.65

Finally, the equality analysis, which evaluates specific connections between nodes, also indicated that there was no difference between the two networks.

3.3. Analysis of the Predictive Factors of Suicidal Ideation

Initially, no evidence of collinearity was found among the factors, given that all tolerance values exceeded 0.1 and the corresponding VIF scores remained below the threshold of 5 for all variables included (see Appendix A, Table A6).

The model fit indicated that at least one parameter of the model was significant ($\chi^2(11) = 205{,}989$, $p < 0.01$) and explained 39% (Nagelkerke $R^2 = 0.39$) of the variance in suicidal ideation.

The results of the binary logistic regression are shown in Table 4. The dimensions of depression ($\beta = 1.60$; $p = < 0.01$) and hostility ($\beta = 0.59$; $p = < 0.01$) were the only variables that were independently associated with suicidal ideation.

Table 4. Binary logistic regression (n = 625).

Model 1	β	Error	df	Sig.
Sex	−0.159	0.240	1	0.507
Age	0.017	0.010	1	0.091
Somatization	−0.438	0.204	1	0.032 *
Obsessive-Compulsive	−0.043	0.188	1	0.819
Interpersonal Susceptibility	0.133	0.204	1	0.516
Depression	0.110	0.014	1	<0.01 ***
Anxiety	0.056	0.228	1	0.804
Hostility	0.698	0.154	1	<0.01 ***
Phobic Anxiety	0.004	0.198	1	0.982
Paranoid Ideation	−0.422	0.204	1	0.039 *
Psychoticism	−3.864	0.272	1	0.027 *

Note: * $p < 0.05$ *** $p < 0.001$, β = beta, Sig. = significance level.

4. Discussion

The main objective of this study was to analyze in an outpatient setting how psychopathological networks are configured in individuals with suicidal ideation and to explore the differences compared with those without suicidal ideation.

The initial bivariate contrasts confirmed that there were significant differences in symptoms between the two groups. As expected, patients with suicidal ideation presented more intense psychopathological symptoms at the start of therapy. This finding is consistent with much of the literature, which indicates a strong relationship between the presence of psychological disorders and the likelihood of experiencing suicidal ideation, attempts, and behaviors (May & Klonsky, 2016; San Too et al., 2019). Although the scores were consistently higher in all dimensions evaluated, depressive symptoms were clearly more pronounced in the suicidal ideation group (2.26 versus 1.40). However, what stood out the most were the significant differences in the dimensions of interpersonal susceptibility and hostility. Both dimensions have a strong relational component, suggesting that social factors play a key role in this phenomenon (Barker et al., 2022; Chu et al., 2017; Coppersmith et al., 2022; McClelland et al., 2020).

The results of the network analysis for the general sample showed that the most central symptoms for individuals in a clinical outpatient context were depression, anxiety, interpersonal susceptibility, and thoughts of social alienation. However, when analyzing only the network for individuals with suicidal ideation, the most central symptoms were anxiety, thoughts of social alienation, and interpersonal susceptibility. The most central node in terms of centrality strength and expected influence was anxiety, above other symptoms traditionally associated with suicidal behavior, such as depression (D. De Beurs et al., 2019; Franklin et al., 2017). This suggests that anxious symptoms are strongly connected to other symptoms and may represent key targets for clinical attention (McNally et al., 2015), although the cross-sectional nature of the data precludes assumptions about influence or directionality. This finding aligns with the logic of undirected network models, where changes in one symptom may be reflected in related symptoms; however, this study does not provide evidence of causal or directional effects. The fact that anxiety occupies such a central position further reinforces the idea that it is a highly disruptive process (Stanley et al., 2018) with wide-ranging implications across different areas of the individual (Olatunji et al., 2007), particularly in the population with suicidal ideation. In fact, anxious traits were also central in a recent network analysis study on suicidal ideation and emotional lability, aligning with the findings of this study. These authors (Núñez et al., 2020) proposed new hypotheses on how anxiety could lead to depression, rather than depression leading to anxious symptoms, as suggested by other studies (Cramer et al., 2010).

These findings connect directly with the current transdiagnostic view of psychological disorders. While the relationship with depressive disorders is clear (Beard et al., 2016; Casey et al., 2008), the psychological factors contributing to the development of suicidal ideation go beyond depressive symptoms (Klonsky et al., 2016). This was evident in the dimensions with high centrality, such as psychoticism and interpersonal susceptibility. Some items related to psychoticism, such as "Feeling lonely even when I am with others" and "Feeling always distant, with no sense of intimacy with anyone", and items related to interpersonal susceptibility, such as "Feeling that others don't understand me" and "Feeling inferior to others", are considered clear risk factors for the development of suicidal ideation (Klonsky & May, 2015; Van Orden et al., 2010). These symptoms affect key risk factors such as sense of disconnection and loneliness, which again highlights the importance of the social component in this phenomenon.

This point is particularly relevant when interpreting psychometric tests in clinical settings, such as the SCL-90-R. These instruments are frequently used as screening tests in initial evaluations to help guide intervention, but suicidal risk can be overlooked if the connections between other dimensions not traditionally linked to suicide are not established.

The comparison between the psychopathological networks of individuals with and without suicidal ideation yielded unexpected conclusions. Statistically significant differences in the network configuration between the two groups were not observed. Contrarily to expectations, although patients with suicidal ideation had more intense symptoms across all psychopathological dimensions, the relationships between these dimensions were very similar in both groups.

This result suggests that, in clinical outpatient settings, although the initial severity of symptoms is greater in patients with suicidal ideation, the dimensions affected and the relationships between them are similar to those of individuals without ideation. This finding aligns with the perspective that suicide should not be viewed as a phenomenologically distinct phenomenon, but rather as a consequence of more intense distress, possibly experienced with greater anguish or a sense of being trapped (O'Connor & Kirtley, 2018). Moreover, this does not contradict the presence of general differentiating factors between the two populations, such as prior diathesis or vulnerability (Mann et al., 1999) or specific life events related to suicide and acquired capability (Joiner, 2005). These data reinforce the notion of dimensionality in the phenomenon, both in the suicidal continuum and its multiple manifestations (Barnow & Linden, 2000; Joiner et al., 2005; Sveticic & De Leo, 2012). Although the networks were similar in their structure and associative strength, there was evidence of systematically higher symptom intensity in patients with suicidal ideation.

To generate more evidence regarding the relationship between psychopathology and suicidal ideation, a binary logistic regression analysis was conducted, controlling for age and sex. Depressive symptoms, hostility, somatization, paranoid ideation, and psychoticism emerged as significant predictors of suicidal ideation, explaining 37% of the variance in the final model. The presence of depressive symptoms is consistent with previous studies (May & Klonsky, 2016; Tsai et al., 2021). However, the strongest risk factor was hostility, increasing the likelihood of suicidal ideation even after controlling for depressive symptoms. This suggests that hostility contributes uniquely to suicide risk, beyond the effects of depression. The fact that hostility showed such a strong effect highlights the role of interpersonal difficulties in suicidal ideation. This aligns with previous research linking hostility and aggressiveness to suicidal behavior (Gvion & Apter, 2011; Gvion & Levi-Belz, 2018; Lemogne et al., 2011; Menon et al., 2015), underscoring that suicide risk is not solely a matter of emotional distress but also involves perceived conflicts with others.

Beyond affective and interpersonal dimensions, the model also identified somatization, paranoid ideation, and psychoticism as relevant predictors, suggesting that additional forms of psychological dysregulation may elevate suicide risk through distinct mechanisms. Somatization may reflect unprocessed emotional pain manifested in physical symptoms, contributing to a sense of helplessness and unarticulated suffering that increases suicide vulnerability (Torres et al., 2021). Paranoid ideation, marked by mistrust and perceived threats from others, may lead to increased social withdrawal and heightened feelings of persecution, thereby reinforcing alienation and a sense of thwarted belongingness (Joiner, 2005). Finally, psychoticism—characterized by disorganized thinking and perceptual disturbances—may impair reality testing and intensify internal chaos, thereby diminishing coping capacity and increasing suicide risk (Yates et al., 2019).

While depressive symptoms remain clear predictors of suicidal ideation, these additional domains emphasize the multifaceted nature of suicide risk. Somatic complaints may mask underlying emotional distress, paranoid ideation can reinforce isolation, and psychotic features may erode one's connection to reality—all factors that intersect with existing explanatory models of suicidal ideation and behavior (Joiner, 2005; Klonsky & May, 2015; O'Connor & Kirtley, 2018; Van Orden et al., 2010).

It is important to note that network and regression analyses address different, yet complementary, research questions. While network analysis focuses on the interrelations and connectivity between symptoms within a system—highlighting anxiety as a central symptom in this sample—regression models aim to identify which variables independently predict an outcome, in this case, suicidal ideation. The fact that hostility emerged as a significant predictor in the regression analysis does not contradict the centrality of anxiety in the network analysis; rather, it reflects that anxiety may be influential within the network structure, while hostility exerts a stronger predictive effect on suicidal ideation when controlling for other variables. Including both methods allows for a more comprehensive understanding of the psychopathological mechanisms underlying suicidal ideation.

Regarding the limitations of the study, the methodology had certain restrictions due to its developmental stage (Bringmann & Eronen, 2018; Brusco et al., 2019; Guloksuz et al., 2017; Jones et al., 2017; McNally et al., 2017), so the results should be interpreted with caution. Further analyses are needed to address issues related to the stability of the networks, as the current value was above the necessary threshold of 0.50 but below 0.70, which some authors consider adequate (Bringmann & Eronen, 2018).

The assessment of suicidal ideation at a single time point, without complementary information on prior or future ideation, limits the ability to explore this symptom's temporal dynamics. This cross-sectional approach constrains interpretations related to the onset, persistence, or fluctuation of suicidal thoughts. Future longitudinal studies or pre-/post-treatment designs would allow for a more nuanced understanding of how suicidal ideation evolves in clinical outpatient populations.

A further concern is the mismatch between the timeframes of the instruments used, specifically, the BDI-II and the SCL-90-R, which assess symptoms over different reference periods. Although this discrepancy is relatively minor, it may have introduced additional measurement variability and complicate direct comparisons between the constructs evaluated by each instrument.

The gender composition of the sample also warrants consideration, with a predominance of women (66%). This imbalance may limit the generalizability of the results to populations with a higher representation of men. However, given the higher prevalence of suicidal ideation among women in epidemiological research, this distribution reflects patterns typically observed in clinical samples and is thus not unexpected in the present context.

A significant constraint lies in the absence of diagnostic data related to specific mental disorders, which prevented subgroup analyses by diagnostic category. This limits the interpretability of how symptom networks may differ according to underlying psychopathological profiles. Similarly, important clinical variables—such as history of suicide attempts, current psychopharmacological treatment, and substance use—were not collected. These factors are recognized as critical in assessing suicidal risk, and their absence reduces the depth and clinical applicability of the findings. Incorporating such variables in future research would enhance the contextualization and relevance of network structures.

An additional methodological issue involves the dichotomization of suicidal ideation based solely on item 9 of the BDI-II. While the use of this item is supported by prior research, and its predictive validity has been established (Green et al., 2015), this binary classification may lead to loss of nuance and restrict variability within subgroups. The two-week timeframe used may fail to capture individuals with relevant SI histories outside that window. Moreover, the case–control design applied may be subject to Berkson's bias (de Ron et al., 2021), potentially affecting the representativeness and robustness of the estimated networks.

Future studies exploring differences in more specific subgroups could establish the dynamics between the dimensions addressed in this study. Furthermore, the implementation of network analysis based on the items of these dimensions could provide a deeper understanding of how they relate to each other and the directions of these relationships. In addition, incorporating complementary assessment tools may help differentiate psychopathological dimensions more precisely and further explore their unique contributions to suicide risk. This approach would ultimately refine the understanding of how specific psychological factors interact in the prediction of suicidal behavior.

Finally, this study provides updated evidence of the suicide phenomenon in clinical care contexts, serving as a starting point and a framework for future research on the subject, overcoming the previously mentioned limitations. This is the first study to use network analysis to examine the psychopathological symptoms of individuals with suicidal ideation in an outpatient clinical setting. Moreover, an important strength of this study is the use of the SCL-90-R, a widely employed instrument in routine clinical practice. This enhances the ecological validity of the findings, as the results are based on a tool frequently used in real-world consultations, making them more applicable to everyday clinical settings. Additionally, it is interesting to note that the distribution of means for the SCL-90-R dimensions in the present study closely resembled the study by Carrasco et al. (2003), highlighting the symptomatic similarities between clinical outpatient contexts, despite the time that has elapsed, and providing us with an updated reference of the main dimensions affected in a clinical outpatient context. Although the findings should be generalized cautiously to other populations, they have relevant clinical implications. Understanding how psychopathological symptoms relate to suicidal ideation, as well as the relevance of anxious and interpersonal symptoms in configuring the psychopathological networks of suicidal patients, can assist therapists in their evaluations/interventions and provide a therapeutic target for the "deactivation" of adjacent symptoms causing distress to the person. Furthermore, by using item 9 of the BDI-II, which assesses suicidal ideation within the past two weeks, the study deliberately focused on active or current suicidal ideation. This temporal frame enhances the clinical utility of the findings, as it allows for the identification of proximal risk factors and supports timely intervention in routine practice.

Author Contributions: Conceptualization, E.H., I.F.-A., and C.L.; methodology, E.H., T.P.-G., M.R., and I.F.-A.; software, E.H. and M.R.; formal analysis, E.H., M.R., and I.F.-A.; investigation, E.H., I.F.-A., and C.L.; resources, E.H.; data curation, E.H., M.R., and I.F.-A.; writing—original draft preparation, E.H., T.P.-G., and M.R.; writing—review and editing, E.H., T.P.-G., I.F.-A., and C.L.; visualization, E.H. and M.R.; supervision, E.H., I.F.-A., and C.L.; project administration, E.H., I.F.-A., and C.L.; funding acquisition, E.H. All authors have read and agreed to the published version of the manuscript.

Funding: This research received no external funding.

Institutional Review Board Statement: The study was conducted in accordance with the Declaration of Helsinki and approved by the Institutional Review Board of Clínica Universitaria de Psicología, Universidad Complutense de Madrid (approval code: CUP2016-01, 23 September 2016).

Informed Consent Statement: Informed consent was obtained from all subjects involved in the study.

Data Availability Statement: The data presented in this study are available on request from the corresponding author. The data are not publicly available due to privacy and ethical restrictions.

Conflicts of Interest: The authors declare no conflicts of interest.

Appendix A

Table A1. Bivariate correlations of the networks of patients without suicidal ideation (above the diagonal, outside brackets) and with suicidal ideation (above the diagonal, in brackets).

Variables	1	2	3	4	5	6	7	8	9
1. Somatization	1	0.46 *** (0.55 ***)	0.39 *** (0.33 ***)	0.56 *** (0.52 ***)	0.72 *** (0.66 ***)	0.35 *** (0.44 ***)	0.51 *** (0.40 ***)	0.41 *** (0.27 ***)	0.49 *** (0.47 ***)
2. Obsessive-compulsive	0.46 *** (0.55 ***)	1	0.63 *** (0.62 ***)	0.68 *** (0.68 ***)	0.54 *** (0.65 ***)	0.39 *** (0.39 ***)	0.45 *** (0.48 ***)	0.53 *** (0.45 ***)	0.58 *** (0.63 ***)
3. Interpersonal sensitivity	0.39 *** (0.33***)	0.63 *** (0.62 ***)	1	0.66 *** (0.64 ***)	0.47 *** (0.49 ***)	0.36 *** (0.42 ***)	0.54 *** (0.35 ***)	0.70 *** (0.66 ***)	0.67 *** (0.67 ***)
4. Depression	0.56 *** (0.52 ***)	0.68 *** (0.68 ***)	0.66 *** (0.64 ***)	1	0.63 *** (0.60 ***)	0.39 *** (0.43 ***)	0.48 *** (0.40 ***)	0.55 *** (0.45 ***)	0.65 *** (0.63 ***)
5. Anxiety	0.72 *** (0.66 ***)	0.54 *** (0.65 ***)	0.47 *** (0.49 ***)	0.63 *** (0.60 ***)	1	0.39 *** (0.43 ***)	0.65 *** (0.60 ***)	0.45 *** (0.40 ***)	0.60 *** (0.59 ***)
6. Hostility	0.35 *** (0.44 ***)	0.39 *** (0.39 ***)	0.36 *** (0.42 ***)	0.39 *** (0.43 ***)	0.39 *** (0.43 ***)	1	0.26 *** (0.20 ***)	0.46 *** (0.52 ***)	0.41 *** (0.49 ***)
7. Phobic anxiety	0.51 *** (0.40 ***)	0.45 *** (0.48 ***)	0.54 *** (0.35 ***)	0.48 *** (0.40 ***)	0.65 *** (0.60 ***)	0.26 *** (0.20 **)	1	0.50 *** (0.29 ***)	0.52 *** (0.44 ***)
8. Paranoid ideation	0.41 *** (0.27 ***)	0.53 *** (0.45 ***)	0.70 *** (0.66 ***)	0.55 *** (0.45 ***)	0.45 *** (0.40 ***)	0.46 *** (0.52 ***)	0.50 *** (0.29 ***)	1	0.65 *** (0.58 ***)
9. Psychoticism	0.49 *** (0.47 ***)	0.58 *** (0.63 ***)	0.67 *** (0.67 ***)	0.65 *** (0.63 ***)	0.60 *** (0.59 ***)	0.41 *** (0.49 ***)	0.52 *** (0.44 ***)	0.65 *** (0.58 ***)	1

Note: ** $p < 0.05$ and *** $p < 0.001$.

Table A2. Centrality measures for each node across the three networks (global, individuals with suicidal ideation, and individuals without suicidal ideation).

Symptom Dimension	Group	Strength	Closeness	Betweenness	Expected Influence
Somatization	Nonsuicidal Suicidal Global	0.85 0.85 0.76	0.02 0.02 0.01	1.79 5.37 12.00	0.74 0.72 0.75
Obsessive-Compulsive	Nonsuicidal Suicidal Global	0.83 1.00 0.90	0.02 0.02 0.01	0.90 6.28 0.00	0.81 0.99 0.91
Interpersonal Sensitivity	Nonsuicidal Suicidal Global	1.32 1.06 1.05	0.02 0.02 0.01	11.75 9.14 8.00	1.06 0.99 1.06
Depression	Nonsuicidal Suicidal Global	1.07 0.92 0.96	0.02 0.02 0.01	5.90 3.86 14.00	1.02 0.9 0.97
Anxiety	Nonsuicidal Suicidal Global	1.41 1.17 1.23	0.02 0.02 0.01	12.96 12.80 22.00	1.23 1.17 1.24
Hostility	Nonsuicidal Suicidal Global	0.60 0.70 0.63	0.01 0.01 0.01	0.11 3.71 0.00	0.45 0.62 0.63
Phobic Anxiety	Nonsuicidal Suicidal Global	0.83 0.60 0.60	0.02 0.01 0.01	3.71 0.50 0.00	0.65 0.51 0.57
Paranoid Ideation	Nonsuicidal Suicidal Global	1.03 0.84 0.87	0.02 0.02 0.01	7.92 5.16 4.00	0.97 0.78 0.87
Psychoticism	Nonsuicidal Suicidal Global	0.97 1.02 1.11	0.02 0.02 0.01	2.75 4.52 10.00	0.95 1.02 1.12
Suicide	Global	0.46	0.01	2.00	0.45

Table A3. Bootstrap edge weights (global).

Node 1	Node 2	Edge Weight (Mean)	SE	p
Phobic Anxiety	Paranoid Ideation	−0.009	0.027	0.741
Phobic Anxiety	Psychoticism	−0.031	0.033	0.339
Anxiety	Phobic Anxiety	0.232	0.048	<0.001
Anxiety	Hostility	−0.025	0.045	0.573
Anxiety	Paranoid Ideation	−0.128	0.037	<0.001
Anxiety	Psychoticism	−0.003	0.023	0.897
Depression	Phobic Anxiety	−0.170	0.045	<0.001
Depression	Anxiety	−0.043	0.050	0.39
Depression	Hostility	−0.066	0.056	0.239
Depression	Paranoid Ideation	−0.136	0.041	<0.001
Depression	Psychoticism	−0.017	0.031	0.579
Hostility	Phobic Anxiety	−0.156	0.044	<0.001
Hostility	Paranoid Ideation	0.139	0.041	<0.001
Hostility	Psychoticism	0.007	0.034	0.842
Paranoid Ideation	Psychoticism	0.070	0.039	0.069
Obsessive-Compulsive	Phobic Anxiety	−0.058	0.034	0.084
Obsessive-Compulsive	Anxiety	−0.057	0.043	0.186
Obsessive-Compulsive	Depression	0.025	0.037	0.5
Obsessive-Compulsive	Hostility	−0.076	0.043	0.077
Obsessive-Compulsive	Paranoid Ideation	−0.095	0.037	0.011
Obsessive-Compulsive	Psychoticism	−0.041	0.033	0.213
Somatization	Phobic Anxiety	−0.069	0.042	0.106
Somatization	Anxiety	0.147	0.059	0.013
Somatization	Depression	−0.141	0.058	0.015
Somatization	Hostility	−0.046	0.046	0.314
Somatization	Paranoid Ideation	−0.121	0.038	0.001
Somatization	Obsessive-Compulsive	−0.138	0.045	0.002
Somatization	Psychoticism	−0.143	0.043	<0.001
Somatization	Interpersonal Sensitivity	−0.272	0.041	<0.001
Interpersonal Sensitivity	Phobic Anxiety	0.019	0.032	0.546
Interpersonal Sensitivity	Anxiety	−0.151	0.045	<0.001
Interpersonal Sensitivity	Depression	0.035	0.042	0.403
Interpersonal Sensitivity	Hostility	−0.099	0.043	0.02
Interpersonal Sensitivity	Paranoid Ideation	0.243	0.038	<0.001
Interpersonal Sensitivity	Psychoticism	0.057	0.040	0.152

Note: Edge weights represent the estimated partial correlations between nodes. Standard errors and p-values were derived from nonparametric bootstrap resampling (1000 samples); SE = standard error, p = significance.

Table A4. Bootstrap edge weights (nonsuicidal network, n = 394).

Node 1	Node 2	Edge Weight (Mean)	SE	p
Phobic Anxiety	Paranoid Ideation	0.103	0.058	0.075
Phobic Anxiety	Psychoticism	0.040	0.039	0.313
Anxiety	Phobic Anxiety	0.355	0.049	<0.001
Anxiety	Hostility	0.078	0.048	0.101
Anxiety	Paranoid Ideation	−0.035	0.045	0.434
Anxiety	Psychoticism	0.169	0.044	<0.001
Depression	Phobic Anxiety	−0.022	0.037	0.56
Depression	Anxiety	0.159	0.047	<0.001
Depression	Hostility	0.035	0.039	0.377
Depression	Paranoid Ideation	0.014	0.030	0.651
Depression	Psychoticism	0.158	0.052	0.002
Hostility	Phobic Anxiety	−0.059	0.050	0.239
Hostility	Paranoid Ideation	0.215	0.045	<0.001
Hostility	Psychoticism	0.050	0.048	0.3
Paranoid Ideation	Psychoticism	0.244	0.049	<0.001
Obsessive-Compulsive	Phobic Anxiety	0.008	0.024	0.74
Obsessive-Compulsive	Anxiety	0.084	0.047	0.075
Obsessive-Compulsive	Depression	0.300	0.045	<0.001
Obsessive-Compulsive	Hostility	0.087	0.049	0.077
Obsessive-Compulsive	Paranoid Ideation	0.033	0.037	0.374
Obsessive-Compulsive	Psychoticism	0.071	0.048	0.144
Obsessive-Compulsive	Interpersonal Sensitivity	0.212	0.047	<0.001
Somatization	Phobic Anxiety	0.053	0.044	0.234
Somatization	Anxiety	0.455	0.043	<0.001
Somatization	Depression	0.148	0.053	0.005
Somatization	Hostility	0.059	0.049	0.23
Somatization	Paranoid Ideation	0.026	0.034	0.449
Somatization	Obsessive-Compulsive	0.030	0.039	0.446
Somatization	Psychoticism	0.019	0.035	0.585
Somatization	Interpersonal Sensitivity	−0.050	0.046	0.283
Interpersonal Sensitivity	Phobic Anxiety	0.182	0.055	0.001
Interpersonal Sensitivity	Anxiety	−0.071	0.049	0.145
Interpersonal Sensitivity	Depression	0.228	0.052	<0.001
Interpersonal Sensitivity	Hostility	−0.011	0.031	0.72
Interpersonal Sensitivity	Paranoid Ideation	0.352	0.043	<0.001
Interpersonal Sensitivity	Psychoticism	0.209	0.052	<0.001

Note: Edge weights represent the estimated partial correlations between nodes. Standard errors and p-values were derived from nonparametric bootstrap resampling (1000 samples); SE = standard error, *p* = significance.

Table A5. Bootstrap edge weights (suicidal network, n = 203).

Node 1	Node 2	Edge Weight (Mean)	SE	p
Phobic Anxiety	Paranoid Ideation	0.017	0.037	0.648
Phobic Anxiety	Psychoticism	0.072	0.059	0.22
Anxiety	Phobic Anxiety	0.325	0.066	<0.001
Anxiety	Hostility	0.062	0.057	0.273
Anxiety	Paranoid Ideation	0.008	0.024	0.73
Anxiety	Psychoticism	0.116	0.056	0.038
Depression	Phobic Anxiety	0.011	0.031	0.733
Depression	Anxiety	0.107	0.058	0.066
Depression	Hostility	0.043	0.044	0.329
Depression	Paranoid Ideation	0.002	0.024	0.929
Depression	Psychoticism	0.155	0.060	0.009
Hostility	Phobic Anxiety	−0.042	0.061	0.49
Hostility	Paranoid Ideation	0.251	0.070	<0.001
Hostility	Psychoticism	0.122	0.064	0.058
Paranoid Ideation	Psychoticism	0.160	0.061	0.008
Obsessive-Compulsive	Phobic Anxiety	0.097	0.058	0.091
Obsessive-Compulsive	Anxiety	0.174	0.065	0.007
Obsessive-Compulsive	Depression	0.279	0.056	<0.001
Obsessive-Compulsive	Hostility	0.007	0.025	0.796
Obsessive-Compulsive	Paranoid Ideation	0.015	0.037	0.683
Obsessive-Compulsive	Psychoticism	0.128	0.052	0.014
Obsessive-Compulsive	Interpersonal Sensitivity	0.168	0.053	0.002
Somatization	Phobic Anxiety	0.019	0.035	0.592
Somatization	Anxiety	0.359	0.049	<0.001
Somatization	Depression	0.098	0.063	0.122
Somatization	Hostility	0.155	0.067	0.02
Somatization	Paranoid Ideation	−0.028	0.048	0.563
Somatization	Obsessive-Compulsive	0.126	0.069	0.069
Somatization	Psychoticism	0.032	0.043	0.459
Somatization	Interpersonal Sensitivity	−0.039	0.058	0.503
Interpersonal Sensitivity	Phobic Anxiety	0.010	0.029	0.721
Interpersonal Sensitivity	Anxiety	0.014	0.029	0.628
Interpersonal Sensitivity	Depression	0.213	0.062	<0.001
Interpersonal Sensitivity	Hostility	0.012	0.031	0.692
Interpersonal Sensitivity	Paranoid Ideation	0.358	0.056	<0.001
Interpersonal Sensitivity	Psychoticism	0.242	0.048	<0.001

Note: Edge weights represent the estimated partial correlations between nodes. Standard errors and *p*-values were derived from nonparametric bootstrap resampling (1000 samples); SE = standard error, *p* = significance.

Table A6. Summary of multicollinearity analysis (n = 621).

N = 621	Standardized Coefficients β	t	Sig.	Collinearity Statistics	
				Tolerance	VIF
Sex	−0.036	−0.950	0.342	0.922	1.085
Age	0.002	1.597	0.111	0.916	1.091
Somatization	−0.071	−2.192	0.029	0.421	2.375
Obsessive-Compulsive	0.002	0.055	0.956	0.407	2.456
Interpersonal Susceptibility	0.036	1.124	0.262	0.338	2.962
Depression	0.019	7.549	9.573	0.000	0.517
Anxiety	0.028	−0.256	0.760	0.448	0.313
Hostility	0.127	3.052	5.188	0.000	0.630
Phobic Anxiety	0.001	−0.680	0.033	0.974	0.527
Paranoid Ideation	−0.050	−1.179	−1.578	0.115	0.422
Psychoticism	0.028	1.695	0.091	0.318	3.141

Note. N = sample size; β = standardized coefficient; t = t-value; Sig. = significance level (*p*-value); VIF = variance inflation factor; *p* values indicate significance levels.

References

Al-Halabí, S., & Fonseca-Pedrero, E. (2023). *Manual de psicología de la conducta suicida*. Pirámide.

Arria, A. M., O'Grady, K. E., Caldeira, K. M., Vincent, K. B., Wilcox, H. C., & Wish, E. D. (2009). Suicide ideation among college students: A multivariate analysis. *Archives of Suicide Research, 13*(3), 230–246. [CrossRef]

Barker, J., Oakes-Rogers, S., & Leddy, A. (2022). What distinguishes high and low-lethality suicide attempts in older adults? A systematic review and meta-analysis. *Journal of Psychiatric Research, 154*, 91–101. [CrossRef]

Barnow, S., & Linden, M. (2000). Epidemiology and psychiatric morbidity of suicidal ideation among the elderly. *Crisis: The Journal of Crisis Intervention and Suicide Prevention, 21*(4), 171. [CrossRef] [PubMed]

Beard, C., Millner, A. J., Forgeard, M. J. C., Fried, E. I., Hsu, K. J., Treadway, M. T., Leonard, C. V., Kertz, S. J., & Björgvinsson, T. (2016). Network analysis of depression and anxiety symptom relationships in a psychiatric sample. *Psychological Medicine, 46*(16), 3359–3369. [CrossRef] [PubMed]

Beck, A. T., Steer, R. A., & Brown, G. (1996). *Beck Depression Inventory–II (BDI-II)*. APA PsycTests.

Blakely, T. A., Collings, S. C., & Atkinson, J. (2003). Unemployment and suicide. *Evidence for a causal association?* Journal of Epidemiology & Community Health, 57(8), 594–600. [CrossRef]

Borsboom, D. (2017). Una teoría de redes de los trastornos mentales. *World Psychiatry, 16*(1), 5–13. [CrossRef]

Borsboom, D., & Cramer, A. O. (2013). Network analysis: An integrative approach to the structure of psychopathology. *Annual Review of Clinical Psychology, 9*(1), 91–121. [CrossRef]

Bringmann, L., & Eronen, M. (2018). Don't blame the model: Reconsidering the network approach to psychopathology. *Psychological Review, 125*(4), 606. [CrossRef]

Brusco, M. J., Steinley, D., Hoffman, M., Davis-Stober, C., & Wasserman, S. (2019). On Ising models and algorithms for the construction of symptom networks in psychopathological research. *Psychological Methods, 24*(6), 735. [CrossRef]

Burger, J., Isvoranu, A.-M., Lunansky, G., Haslbeck, J. M. B., Epskamp, S., Hoekstra, R. H. A., Fried, E. I., Borsboom, D., & Blanken, T. F. (2022). Reporting standards for psychological network analyses in cross-sectional data. *Psychological Methods, 28*(4), 806–824. [CrossRef]

Carrasco, M., Ángel, Sánchez Moral, V., Ciccotelli, H., & del Barrio, M. V. (2003). Symptom check list SCL-90-Revised: Analysis in psychiatric patients. *Acción Psicológica, 2*(2), 149–161. [CrossRef]

Casey, P., Dunn, G., Kelly, B. D., Lehtinen, V., Dalgard, O. S., Dowrick, C., & Ayuso-Mateos, J. L. (2008). The prevalence of suicidal ideation in the general population: Results from the Outcome of Depression International Network (ODIN) study. *Social Psychiatry and Psychiatric Epidemiology, 43*(4), 299–304. [CrossRef] [PubMed]

Castillejos, M. C., Huertas, P., Martin, P., & Moreno Kuestner, B. (2021). Prevalence of suicidality in the European general population: A systematic review and meta-analysis. *Archives of Suicide Research, 25*(4), 810–828. [CrossRef]

Chu, C., Buchman-Schmitt, J. M., Stanley, I. H., Hom, M. A., Tucker, R. P., Hagan, C. R., Rogers, M. L., Podlogar, M. C., Chiurliza, B., Ringer, F. B., Michaels, M. S., Patros, C. H. G., & Joiner, T. E., Jr. (2017). The interpersonal theory of suicide: A systematic review and meta-analysis of a decade of cross-national research. *Psychological Bulletin, 143*(12), 1313. [CrossRef]

Coppersmith, D. D. L., Fortgang, R. G., Kleiman, E. M., Millner, A. J., Yeager, A. L., Mair, P., & Nock, M. K. (2022). Effect of frequent assessment of suicidal thinking on its incidence and severity: High-resolution real-time monitoring study. *The British Journal of Psychiatry, 220*(1), 41–43. [CrossRef] [PubMed]

Cramer, A. O. J., Waldorp, L. J., van der Maas, H. L. J., & Borsboom, D. (2010). Comorbidity: A network perspective. *Behavioral and Brain Sciences, 33*(2–3), 137–150. [CrossRef] [PubMed]

Crosby, A. E., Ortega, L., & Melanson, C. (2011). *Self-directed violence surveillance: Uniform definitions and recommended data elements.* Centers for Disease Control and Prevention, National Center for Injury Prevention and Control, Division of Violence Prevention.

De Beurs, D., Fried, E., Wetherall, K., Cleare, S., O'Connor, D., Ferguson, E., O'Carroll, R. E., & O'Connor, R. C. (2019). Exploring the psychology of suicidal ideation: A theory driven network analysis. *Behaviour Research and Therapy, 120,* 103419. [CrossRef]

De Beurs, D. P., Van Borkulo, C. D., & O'Connor, R. C. (2017). Association between suicidal symptoms and repeat suicidal behaviour within a sample of hospital-treated suicide attempters. *BJPsych Open, 3*(3), 120–126. [CrossRef]

Dehara, M., Wells, M. B., Sjöqvist, H., Kosidou, K., Dalman, C., & Sörberg Wallin, A. (2021). Parenthood is associated with lower suicide risk: A register-based cohort study of 1.5 million Swedes. *Acta Psychiatrica Scandinavica, 143*(3), 206–215. [CrossRef]

De Leo, D., Draper, B. M., Snowdon, J., & Kõlves, K. (2013). Suicides in older adults: A case–control psychological autopsy study in Australia. *Journal of Psychiatric Research, 47*(7), 980–988. [CrossRef]

Derogatis, L. R. (2001). *Cuestionario de 90 síntomas (SCL-90-R).* TEA Ediciones.

de Ron, J., Fried, E. I., & Epskamp, S. (2021). Psychological networks in clinical populations: Investigating the consequences of Berkson's bias. *Psychological Medicine, 51*(1), 168–176. [CrossRef]

Ducasse, D., Lopez-Castroman, J., Dassa, D., Brand-Arpon, V., Dupuy-Maurin, K., Lacourt, L., Guillaume, S., Courtet, P., & Olié, E. (2020). Exploring the boundaries between borderline personality disorder and suicidal behavior disorder. *European Archives of Psychiatry and Clinical Neuroscience, 270*(8), 959–967. [CrossRef] [PubMed]

Epskamp, S. (2017). *Network psychometrics* [Doctoral dissertation, University of Amsterdam].

Epskamp, S., Borsboom, D., & Fried, E. I. (2018). Estimating psychological networks and their accuracy: A tutorial paper. *Behavior Research Methods, 50*(1), 195–212. [CrossRef] [PubMed]

Epskamp, S., Cramer, A. O., Waldorp, L. J., Schmittmann, V. D., & Borsboom, D. (2012). qgraph: Network visualizations of relationships in psychometric data. *Journal of Statistical Software, 48,* 1–18. [CrossRef]

Epskamp, S., & Fried, E. I. (2018). A tutorial on regularized partial correlation networks. *Psychological Methods, 23*(4), 617–634. [CrossRef]

Fonseca-Pedrero, E. (2017). Análisis de redes: ¿una nueva forma de comprender la psicopatología? *Revista de Psiquiatría y Salud Mental, 10*(4), 206–215. [CrossRef]

Fonseca-Pedrero, E. (2018). Análisis de redes en psicología. *Papeles del Psicólogo, 39*(1), 1–12. [CrossRef]

Fonseca-Pedrero, E. (2022, April 27). *Análisis de redes [Sesión aplicada].* Foro Precision Psychology. Available online: https://www.youtube.com/watch?v=Z_3eNeSXEhQ (accessed on 19 January 2025).

Fonseca-Pedrero, E., Al-Halabí, S., Pérez-Albéniz, A., & Debbané, M. (2022). Risk and protective factors in adolescent suicidal behaviour: A network analysis. *International Journal of Environmental Research and Public Health, 19*(3), 1784. [CrossRef]

Fonseca-Pedrero, E., Díez-Gómez, A., de la Barrera, U., Sebastián-Enesco, C., Ortuño-Sierra, J., Montoya-Castilla, I., Lucas-Molina, B., Inchausti, F., & Perez-Albeniz, A. (2020a). Suicidal behaviour in adolescents: A network analysis. *Spanish Journal of Psychiatry and Mental Health, 17*(1), 3–10. [CrossRef]

Fonseca-Pedrero, E., Díez-Gómez, A., Sebastián-Enesco, C., & Pérez-Albéniz, A. (2020b). Comprensión de las dificultades emocionales y conductuales y el comportamiento prosocial desde el prisma del análisis de redes. *Redes. Revista Hispana Para el Análisis de Redes Sociales, 31*(1), 19–29. [CrossRef]

Franklin, J. C., Ribeiro, J. D., Fox, K. R., Bentley, K. H., Kleiman, E. M., Huang, X., Musacchio, K. M., Jaroszewski, A. C., Chang, B. P., & Nock, M. K. (2017). Risk factors for suicidal thoughts and behaviors: A meta-analysis of 50 years of research. *Psychological bulletin, 143*(2), 187. [CrossRef] [PubMed]

Fried, E. I., Epskamp, S., Nesse, R. M., Tuerlinckx, F., & Borsboom, D. (2016). What are 'good' depression symptoms? Comparing the centrality of DSM and non-DSM symptoms of depression in a network analysis. *Journal of Affective Disorders, 189,* 314–320. [CrossRef]

Glenn, C. R., Kleiman, E. M., Kandlur, R., Esposito, E. C., & Liu, R. T. (2022). Thwarted belongingness mediates interpersonal stress and suicidal thoughts: An intensive longitudinal study with high-risk adolescents. *Journal of Clinical Child & Adolescent Psychology, 51*(3), 295–311. [CrossRef]

González de Rivera, J. L., De las Cuevas, C., Rodríguez, M., & Rodríguez, F. (2002). *Cuestionario de 90 síntomas SCL-90-R de Derogatis, L.* Adaptación española. TEA Ediciones.

Green, K. L., Brown, G. K., Jager-Hyman, S., Cha, J., Steer, R. A., & Beck, A. T. (2015). The predictive validity of the beck depression inventory suicide item. *The Journal of Clinical Psychiatry*, *76*(12), 15048. [CrossRef]

Guloksuz, S., Pries, L. K., & Van Os, J. (2017). Application of network methods for understanding mental disorders: Pitfalls and promise. *Psychological Medicine*, *47*(16), 2743–2752. [CrossRef]

Gvion, Y., & Apter, A. (2011). Aggression, impulsivity, and suicide behavior: A review of the literature. *Archives of Suicide Research*, *15*(2), 93–112. [CrossRef] [PubMed]

Gvion, Y., & Levi-Belz, Y. (2018). Serious suicide attempts: Systematic review of psychological risk factors. *Frontiers in Psychiatry*, *9*, 56. [CrossRef]

Hevey, D. (2018). Network analysis: A brief overview and tutorial. *Health Psychology and Behavioral Medicine*, *6*(1), 301–328. [CrossRef]

Hom, M. A., Stanley, I. H., Rogers, M. L., Gallyer, A. J., Dougherty, S. P., Davis, L., & Joiner, T. E. (2018). Investigating the iatrogenic effects of repeated suicidal ideation screening on suicidal and depression symptoms: A staggered sequential study. *Journal of Affective Disorders*, *232*, 139–142. [CrossRef]

Hubers, A. A. M., Moaddine, S., Peersmann, S. H. M., Stijnen, T., van Duijn, E., van der Mast, R., Dekkers, O. M., & Giltay, E. J. (2018). Suicidal ideation and subsequent completed suicide in both psychiatric and non-psychiatric populations: A meta-analysis. *Epidemiology and Psychiatric Sciences*, *27*(2), 186–198. [CrossRef]

Instituto Nacional de Estadística. (2024). *Defunciones según la causa de muerte*. Available online: https://www.ine.es (accessed on 16 January 2025).

Joiner, T. E. (2005). *Why people die by suicide*. Harvard University Press.

Joiner, T. E., Jr., Conwell, Y., Fitzpatrick, K. K., Witte, T. K., Schmidt, N. B., Berlim, M. T., Fleck, M. P. A., & Rudd, M. D. (2005). Four studies on how past and current suicidality relate even when "everything but the kitchen sink" is covaried. *Journal of Abnormal Psychology*, *114*(2), 291–303. [CrossRef] [PubMed]

Jones, P. J., Heeren, A., & McNally, R. J. (2017). Commentary: A network theory of mental disorders. *Frontiers in Psychology*, *8*, 1305. [CrossRef] [PubMed]

Jones, P. J., Mair, P., & McNally, R. J. (2018). Visualizing psychological networks: A tutorial in R. *Frontiers in Psychology*, *9*, 1742. [CrossRef]

Kim, J. L., Kim, J. M., Choi, Y., Lee, T. H., & Park, E. C. (2016). Effect of socioeconomic status on the linkage between suicidal ideation and suicide attempts. *Suicide and Life-Threatening Behavior*, *46*(5), 588–597. [CrossRef]

Klonsky, E. D., & May, A. M. (2015). The Three-step Theory (3ST): A new theory of suicide rooted in the "ideation-to-action" framework. *International Journal of Cognitive Therapy*, *8*(2), 114–129. [CrossRef]

Klonsky, E. D., May, A. M., & Saffer, B. Y. (2016). Suicide, suicide attempts, and suicidal ideation. *Annual Review of Clinical Psychology*, *12*, 307–330. [CrossRef] [PubMed]

Labrador, F. J., Estupiñá, F. J., & García Vera, M. P. (2010). Demanda de atención psicológica en la práctica clínica: Tratamientos y resultados. *Psicothema*, *22*(4), 619–626.

Large, M., Corderoy, A., & McHugh, C. (2020). Is suicidal behaviour a stronger predictor of later suicide than suicidal idea-tion? A systematic review and meta-analysis. *Australian & New Zealand Journal of Psychiatry*, *55*(3), 254–267. [CrossRef]

Lemogne, C., Fossati, P., Limosin, F., Nabi, H., Encrenaz, G., Bonenfant, S., & Consoli, S. M. (2011). Cognitive hostility and suicide. *Acta Psychiatrica Scandinavica*, *124*(1), 62–69. [CrossRef]

Lorant, V., De Gelder, R., Kapadia, D., Borrell, C., Kalediene, R., Kovács, K., Leinsalu, M., Martikainen, P., Menvielle, G., Regidor, E., Rodríguez-Sanz, M., Wojtyniak, B., Strand, B. H., Bopp, M., & Mackenbach, J. P. (2018). Socioeconomic inequalities in suicide in Europe: The widening gap. *The British Journal of Psychiatry*, *212*(6), 356–361. [CrossRef]

Mann, J. J., Waternaux, C., Haas, G. L., & Malone, K. M. (1999). Toward a clinical model of suicidal behavior in psychiatric patients. *The American Journal of Psychiatry*, *156*(2), 181–189. [CrossRef] [PubMed]

May, A. M., & Klonsky, E. D. (2016). What distinguishes suicide attempters from suicide ideators meta-analysis of potential factors. *Clinical Psychology: Science and Practice*, *23*(1), 5–20. [CrossRef]

McClelland, H., Evans, J. J., Nowland, R., Ferguson, E., & O'Connor, R. C. (2020). Loneliness as a predictor of suicidal ideation and behaviour: A systematic review and meta-analysis of prospective studies. *Journal of Affective Disorders*, *274*, 880–896. [CrossRef]

McNally, R. J., Mair, P., Mugno, B. L., & Riemann, B. C. (2017). Co-morbid obsessive–compulsive disorder and depression: A Bayesian network approach. *Psychological Medicine*, *47*(7), 1204–1214. [CrossRef]

McNally, R. J., Robinaugh, D. J., Wu, G. W., Wang, L., Deserno, M. K., & Borsboom, D. (2015). Mental disorders as causal systems: A network approach to posttraumatic stress disorder. *Clinical Psychological Science*, *3*(6), 836–849. [CrossRef]

Menon, V., Sarkar, S., Kattimani, S., & Mathan, K. (2015). Do personality traits such as impulsivity and hostility-aggressiveness predict severity of intent in attempted suicide? Findings from a record based study in South India. *Indian Journal of Psychological Medicine*, *37*(4), 393–398. [CrossRef] [PubMed]

Milner, A., Hjelmeland, H. M., Arensman, E., & De Leo, D. (2013a). Social-environmental factors and suicide mortality: A narrative review of over 200 Articles. *Sociology Mind, 3*(2), 137–148. [CrossRef]

Milner, A., Page, A., & LaMontagne, A. D. (2013b). Long-term unemployment and suicide: A systematic review and meta-analysis. *PLoS ONE, 8*(1), e51333. [CrossRef]

Moore, F. R., Doughty, H., Neumann, T., McClelland, H., Allott, C., & O'Connor, R. C. (2022). Impulsivity, aggression, and suicidality relationship in adults: A systematic review and meta-analysis. *EClinicalMedicine, 45*, 101307. [CrossRef]

Nock, M. K., Borges, G., Bromet, E. J., Alonso, J., Angermeyer, M., Beautrais, A., Bruffaerts, R., Chiu, W. T., de Girolamo, G., Gluzman, S., de Graaf, R., Gureje, O., Haro, J. M., Huang, Y., Karam, E., Kessler, R. C., Lepine, J. P., Levinson, D., Medina-Mora, M. E., ... Williams, D. (2008). Cross-national prevalence and risk factors for suicidal ideation, plans and attempts. *The British Journal of Psychiatry, 192*(2), 98–105. [CrossRef]

Nock, M. K., Hwang, I., Sampson, N., Kessler, R. C., Angermeyer, M., Beautrais, A., Borges, G., Bromet, E., Bruffaerts, R., de Girolamo, G., de Graaf, R., Florescu, S., Gureje, O., Haro, J. M., Hu, C., Huang, Y., Karam, E. G., Kawakami, N., Kovess, V., & Williams, D. R. (2009). Cross-national analysis of the associations among mental disorders and suicidal behavior: Findings from the WHO World Mental Health Surveys. *PLoS Medicine, 6*(8), e1000123. [CrossRef] [PubMed]

Nock, M. K., Hwang, I., Sampson, N. A., & Kessler, R. C. (2010). Mental disorders, comorbidity and suicidal behavior: Results from the National Comorbidity Survey Replication. *Molecular Psychiatry, 15*(8), 868–876. [CrossRef]

Núñez, D., Ulloa, J. L., Guillaume, S., Olie, E., Alacreu-Crespo, A., & Courtet, P. (2020). Suicidal ideation and affect lability in single and multiple suicidal attempters with major depressive disorder: An exploratory network analysis. *Journal of Affective Disorders, 272*, 371–379. [CrossRef]

O'Connor, R. C., & Kirtley, O. J. (2018). The integrated motivational–volitional model of suicidal behaviour. *Philosophical Transactions of the Royal Society B: Biological Sciences, 373*(1754), 20170268. [CrossRef] [PubMed]

Olatunji, B. O., Cisler, J. M., & Tolin, D. F. (2007). Quality of life in the anxiety disorders: A meta-analytic review. *Clinical Psychology Review, 27*(5), 572–581. [CrossRef] [PubMed]

Pelizza, L., Poletti, M., Azzali, S., Paterlini, F., Garlassi, S., Scazza, I., Chiri, L. R., Pupo, S., Pompili, M., & Raballo, A. (2020). Suicide risk in young people at Ultra-High Risk (UHR) of psychosis: Findings from a 2-year longitudinal study. *Schizophrenia Research, 220*, 98–105. [CrossRef]

Posner, K., Brown, G. K., Stanley, B., Brent, D. A., Yershova, K. V., Oquendo, M. A., Currier, G. W., Melvin, G. A., Greenhill, L., Shen, S., & Mann, J. J. (2011). The Columbia–Suicide Severity Rating Scale: Initial validity and internal consistency findings from three multisite studies with adolescents and adults. *American Journal of Psychiatry, 168*(12), 1266–1277. [CrossRef]

Rath, D., De Beurs, D., Hallensleben, N., Spangenberg, L., Glaesmer, H., & Forkmann, T. (2019). Modelling suicide ideation from beep to beep: Application of network analysis to ecological momentary assessment data. *Internet Interventions, 18*, 100292. [CrossRef]

Robinaugh, D. J., Millner, A. J., & McNally, R. J. (2016). Identifying highly influential nodes in the complicated grief network. *Journal of Abnormal Psychology, 125*(6), 747. [CrossRef]

Sadock, V. A., Kaplan, H. I., & Ruiz, P. (2015). *Sinopsis de psiquiatría: Ciencias de la conducta, psiquiatría clínica* (11th ed.). Wolters Kluwer.

San Too, L., Spittal, M. J., Bugeja, L., Reifels, L., Butterworth, P., & Pirkis, J. (2019). The association between mental disorders and suicide: A systematic review and meta-analysis of record linkage studies. *Journal of Affective Disorders, 259*, 302–314. [CrossRef]

Shah, A. (2011). Are elderly dependency ratios associated with general population suicide rates? *International Journal of Social Psychiatry, 57*(3), 277–283. [CrossRef] [PubMed]

Stanley, I. H., Boffa, J. W., Rogers, M. L., Hom, M. A., Albanese, B. J., Chu, C., Capron, D. W., Schmidt, N. B., & Joiner, T. E. (2018). Anxiety sensitivity and suicidal ideation/suicide risk: A meta-analysis. *Journal of Consulting and Clinical Psychology, 86*(11), 946. [CrossRef] [PubMed]

Sveticic, J., & De Leo, D. (2012). The hypothesis of a continuum in suicidality: A discussion on its validity and practical implications. *Mental Illness, 4*(2), 73–78. [CrossRef]

Taylor, P. J., Gooding, P. A., Wood, A. M., Johnson, J., Pratt, D., & Tarrier, N. (2010). Defeat and entrapment in schizophrenia: The relationship with suicidal ideation and positive psychotic symptoms. *Psychiatry Research, 178*(2), 244–248. [CrossRef] [PubMed]

Taylor, P. J., Hutton, P., & Wood, L. (2015). Are people at risk of psychosis also at risk of suicide and self-harm? A systematic review and meta-analysis. *Psychological Medicine, 45*(5), 911–926. [CrossRef]

Torres, M. E., Löwe, B., Schmitz, S., Pienta, J. N., Van Der Feltz-Cornelis, C., & Fiedorowicz, J. G. (2021). Suicide and suicidality in somatic symptom and related disorders: A systematic review. *Journal of Psychosomatic Research, 140*, 110290. [CrossRef]

Tsai, M., Lari, H., Saffy, S., & Klonsky, E. D. (2021). Examining the three-step theory (3ST) of suicide in a prospective study of adult psychiatric inpatients. *Behavior Therapy, 52*(3), 673–685. [CrossRef]

Van Borkulo, C. D., van Bork, R., Boschloo, L., Kossakowski, J. J., Tio, P., Schoevers, R. A., Borsboom, D., & Waldorp, L. J. (2022). Comparing network structures on three aspects: A permutation test. *Psychological Methods, 28*(6), 1273–1285. [CrossRef]

Van Orden, K. A., Witte, T. K., Cukrowicz, K. C., Braithwaite, S. R., Selby, E. A., & Joiner, T. E., Jr. (2010). The interpersonal theory of suicide. *Psychological Review, 117*(2), 575. [CrossRef]

Westefeld, J. S., Casper, D., Galligan, P., Gibbons, S., Lustgarten, S., Rice, A., Rowe-Johnson, M., & Yeates, K. (2015). Suicide and older adults: Risk factors and recommendations. *Journal of Loss and Trauma, 20*(6), 491–508. [CrossRef]

World Health Organization. (2014). *Preventing suicide: A global imperative.* World Health Organization.

World Medical Association. (2013). Helsinki declaration: World medical association declaration of Helsinki: Ethical principles for medical research involving human subjects. *JAMA, 310*(20), 2191–2194. [CrossRef] [PubMed]

Yates, K., Lång, U., Cederlöf, M., Boland, F., Taylor, P., Cannon, M., McNicholas, F., DeVylder, J., & Kelleher, I. (2019). Association of psychotic experiences with subsequent risk of suicidal ideation, suicide attempts, and suicide deaths: A systematic review and meta-analysis of longitudinal population studies. *JAMA Psychiatry, 76*(2), 180–189. [CrossRef] [PubMed]

behavioral sciences

MDPI

Article

Concurrent Validity of Digital Measures of Psychological Dimensions Associated with Suicidality Using AuxiliApp

Miguel Zacarías Pérez Sosa [1,2], Diego de-la-Vega-Sánchez [1,2,*], Sergio Sanz-Gómez [2], Adrián Alacreu-Crespo [3], Pedro Moreno-Gea [4], Pilar A. Saiz [5,6,7,8], Julio Seoane Rey [9], José Giner [2] and Lucas Giner [2]

1 Hospital Universitario Virgen Macarena, 41009 Sevilla, Spain; miguelzacarias88.ull@gmail.com
2 Departamento de Psiquiatría, Universidad de Sevilla, 41013 Sevilla, Spain; ssanz1@us.es (S.S.-G.); jginer@us.es (J.G.); lginer@us.es (L.G.)
3 Departamento de Psicología y Sociología, Universidad de Zaragoza, 50009 Zaragoza, Spain; aalacreu@unizar.es
4 Psiquiatria, 30204 Cartagena, Spain; pmoreno@psiquiatria.com
5 Departamento de Psiquiatría, Universidad de Oviedo, 33003 Oviedo, Spain; frank@uniovi.es
6 Centro de Investigación Biomédica en Red en Salud Mental (CIBERSAM), Instituto de Salud Carlos III, 28029 Madrid, Spain
7 Instituto de Investigación Sanitaria del Principado de Asturias (ISPA), 33011 Oviedo, Spain
8 Servicio de Salud del Principado de Asturias (SESPA), 33011 Oviedo, Spain
9 Departamento de Psicología Social, Universidad de Valencia, 46010 Valencia, Spain; seoane@uv.es
* Correspondence: dvega2@us.es

Abstract

Suicide is a major public health concern, and accurate risk assessment is essential for prevention. Slider-format questions offer a quick, intuitive, and accessible method to evaluate suicide-related dimensions. This study examines the reliability of slider-based items compared to standardized psychometric instruments when delivered via a mobile app. A total of 299 university students completed a digital self-report questionnaire using the AuxiliApp mobile platform. Participants answered validated scales assessing depression, psychological pain, suicidal ideation, anger, impulsivity, loneliness, and reasons for living, each presented in both traditional Likert and novel slider formats. Pearson correlations were used to evaluate the relationship between traditional and slider-based scores. All correlations were statistically significant ($p < 0.001$). Moderate correlations were found in most domains, including depression, psychological pain, suicidal ideation, loneliness, and key aspects of impulsivity and anger. Lower correlations appeared in subscales related to anger control and protective beliefs against suicide. Slider-based items demonstrated acceptable psychometric equivalence and concurrent validity compared to traditional scales. Their brevity and compatibility with mobile devices support their use in telehealth and digital mental health screening. While not a replacement for clinical evaluation, they may facilitate early detection and ongoing monitoring in at-risk populations.

Keywords: suicide; suicide prevention; risk assessment; digital technology; mHealth

1. Introduction

Suicide remains a critical global public health issue, accounting for a significant number of deaths worldwide. According to the World Health Organization (WHO), nearly 800,000 people die by suicide each year, representing approximately 1.4% of all deaths globally (Wang et al., 2016). This issue is particularly pressing among young adults (World

Health Organization, 2021). Numerous risk factors have been identified in association with suicidal behavior, including the presence of a mental disorder—87.3% of individuals who die by suicide are estimated to have been diagnosed with a mental illness prior to their death (Arsenault-Lapierre et al., 2004)—as well as traits such as impulsivity, aggressiveness, and emotional instability (Chamorro et al., 2012; Critchfield et al., 2004; Lin & Zhang, 2017).

Impulsivity—defined as a predisposition to act without forethought or planning, often resulting in adverse consequences for oneself or others—has been consistently associated with suicidal behaviors (Herpertz et al., 1995; Simeon et al., 1992; Swann et al., 2020; Moore et al., 2023), including self-harm (Hamza et al., 2015; Hamza & Willoughby, 2019), suicide attempts (Auerbach et al., 2017; Cole et al., 2019; Costanza et al., 2020; Liu et al., 2017), and deaths by suicide (Alasaarela et al., 2017; Dalca et al., 2013; Caro-Cañizares et al., 2024), particularly among younger populations (Alasaarela et al., 2017; Auerbach et al., 2017). This association is robust across various populations, including psychiatric inpatients, those with substance use disorders, and individuals with trauma histories, and its effect is especially pronounced when measured close in time to suicidal behavior (Horesh et al., 1997; Kotler et al., 2001). Neurobiological links also highlight impulsivity and aggression as associated with altered brain function in regions responsible for emotion regulation, potentially serving as biological markers for suicide risk (Lee et al., 2024; Swann et al., 2020).

Anger has also been linked to suicidal behavior (Hawkins et al., 2014; Maino et al., 2019; Rogers et al., 2017; Moore et al., 2023), especially in individuals with post-traumatic stress disorder (Dillon et al., 2020; Wilks et al., 2019; Kotler et al., 2001) and among adolescents and young adults (Nock et al., 2013; Park et al., 2010), particularly young males (Daniel et al., 2009; Esposito et al., 2003). Associations have also been observed in populations with borderline personality disorder (Evren et al., 2011; Mercer et al., 2009; Stringer et al., 2013; Giegling et al., 2009) and major depressive disorder (Painuly et al., 2007). While anger alone may be less specific to suicide risk than impulsivity, its presence is often elevated in those with mental health issues (Horesh et al., 1997; Caro-Cañizares et al., 2024). Crucially, high levels of both anger and impulsivity can act synergistically, further increasing suicide risk beyond the effect of either trait alone, mediating the impact of stressful life events on suicide risk (Horesh et al., 1997; Moore et al., 2023; Caro-Cañizares et al., 2024).

Other psychological dimensions related to suicide risk include psychological pain (Holden et al., 2001; Troister & Holden, 2012, 2013), loneliness (Ernst et al., 2021; Killgore et al., 2020), and the absence of reasons for living (Chen et al., 2020; Rozek et al., 2021). To identify individuals at elevated risk of suicide, clinicians and researchers rely on assessment tools that evaluate these dimensions. The Beck inventories, for example, have been used to detect individuals at risk through scales assessing depression (Green et al., 2015; Troister et al., 2015), hopelessness (T. Beck et al., 1990; Rueda-Jaimes et al., 2018; Sánchez-Teruel et al., 2020; Sueki, 2022), and suicidal intent (Harriss & Hawton, 2005; Stefansson et al., 2012; Sun et al., 2015; Zhang & Jia, 2007).

Several strategies have demonstrated efficacy in the prevention of suicidal behavior. These include early detection of suicidal ideation and behavior, the implementation of individualized safety plans during crises, timely access to specialized mental healthcare—especially following critical events such as hospital discharge—continuity of care, and the presence of strong social and family support networks (Turecki et al., 2019; Zalsman et al., 2016). The COVID-19 pandemic appears to have exacerbated suicide risk through two primary mechanisms: by intensifying known risk factors such as psychological distress, social isolation, and hopelessness; and by undermining the functioning of public health systems (Dubé et al., 2021; Reger et al., 2020). In response to these systemic strains and growing needs within the population, it is imperative to reconsider and innovate our approaches to suicide prevention.

New technologies and telemedicine are rapidly transforming healthcare delivery, offering unprecedented opportunities to reach individuals who might otherwise lack access to mental health services (Hilty et al., 2022; Lindsay et al., 2024; Olié et al., 2021). The COVID-19 pandemic significantly accelerated the adoption of telehealth, demonstrating its feasibility and utility for a wide range of psychiatric interventions, including psychotherapy, medication management, and crisis support (Heidari et al., 2023; Alemu et al., 2023). Mobile applications, in particular, provide a ubiquitous and convenient platform for self-monitoring, psychoeducation, and even early detection of mental health concerns, including those related to suicide risk (Areán et al., 2021). These tools can bridge geographical barriers, reduce stigma, and offer discreet support, making them invaluable assets in modern mental health frameworks (Melia et al., 2020). However, it is important to note that a systematic review of mobile applications for depression and suicide prevention revealed that only a small fraction incorporated evidence-based strategies to address suicidal behavior (Torous & Roberts, 2017). This highlights a critical gap in the application of digital technologies for suicide prevention.

Accurate and timely identification of individuals at risk is paramount for effective prevention strategies. Traditional methods of psychological assessment, though well-established, can sometimes be lengthy, resource-intensive, or less engaging, particularly for younger, digitally native populations. In this context, the development and validation of innovative assessment tools adapted to digital platforms are crucial for enhancing accessibility, efficiency, and user engagement in mental healthcare. Numerous studies have shown that participants tend to feel more comfortable completing electronic questionnaires than traditional paper-based ones. Electronic formats enhance accessibility and optimize time efficiency, while demonstrating acceptable psychometric equivalence, provided that standardized protocols are followed and the tools are properly validated (Barrigón et al., 2017).

Visual analog scales (VAS), or slider-type questions, offer a continuous graphical format that allows individuals to indicate the position that best reflects their subjective experience. These scales are generally quicker, simpler, and more intuitive to complete. Research has demonstrated robust correlations between VAS and traditional measures in domains such as affective and psychotic symptoms. For example, Palmier-Claus and colleagues (Palmier-Claus et al., 2012) validated an analog-format self-report tool named ClinTouch, comparing it with the PANSS and Calgary scales, finding moderate to strong associations for several parameters. Similarly, a review examining digital self-report questionnaires in patients with depression and mania (Faurholt-Jepsen et al., 2016) found that instruments evaluated in depression studies demonstrated good validity and reliability when compared with established clinical scales.

Given the nascent development and empirical investigation of slider-format questions for these specific psychological constructs in mobile health applications, this study aims to compare the psychometric equivalence and utility of traditional paper-based scales with matched slider-format questions assessing dimensions related to suicide risk, including suicidal intent, impulsivity, aggressiveness, anger, depression, reasons for living, loneliness, and psychological pain. This study adopts an exploratory research design to examine the psychometric equivalence between these novel digital items and established standardized scales, all administered within a mobile application.

2. Materials and Methods

This study employed a quantitative, cross-sectional, and correlational design aimed at assessing the psychometric equivalence of slider-format questions against established standardized scales when administered via a mobile application. Data collection was synchronous, meaning all data for each participant were collected at a single point in time.

2.1. Participants

A total of 299 university students from various universities across Spain participated in the study. The mean age of the sample was M = 19.86, SD = 1.86 years, and 71.2% of the participants were women. A total of 73.9% of participants were enrolled at the University of Seville, while the remaining 26.1% attended the University of Oviedo. Most participants (121) were studying medicine (50.5%), followed by nursing and physiotherapy (42.8%), and criminology (6.7%). The recruitment of participants was conducted using a non-probabilistic convenience sampling method, involving invitations distributed through university channels and social media across the country.

Inclusion criteria for participation were being a university student, being 18 years of age or older, being healthy volunteers, providing informed consent, having access to a mobile device with internet connection, and ability to comprehend and respond to questionnaires in Spanish. Exclusion criteria for participation were failure to complete all study questionnaires, providing inconsistent or invalid responses (e.g., straight-lining, obvious random responses).

The study was conducted entirely in Spanish.

2.2. Sample Size and Power Analysis

A formal power analysis was not conducted prior to data collection. This study adopted an exploratory research design to investigate the psychometric equivalence of a novel assessment format for suicide-related dimensions. The sample size was primarily determined by convenience and participant availability within the university setting, aiming to recruit a sufficient number of participants to explore the relationships between the measures. While a power analysis was not performed, the collected sample size of 299 participants was considered appropriate for detecting correlations of moderate effect size ($r > 0.3$) given the nature of the study and in line with typical sample sizes in instrument validation research.

2.3. Ethical Considerations

The study protocol, titled 'Validación de escalas de valoración del riesgo de suicidio en versión analógica', was reviewed and received a favorable dictamen from the Comité Coordinador de Ética de la Investigación Biomédica de Andalucía on 29 May 2017, under protocol version V1. All participants provided informed consent digitally prior to their participation. They were fully informed about the study's objectives, procedures, potential risks, and benefits, as well as their right to withdraw at any time without penalty. Participant data were handled with strict confidentiality and anonymity, in accordance with ethical guidelines.

2.4. Procedure

The study was conducted entirely through AuxiliApp, a proprietary mobile application designed for mental health assessment and support. All participants completed a self-administered digital questionnaire via this mobile platform. Data collection was therefore 100% digital, ensuring consistency in the administration format.

Regarding the administration flow, participants first completed the entire battery of original, multi-item validated scales, administered digitally within the AuxiliApp (see Figure 1). Each of these original scales preserved its specific, original response format (e.g., categories, numerical ranges, or yes/no options as per its design). Following the completion of all original scales, participants then proceeded to complete a collection of single slider-format items, each carefully selected by the research team as most representative for a specific construct (e.g., mood, loneliness, impulsivity). These slider items universally utilized a 0–10 continuous scale. All assessments were conducted sequentially within a single digital session on the AuxiliApp (https://psiquiatria.com/publico/index.php; accessed on 20 December 2024), ensuring a consistent testing environment for all participants. This sequential administration within a single session allowed for the assessment of convergent validity between the traditional multi-item scales and their novel slider-format counterparts, thereby evaluating the psychometric equivalence of these different assessment formats for the same constructs.

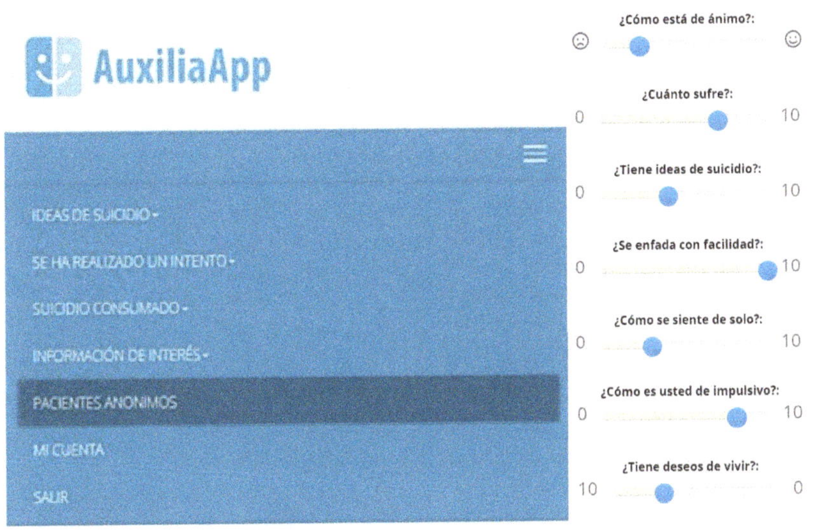

Figure 1. Main menu of the AuxiliApp web version.

The development of the slider-format items for AuxiliApp was a meticulous process undertaken by the research team. The team comprises university professors and distinguished academics with extensive expertise in suicidology, psychometrics, and instrument development. Notably, several members, including Professors Sáiz Martínez, Pilar, Seoane Rey, Julio, Giner Ubago, and José (all full professors), have a proven track record in both developing novel psychological instruments (e.g., the Oviedo Sleep Questionnaire; Paz García-Portilla et al., 2009 and rigorously adapting numerous internationally recognized scales into Spanish (e.g., Social Anxiety and Distress Scale, Sheehan Disability Inventory; Bobes García et al., 1999; MINI International Neuropsychiatric Interview; Ferrando et al., 1998; EuropASI; Bobes et al., 1996; Clinician Administered PTSD Scale (CAPS); Grupo Español de Trabajo para la Evaluación por Estrés Postraumático, 2000, among others).

The decision-making process for item selection and their subsequent adaptation to the slider format was achieved through multiple consensus meetings among the research team. These discussions leveraged the team's collective clinical and psychometric expertise, informed by a thorough review of existing scientific literature on digital assessment and the psychometric properties of the original scales. The primary objective was to create digital equivalents that maintained the psychometric integrity and semantic content of established, validated instruments.

Specifically, the slider-format items were conceived as a direct, literal, one-to-one adaptation of the original items from the selected standardized scales. Minor linguistic adjustments were applied to enhance clarity and natural flow within a digital self-report context, while scrupulously preserving the semantic meaning of the original questions. For instance, an item like "I keep calm" from the original STAXI scale was rephrased to "¿Mantiene la calma?" (Do you keep calm?) or "I get angry easily" to "¿Se enfada con facilidad?" (Do you get angry easily?) in the slider format. These adaptations were solely aimed at optimizing readability and user experience within the app without altering the underlying construct being measured.

The rationale for reversing certain items was grounded in psychometric principles. For the majority of scales, a higher numerical score consistently indicates a greater severity or presence of a symptom. For items or subscales designed to measure the absence of a symptom or the presence of a protective factor (e.g., reasons for living), the response scale for the slider was intentionally reversed. This ensured that, for all measured dimensions, a higher numerical value assigned by the slider consistently reflected a greater level of the measured construct (e.g., more reasons for living), thereby maintaining a uniform interpretative direction for all data analysis.

2.5. Instruments

All instruments were administered digitally through AuxiliApp, presenting two distinct formats: the original validated Likert-type scale format and a novel slider-format adaptation. Participants completed both versions for each dimension. The dimensions assessed were suicidal intent, impulsivity, aggressiveness, anger, depression, reasons for living, loneliness, and psychological pain.

- Beck Depression Inventory-II (BDI-II): Assesses the severity of depressive symptoms (A. T. Beck et al., 1960; Spanish adaptation by Sanz et al., 2003, which reported an excellent internal consistency of $\alpha = 0.89$ in the general population). The scale consists of 21 items rated on a 4-point scale from 0 to 3, covering emotional, cognitive, and somatic aspects of depression, such as hopelessness, guilt, and physical discomfort.
- Psychache Scale: Measures psychological pain using 13 items rated on a 5-point Likert scale (Holden et al., 2001; Spanish adaptation by Ordóñez-Carrasco et al., 2022, which reported an excellent internal consistency of $\alpha = 0.90$). Higher scores indicate greater levels of psychological distress.
- Paykel Suicide Scale (PSS): Assesses the severity and frequency of suicidal ideation. For this study, we utilized a Spanish adaptation for adolescents (Fonseca-Pedrero et al., 2018; see also Baños-Chaparro & Ramos-Vera, 2020, who reported an excellent internal consistency of $\alpha = 0.94$ in a Peruvian adolescent sample).
- State-Trait Anger Expression Inventory-2 (STAXI-2): Evaluates the experience, expression, and control of anger (Spielberger et al., 1983; Spanish adaptation by Miguel-Tobal et al., 2001). The scale comprises several subscales, including State Anger, Trait Anger, Anger Expression-Out, Anger Expression-In, Anger Control-Out, and Anger Control-In. Psychometric studies of its Spanish version have demonstrated good internal consistency, with Cronbach's alpha values ranging from 0.70 to 0.90 for its various subscales (e.g., García-Batista et al., 2018).
- UCLA Loneliness Scale: Designed to assess perceived loneliness and social isolation. It contains 20 items rated on a 4-point scale, with higher scores indicating more frequent

experiences of loneliness (Russell, 1996; Spanish adaptation by Vázquez Morejón & Jiménez García-Bóveda, 1994; see also Velarde-Mayol et al., 2016) has shown high reliability, with an excellent internal consistency of $\alpha = 0.90$.

- Barratt Impulsiveness Scale (BIS): A widely used self-report measure of impulsivity (Patton et al., 1995). For this study, the Spanish adaptation for adolescents (Martínez-Loredo et al., 2015) was utilized, which has demonstrated good psychometric properties, including excellent internal consistency for the total scale ($\alpha = 0.89$) and good consistency for its subscales (Attentional Impulsivity: $\alpha = 0.70$; Non-planning Impulsivity: $\alpha = 0.81$; Motor Impulsivity: $\alpha = 0.79$).
- Reasons for Living Inventory (RFL): Measures an individual's perceived reasons for not committing suicide (Linehan et al., 1983). The Spanish adaptation (Oquendo et al., 2000) has shown excellent internal consistency, with a Cronbach's alpha of $\alpha = 0.94$ for the total scale, and values ranging from 0.70 to 0.89 for its various subscales (Survival and Coping Beliefs, Responsibility to Family, Child Concerns, Fear of Suicide, Fear of Social Disapproval, and Moral/Religious Objections).

These instruments were selected for their relevance to suicide risk and their established psychometric properties. Each was paired with a slider-format item designed to assess the same construct in a more concise and accessible visually intuitive format within the AuxiliApp.

2.6. Statistical Analysis

Pearson product–moment correlation coefficients were calculated to assess the convergent validity between scores obtained from traditional multi-item scales and their corresponding slider-format items for each relevant construct (Cohen et al., 2003). This analysis aimed to evaluate the psychometric equivalence of the novel slider format against established measures.

Regarding the distribution of continuous variables, Pearson's correlation coefficient was used due to its ability to measure the linear relationship between variables. Given the continuous nature of the data and the sample sizes for each correlation (ranging from N = 56 for the Beck Depression Inventory to N = 274 for the Reasons for Living Inventory), this statistic was considered appropriate for the purposes of this study, relying on the robustness of Pearson's r in samples of this size.

3. Results

Prior to presenting the main analyses, it is important to address the varying sample sizes across the instruments. While the majority of the scales included in AuxiliApp were completed by over 200 participants, the Beck Depression Inventory-II (BDI-II) had a substantially smaller valid sample size of N = 56. This discrepancy was primarily attributed to participant dropout or incomplete responses, likely due to the BDI-II being administered towards the end of a comprehensive battery of questionnaires. Given the extended length of the overall assessment, it is plausible that some participants discontinued the survey before completing this final instrument. All subsequent analyses involving the BDI-II are based on this sample size, and this limitation is acknowledged.

All Pearson correlations between the traditional scale scores and their corresponding slider-format items were statistically significant ($p < 0.001$). According to Guilford's criteria (Guilford, 1956), most correlations were moderate (r = 0.40–0.70), while a subset were low (r = 0.20–0.40), particularly in subscales related to anger expression and family-based protective beliefs.

Moderate correlations were observed between the slider items and the traditional instruments assessing depression (BDI-II, r = −0.541), psychological pain (Psychache

Scale, r = 0.598), suicidal ideation (Paykel, r = 0.503), loneliness (UCLA, r = 0.582), and several impulsivity and anger-related dimensions. Specifically, the BIS subscales showed correlations of r = −0.581 (Cognitive/Attentional), r = −0.445 (Non-Planning), and r = 0.426 (Motor). For anger, STAXI-2 subscales showed moderate correlations in State Anger (r = 0.459), Trait Anger (r = 0.558), and Anger Expression-In (r = 0.489).

Lower correlations were found for STAXI-2 subscales of Anger Expression-Out (r = 0.292), External Anger Control (r = 0.354), and Internal Anger Control (r = 0.380). Similarly, within the Reasons for Living Inventory (RFL), the Survival and Coping Beliefs subscale showed a moderate negative correlation (r = −0.589), while the Family Responsibility and Child-Related Concerns (r = −0.382), Fear of Suicide (r = −0.283), Fear of Social Disapproval (r = −0.455), and Moral Objections (r = −0.359) subscales showed low correlations.

In all inversely worded items, higher traditional scale scores (indicating greater symptomatology or protective beliefs) corresponded to lower scores on the associated slider question, accounting for the negative correlations. Overall, the data supports the validity of slider-format questions as a simplified yet valid alternative for assessing core dimensions related to suicide risk.

A detailed comparison of the means and correlations between the traditional and slider-format items is presented in Table 1.

Table 1. Summary of results from traditional format and electronic slider format.

Scale	Slider Question	N	Traditional Format Mean (Min–Max)	Slider Format Mean (Min–Max)	Pearson's r	*p*-Value
* Beck Depression Inventory	How is your mood?	56	5.268 (0–32)	7.197 (0–10)	−0.541	<0.001
Psychache Scale	How much are you suffering?	265	22.694 (13–64)	2.385 (0–9)	0.598	<0.001
Paykel	Do you have suicidal thoughts?	223	0.973 (0–5)	0.883 (0–10)	0.503	<0.001
STAXI-2—State Anger	Do you feel angry?	270	18.622 (15–50)	1.541 (0–8)	0.459	<0.001
STAXI-2—Trait Anger	Do you get angry easily?	270	21.152 (10–37)	4.037 (0–10)	0.558	<0.001
STAXI-2—Anger Expression-Out	Do you express your anger?	270	12.296 (6–23)	4.852 (0–10)	0.292	<0.001
STAXI-2—Anger Expression-In	Do you keep your anger to yourself?	270	12.456 (6–22)	3.889 (0–10)	0.489	<0.001
STAXI-2—External Anger Control	Do you remain calm?	270	17.900 (6–24)	5.756 (0–10)	0.354	<0.001
STAXI-2—Internal Anger Control	Do you count to ten before expressing your anger?	270	14.463 (6–24)	3.118 (0–10)	0.380	<0.001
UCLA Loneliness Scale	How lonely do you feel?	249	12.076 (0–58)	2.531 (0–10)	0.582	<0.001
* BIS—Cognitive/Attentional	Do you find it easy to concentrate?	272	12.658 (2–28)	6.224 (0–10)	−0.581	<0.001
* BIS—Non-Planning	Do you finish what you start?	272	14.158 (2–40)	7.404 (0–10)	−0.445	<0.001
BIS—Motor	How impulsive are you?	272	14.856 (2–39)	5.353 (0–10)	0.426	<0.001
* RFL—Survival and Coping	Do you have a desire to live?	274	19.467 (0–118)	9.310 (0–10)	−0.589	<0.001
* RFL—Family-Related	Does your family motivate you to live?	274	11.912 (0–50)	9.164 (0–10)	−0.382	<0.001
* RFL—Fear of Suicide	Are you afraid of suicide?	274	22.580 (0–35)	5.967 (0–10)	−0.283	<0.001
* RFL—Fear of Disapproval	Are you concerned about what people would think if you died by suicide?	274	10.117 (0–15)	3.817 (0–10)	−0.455	<0.001
RFL—Moral Objections	Do you think suicide is wrong?	274	13.496 (0–20)	7.256 (0–10)	−0.359	<0.001

Note: * The slider question is inversely worded. N = number of participants with complete data for each variable. BDI-II: Beck Depression Inventory-II, Paykel: Paykel Suicidal Ideation Scale, STAXI-2: State-Trait Anger Expression Inventory-2, UCLA: University of California, Los Angeles, BIS: Barratt Impulsiveness Scale, RFL: Reasons For Living Inventory, Min-Max: Minimum-Maximum.

4. Discussion

Our findings indicate that slider-format items can approximate scores from validated instruments with moderate correlations in most domains, including depression, psychological pain, suicidal ideation, loneliness, and core aspects of impulsivity and anger. Specifically, these moderate correlations provide evidence of convergent validity for the slider items across these dimensions. The demonstrated feasibility of digitally assessing constructs like impulsivity and anger, consistently identified as key risk factors for suicidal behavior (Moore et al., 2023; Caro-Cañizares et al., 2024; Lee et al., 2024), underscores the potential of mobile applications to facilitate timely and efficient risk assessments. While lower correlations were observed in some subscales—particularly those assessing nuanced components of anger regulation and certain protective beliefs against suicide—this does not diminish the potential utility of digital sliders, especially considering their brevity, accessibility, and ease of implementation.

The broader relevance of telemedicine has become undeniable, especially during the COVID-19 crisis. The pandemic not only challenged the capacity of healthcare systems, with a reported 90% of countries experiencing disruptions in essential health services (World Health Organization, 2021), but also profoundly reshaped how care is delivered and received. Many individuals refrained from seeking care for non-COVID-related issues (Moynihan et al., 2021), negatively affecting public health outcomes. The pandemic's psychological impact is well documented: there has been a marked increase in the prevalence of mental disorders (Santomauro et al., 2021; Winkler et al., 2020), worsened outcomes for individuals with pre-existing psychiatric conditions (Neelam et al., 2021), and heightened suicide risk (Dubé et al., 2021; John et al., 2021). Some have even described this as a parallel pandemic of mental health (Patten et al., 2021) or predicted that mental illness will represent the next global health crisis (Ornell et al., 2021).

In this context, the integration of new technologies into clinical practice has transitioned from a complementary approach to a necessary evolution in care delivery. International healthcare systems rapidly pivoted from in-person consultations to virtual modalities (Wang et al., 2016), reinforcing the need for tools that are compatible with remote assessment. Accurate and timely identification of individuals at risk is paramount for effective prevention strategies. Traditional methods of psychological assessment, though well-established, can sometimes be lengthy, resource-intensive, or less engaging, particularly for younger, digitally native populations (Marciano & Saboor, 2023).

The present study sought to explore whether simplified, slider-format questions administered via a mobile app could serve as psychometrically equivalent and valid alternatives to traditional psychometric instruments in assessing suicide-related dimensions. The existing literature largely supports the digitalization of self-report measures. Rutherford's meta-analysis (Rutherford et al., 2016) concluded that paper-based and electronic formats can be used interchangeably under appropriate conditions. Other researchers, while more cautious, recognize the advantages of digital adaptation, though they advise against assuming full psychometric equivalence without prior validation (Alfonsson et al., 2014; Barrigón et al., 2017; Gwaltney et al., 2008).

Slider questions provide a practical and highly intuitive format for widespread use across digital platforms, such as mobile phones and tablets. Their continuous visual nature offers a more nuanced response scale than discrete options, eliminating explicit numerical choices and facilitating a direct drag-and-drop interaction common in modern digital interfaces (Roster et al., 2015).

These features, combined with their inherent brevity, enhance user engagement and allow for broader reach, especially in underserved or geographically isolated populations (Melia et al., 2020). Unlike lengthy standardized scales, slider items can be completed quickly and easily, offering a feasible solution for both large-scale screening and ongoing patient monitoring.

Furthermore, the integration of digital tools, such as mobile applications, into mental healthcare delivery has gained significant traction, particularly in the context of suicide prevention. Evidence suggests that web-based and mobile interventions can play a vital role in various aspects of suicide prevention, including delivering psychoeducation, providing crisis support, enhancing coping skills, facilitating self-monitoring of mood and suicidal ideation, and improving access to care for underserved populations (Hilty et al., 2022; Lindsay et al., 2024; Olié et al., 2021; Areán et al., 2021). For instance, apps offering immediate access to helplines or safety planning tools have shown promise in acute crisis situations, while those incorporating cognitive behavioral therapy (CBT) or dialectical behavior therapy (DBT) elements can foster long-term resilience and skill development (Schäfer et al., 2024). While promising, a systematic review of mobile applications for depression and suicide prevention revealed that only a small fraction incorporated evidence-based strategies to address suicidal behavior (Torous & Roberts, 2017), highlighting a critical gap. Our study addresses this by specifically validating a novel, user-friendly assessment format that can enhance the utility and applicability of these technologies in mental health assessment and proactive suicide prevention.

Future Directions

Beyond the current findings, future research should explore more advanced psychometric properties and clinical applications of slider-based assessments. Specifically, assessing whether the psychometric equivalence and reliability of these scales vary among individuals with differing levels of suicidal ideation would be a highly valuable next step. Such subgroup analyses could reveal important nuances in the performance of these digital tools across different risk profiles, further enhancing their precision and clinical utility in targeted suicide prevention efforts. Additionally, longitudinal studies are needed to evaluate the test–retest reliability of slider items over time and their sensitivity to change following interventions, providing further evidence for their dynamic assessment capabilities. The feasibility of integrating such tools into clinical workflows warrants further exploration, particularly in primary care, university health services, and other first-line support environments.

5. Conclusions

In conclusion, this study provides compelling evidence for the psychometric equivalence and utility of slider-format questions integrated into a mobile app for assessing key dimensions related to suicide risk. This novel approach offers a highly intuitive and engaging method for data collection, potentially enhancing user compliance and data quality in self-report assessments. While these simplified tools should not replace comprehensive clinical evaluations, they hold promise for broad applications in early screening, symptom monitoring, and follow-up in mental health contexts. Their digital format aligns well with contemporary telemedicine practices and may help overcome structural and social barriers to care. The primary contribution of this research lies in validating a unique, user-friendly digital assessment format that goes beyond traditional Likert scales, offering a continuous and visually interactive response mechanism. This innovation has significant implications for advancing the field of digital mental health, particularly in suicide prevention, by facilitating rapid, sensitive, and accessible screening and monitoring of risk factors. Our findings support the integration of such innovative digital tools into comprehensive suicide prevention strategies, paving the way for more dynamic and personalized interventions. Continued research is needed to evaluate the clinical utility and diagnostic performance of slider-based assessments across diverse populations and settings.

6. Strengths and Limitations

One of the key strengths of this study lies in its innovative use of slider-format items within a mobile application to assess complex psychological constructs associated with suicide risk. The digital nature of the tool offers advantages in terms of cost-efficiency, accessibility, and scalability, making it well-suited for large-scale implementation and routine screening. Moreover, the inclusion of a young university population—typically comfortable with digital platforms—enhances the ecological validity of the method. A key novelty of this study lies in its comprehensive validation of a broad range of suicide-risk factors using the innovative slider format delivered through a dedicated mental health application (AuxiliApp).

However, this study is not without limitations. First, the sample consisted exclusively of university students, limiting the generalizability of the findings to broader or clinical populations. While this population is highly relevant given the rising rates of mental health concerns and suicide risk in young adults, it is also characterized by a higher level of education and digital literacy, which may have contributed to the observed high usability and acceptance of the mobile application. Consequently, the generalizability of our findings to broader or more diverse populations, including individuals with lower educational attainment, older adults, or those with limited technological proficiency, cannot be assumed. Future research should aim to replicate these findings in more heterogeneous populations to establish the broader applicability of slider-based assessment formats in diverse clinical and general settings. Second, while correlations between slider and traditional items were statistically significant, some remained in the low range, particularly in constructs related to anger control and moral or familial reasons for living. Additionally, the study did not assess predictive validity or compare diagnostic performance, nor did it establish specific clinical cutoffs or diagnostic thresholds for the novel slider format. The current 0–10 scale for slider items, while intuitive, lacks the direct interpretative or diagnostic capability of traditional scales with established severity categories. Finally, inverse wording in some slider items may have introduced interpretive variability.

Author Contributions: Conceptualization, L.G. and J.S.R.; Methodology, M.Z.P.S.; Software, P.M.-G.; Validation, P.M.-G., M.Z.P.S. and D.d.-l.-V.-S.; Formal Analysis, D.d.-l.-V.-S. and P.M.-G.; Investigation, J.S.R. and J.G.; Resources, P.A.S. and L.G.; Data Curation, A.A.-C.; Writing—Original Draft Preparation, M.Z.P.S.; Writing—Review and Editing, M.Z.P.S., D.d.-l.-V.-S., S.S.-G. and A.A.-C.; Visualization, S.S.-G. and A.A.-C.; Supervision, M.Z.P.S.; Project Administration, L.G. and J.S.R.; Funding Acquisition, L.G. All authors have read and agreed to the published version of the manuscript.

Funding: Sergio Sanz-Gómez work is funded by the VI-PPITUS.

Institutional Review Board Statement: The study was conducted according to the guidelines of the Declaration of Helsinki, and approved by the Research Ethics Committee (CEI) of the Virgen Macarena—Virgen del Rocío University Hospitals (Approval number: 20175291893; Date: 29 May 2017).

Informed Consent Statement: Informed consent was obtained from all participants involved in the study. Written informed consent was provided electronically upon entry into the study application, and signing the consent form was a prerequisite for participation. All participants provided informed consent to take part in the study anonymously, without any financial or academic compensation, through the same application used for participation.

Data Availability Statement: The data supporting the findings of this study are available from the corresponding author upon reasonable request.

Acknowledgments: We would like to thank the University of Seville, the University of Oviedo, and the Spanish Foundation of Psychiatry and Mental Health (Fundación Española de Psiquiatría y Salud Mental) for their support.

Conflicts of Interest: Author Pedro Moreno Gea is Chief Editor of Psiquiatria. The remaining authors declare that the research was conducted in the absence of any commercial or financial relationships that could be construed as a potential conflict of interest. The sponsors had no role in the design, execution, interpretation, or writing of the study.

Abbreviations

The following abbreviations are used in this manuscript:

BDI-II	Beck Depression Inventory-II
BIS	Barratt Impulsiveness Scale
CC BY	Creative Commons Attribution license
COVID-19	Coronavirus Disease 2019
GHQ-12	General Health Questionnaire-12
IDS-C	Inventory of Depressive Symptomatology—Clinician-rated
INE	Instituto Nacional de Estadística
mHealth	Mobile Health (salud móvil)
NT	New technologies
PANSS	Positive and Negative Syndrome Scale
PHQ-9	Patient Health Questionnaire-9
QISD-SR 16	Questionnaire for Impulsive and Self-Destructive Behaviors—Self-Report, 16 items
RFL	Reasons for Living Inventory
SPSS	Statistical Package for the Social Sciences
STAXI-2	State-Trait Anger Expression Inventory-2
UCLA	University of California, Los Angeles (en "UCLA Loneliness Scale")
VAS	Visual Analog Scale
VI-PPITUS	VI Plan Propio de Investigación y Transferencia de la Universidad de Sevilla
WHO	World Health Organization

References

Alasaarela, L., Hakko, H., Riala, K., & Riipinen, P. (2017). Association of self-reported impulsivity to nonsuicidal self-injury, suicidality, and mortality in adolescent psychiatric inpatients. *Journal of Nervous and Mental Disease*, *205*(5), 340–345. [CrossRef]

Alemu, Y., Chen, H., Duan, C., Caulley, D., Arriaga, R. I., & Sezgin, E. (2023). Detecting Clinically Relevant Emotional Distress and Functional Impairment in Children and Adolescents: Protocol for an Automated Speech Analysis Algorithm Development Study. *JMIR Research Protocols*, *12*, e46970. [CrossRef] [PubMed]

Alfonsson, S., Maathz, P., & Hursti, T. (2014). Interformat reliability of digital psychiatric self-report questionnaires: A systematic review. *Journal of Medical Internet Research*, *16*(12), e268. [CrossRef] [PubMed]

Areán, P., Pratap, A., Hsin, H., Huppert, T. K., E Hendricks, K., Heagerty, P. J., Cohen, T., Bagge, C., & Comtois, K. A. (2021). Perceived utility and characterization of personal google search histories to detect data patterns proximal to a suicide attempt in individuals who previously attempted suicide: Pilot cohort study. *Journal of Medical Internet Research*, *23*(5), e27918. [CrossRef] [PubMed]

Arsenault-Lapierre, G., Kim, C. D., & Turecki, G. (2004). Psychiatric diagnoses in 3275 suicides: A meta-analysis. *BMC Psychiatry*, *4*, 37. [CrossRef]

Auerbach, R. P., Stewart, J. G., & Johnson, S. L. (2017). Impulsivity and suicidality in adolescents inpatients. *Journal of Abnormal Child Psychology*, *45*(1), 91–103. [CrossRef]

Baños-Chaparro, J., & Ramos-Vera, C. (2020). Validez e invarianza según sexo y edad de la Escala Paykel de Ideación Suicida en adolescentes peruanos. *Interacciones*, *6*(1), e225. [CrossRef]

Barrigón, M. L., Rico-Romano, A. M., Ruiz-Gomez, M., Delgado-Gomez, D., Barahona, I., Aroca, F., & Baca-García, E. (2017). Estudio comparativo de los formatos en lápiz y papel y electrónicos de los cuestionarios GHQ-12, WHO-5 y PHQ-9. *Revista de Psiquiatría y Salud Mental*, *10*(3), 160–167. [CrossRef]

Beck, A. T., Ward, C. H., Mendelson, M., Mock, J., & Erbaugh, J. (1960). An inventory for measuring depression. *Archives of General Psychiatry, 4*(6), 561–571. [CrossRef]

Beck, T., Brown, G., Berchick, J., Stewart, L., Steer, A., Ed, D., & Ph, D. (1990). Relationship between hopelessness and ultimate suicide: A replication with psychiatric outpatients. *American Journal of Psychiatry, 147*, 190–195. [CrossRef]

Bobes, J., González, M. P., Saiz, P. A., & Bousoño, M. (1996). Índice europeo de severidad de la adicción: EuropASI. Versión española. *Actas de la IV Reunión Interregional de Psiquiatría, 1996*, 201–218.

Bobes García, J., Badia Llach, X., Luque, A., García, M., González Rodríguez, M. P., Dal-Ré Saavedra, R., & Grupo de Validación en Español de Cuestionarios de Evaluación de la Fobia Social. (1999). Validación de las versiones en español de los cuestionarios liebowitz social anxiety scale, social anxiety and distress scale y sheehan disability inventory para la evaluación de la fobia social. *Medicina Clínica, 112*(14), 530–538.

Caro-Cañizares, I., Brenlla, M., Carballo, J., Santos, M., Guija, J., & Giner, L. (2024). Suicidal behaviour and stressful life events: The Mediating role of the impulsivity-aggression-hostility triad through psychological autopsy. *Psicothema, 36*(4), 380–388. [CrossRef]

Chamorro, J., Bernardi, S., Potenza, M. N., Grant, J. E., Marsh, R., Wang, S., & Blanco, C. (2012). Impulsivity in the general population: A national study. *Journal of Psychiatric Research, 46*(8), 994–1001. [CrossRef]

Chen, J. I., Osman, A., Freedenthal, S. L., & Gutierrez, P. M. (2020). An examination of the psychometric properties of the reasons for living inventory within a male veteran clinical sample. *Archives of Suicide Research, 24*(Suppl. S1), 204–230. [CrossRef]

Cohen, J., Cohen, P., West, S. G., & Aiken, L. S. (2003). *Applied multiple regression/correlation analysis for the behavioral sciences* (3rd ed.). Lawrence Erlbaum Associates Publishers.

Cole, A. B., Littlefield, A. K., Gauthier, J. M., & Bagge, C. L. (2019). Impulsivity facets and perceived likelihood of future suicide attempt among patients who recently attempted suicide. *Journal of Affective Disorders, 257*, 195–199. [CrossRef] [PubMed]

Costanza, A., Rothen, S., Achab, S., Thorens, G., Baertschi, M., Weber, K., Canuto, A., Richard-Lepouriel, H., Perroud, N., & Zullino, D. (2020). Impulsivity and impulsivity-related endophenotypes in suicidal patients with substance use disorders: An exploratory study. *International Journal of Mental Health and Addiction, 19*, 1729–1744. [CrossRef]

Critchfield, K. L., Levy, K. N., & Clarkin, J. F. (2004). The relationship between impulsivity, aggression, and impulsive-aggression in borderline personality disorder: An empirical analysis of self-report measures. *Journal of Personality Disorders, 18*(6), 555–570. [CrossRef]

Dalca, I. M., McGirr, A., Renaud, J., & Turecki, G. (2013). Gender-specific suicide risk factors: A case-control study of individuals with major depressive disorder. *Journal of Clinical Psychiatry, 74*(12), 1209–1215. [CrossRef]

Daniel, S. S., Goldston, D. B., Erkanli, A., Franklin, J. C., & Mayfield, A. M. (2009). Trait anger, anger expression, and suicide attempts among adolescents and young adults: A prospective study. *Journal of Clinical Child and Adolescent Psychology, 38*(5), 661–671. [CrossRef]

Dillon, K. H., Van Voorhees, E. E., Dennis, P. A., Glenn, J. J., Wilks, C. R., Morland, L. A., Beckham, J. C., & Elbogen, E. B. (2020). Anger mediates the relationship between posttraumatic stress disorder and suicidal ideation in veterans. *Journal of Affective Disorders, 269*, 117–124. [CrossRef] [PubMed]

Dubé, J. P., Smith, M. M., Sherry, S. B., Hewitt, P. L., & Stewart, S. H. (2021). Suicide behaviors during the COVID-19 pandemic: A meta-analysis of 54 studies. *Psychiatry Research, 301*, 113998. [CrossRef] [PubMed]

Ernst, M., Klein, E. M., Beutel, M. E., & Brähler, E. (2021). Gender-specific associations of loneliness and suicidal ideation in a representative population sample: Young, lonely men are particularly at risk. *Journal of Affective Disorders, 294*, 63–70. [CrossRef] [PubMed]

Esposito, C., Spirito, A., Boergers, J., & Donaldson, D. (2003). Affective, behavioral, and cognitive functioning in adolescents with multiple suicide attempts. *Suicide and Life-Threatening Behavior, 33*(4), 389–399. [CrossRef]

Evren, C., Cinar, O., Evren, B., & Celik, S. (2011). History of suicide attempt in male substance-dependent inpatients and relationship to borderline personality features, anger, hostility and aggression. *Psychiatry Research, 190*(1), 126–131. [CrossRef]

Faurholt-Jepsen, M., Munkholm, K., Frost, M., Bardram, J. E., & Kessing, L. V. (2016). Electronic self-monitoring of mood using IT platforms in adult patients with bipolar disorder: A systematic review of the validity and evidence. *BMC Psychiatry, 16*(1), 7. [CrossRef]

Ferrando, L., Bobes, J., Gibert, M., Soto, M., & Soto, O. (1998). *M.I.N.I. mini international neuropsychiatric interview*. Versión en español 5.0.0.DSM-IV. Instituto IAP.

Fonseca-Pedrero, E., Inchausti, F., Pérez-Gutiérrez, L., Aritio Solana, R., Ortuño-Sierra, J., Sánchez-García, M. A., Lucas-Molina, B., Domínguez, C., Foncea, D., Espinosa, V., Gorría, A., Urbiola-Merina, E., Fernández, M., Merina Díaz, C., Gutiérrez, C., Aures, M., Campos, M. S., & Pérez de Albéniz Iturriaga, A. (2018). Ideación suicida en una muestra representativa de adolescentes españoles. *Revista de Psiquiatría y Salud Mental, 11*(2), 76–85. [CrossRef]

García-Batista, Z. E., Guerra-Peña, K., Cano-Vindel, A., Herrera-Martínez, S. X., Flores-Kanter, P. E., & Medrano, L. A. (2018). Evidencias de validez y fiabilidad de las Puntuaciones del STAXI-2 para población general y hospitalaria: Estudio con una muestra de adultos de República Dominicana. *Suma Psicológica, 25*(1), 21–29. [CrossRef]

Giegling, I., Olgiati, P., Hartmann, A., Calati, R., Möller, H., Rujescu, D., & Serretti, A. (2009). Personality and attempted suicide. Analysis of anger, aggression and impulsivity. *Journal of Psychiatric Research, 43*(16), 1262–1271. [CrossRef]

Green, K. L., Brown, G. K., Jager-Hyman, S., Cha, J., Steer, R. A., & Beck, A. T. (2015). The predictive validity of the beck depression inventory suicide item. *The Journal of Clinical Psychiatry, 76*(12), 1683–1686. [CrossRef]

Grupo Español de Trabajo para la Evaluación por Estrés Postraumático. (2000). Evaluación de las propiedades psicométricas de la versión española de cinco cuestionarios para la evaluación del trastorno de estrés postraumático. *Actas Españolas de Psiquiatría, 28*(4), 207–218.

Guilford, J. P. (1956). *Fundamental statistics in psychology and education* (3rd ed.). McGraw-Hill.

Gwaltney, C. J., Shields, A. L., & Shiffman, S. (2008). Equivalence of electronic and paper-and-pencil administration of patient-reported outcome measures: A meta-analytic review. *Value in Health, 11*(2), 322–333. [CrossRef]

Hamza, C. A., & Willoughby, T. (2019). Impulsivity and nonsuicidal self-injury: A longitudinal examination among emerging adults. *Journal of Adolescence, 75*, 37–46. [CrossRef] [PubMed]

Hamza, C. A., Willoughby, T., & Heffer, T. (2015). Impulsivity and nonsuicidal self-injury: A review and meta-analysis. *Clinical Psychology Review, 38*, 13–24. [CrossRef]

Harriss, L., & Hawton, K. (2005). Suicidal intent in deliberate self-harm and the risk of suicide: The predictive power of the suicide intent scale. *Journal of Affective Disorders, 86*(2–3), 225–233. [CrossRef]

Hawkins, K. A., Hames, J. L., Ribeiro, J. D., Silva, C., Joiner, T. E., & Cougle, J. R. (2014). An examination of the relationship between anger and suicide risk through the lens of the interpersonal theory of suicide. *Journal of Psychiatric Research, 50*(1), 59–65. [CrossRef] [PubMed]

Heidari, P., Broadbear, J. H., Brown, R., Dharwadkar, N. P., & Rao, S. (2023). Mental health support for and telehealth use by Australians living with borderline personality disorder during the onset of the COVID-19 pandemic: A national study. *Digital Health, 9*, 20552076231169824. [CrossRef]

Herpertz, S., Steinmeyer, S. M., Marx, D., Oidtmann, A., & Sass, H. (1995). The significance of aggression and impulsivitiy for self-mutilative behavior. *Pharmacopsychiatry, 28*(Suppl. S2), 64–72. [CrossRef]

Hilty, D. M., Armstrong, C. M., A Smout, S., Crawford, A., Maheu, M. M., Drude, K. P., Chan, S., Yellowlees, P. M., & Krupinski, E. A. (2022). Findings and guidelines on provider technology, fatigue, and well-being: Scoping review. *Journal of Medical Internet Research, 24*(5), e34451. [CrossRef]

Holden, R. R., Mehta, K., Cunningham, E. J., & McLeod, L. D. (2001). Development and preliminary validation of a scale of psychache. *Canadian Journal of Behavioural Science, 33*(4), 224–232. [CrossRef]

Horesh, N., Rolnick, T., Iancu, I., Dannon, P., Lepkifker, E., Apter, A., & Kotler, M. (1997). Anger, impulsivity and suicide risk. *Psychotherapy and Psychosomatics, 66*(2), 92–96. [CrossRef] [PubMed]

John, A., Eyles, E., Webb, R. T., Okolie, C., Schmidt, L., Arensman, E., Hawton, K., O'Connor, R. C., Kapur, N., Moran, P., O'Neill, S., McGuinness, L. A., Olorisade, B. K., Dekel, D., Macleod-Hall, C., Cheng, H. Y., Higgins, J. P. T., & Gunnell, D. (2021). The impact of the COVID-19 pandemic on self-harm and suicidal behaviour: Update of living systematic review. *F1000Research, 9*, 1–44. [CrossRef] [PubMed]

Killgore, W. D., Cloonan, S. A., Taylor, E. C., Miller, M. A., & Dailey, N. S. (2020). Three months of loneliness during the COVID-19 lockdown. *Psychiatry Research, 293*, 1–2. [CrossRef]

Kotler, M., Iancu, I., Efroni, R., & Amir, M. (2001). Anger, impulsivity, social support, and suicide risk in patients with posttraumatic stress disorder. *The Journal of Nervous and Mental Disease, 189*(3), 162–167. [CrossRef] [PubMed]

Lee, Y., Gilbert, J., Waldman, L., Zarate, C., & Ballard, E. (2024). Potential association between suicide risk, aggression, impulsivity, and the somatosensory system. *Social Cognitive and Affective Neuroscience, 19*(1), 7. [CrossRef]

Lin, L., & Zhang, J. (2017). Impulsivity, mental disorder, and suicide in rural China. *Archives of Suicide Research, 21*(1), 73–82. [CrossRef]

Lindsay, J. A. B., McGowan, N. M., Henning, T., Harriss, E., & Saunders, K. E. A. (2024). Digital interventions for symptoms of borderline personality disorder: Systematic review and meta-analysis. *Journal of Medical Internet Research, 26*, e54941. [CrossRef]

Linehan, M. M., Goodstein, J. L., Nielsen, S. L., & Chiles, J. A. (1983). Reasons for staying alive when you are thinking of killing yourself: The brief reasons for living inventory. *Journal of Consulting and Clinical Psychology, 51*(2), 276–286. [CrossRef]

Liu, R., Trout, Z., Hernandez, E., Cheek, S., & Gerlus, N. (2017). A behavioral and cognitive neuroscience perspective on impulsivity, suicide, and non-suicidal self-injury: Meta-analysis and recommendations for future research. *Neuroscience & Biobehavioral Reviews, 83*, 440–450.

Maino, M. d. l. P., Morales, S., Echávarri, O., Barros, J., García, A., Moya, C., Szmulewicz, T., Fischman, R., Núñez, C., & Tomicic, A. (2019). Suicide risk configuration system in a clustered clinical sample: A generalized linear model obtained through the LASSO technique. *Revista Brasileira de Psiquiatria, 41*(2), 112–121. [CrossRef]

Marciano, L., & Saboor, S. (2023). Reinventing mental health care in youth through mobile approaches: Current status and future steps. *Frontiers in Psychology, 14*, 1126015. [CrossRef] [PubMed]

Martínez-Loredo, V., Fernández-Hermida, J. R., Fernández-Artamendi, S., Carballo, J. L., & García-Rodríguez, O. (2015). Spanish adaptation and validation of the Barratt Impulsiveness Scale for early adolescents (BIS-11-A). *International Journal of Clinical and Health Psychology, 15*(3), 274–282. [CrossRef]

Melia, R., Francis, K., Hickey, E., Bogue, J., Duggan, J., O'Sullivan, M., & Young, K. (2020). Mobile health technology interventions for suicide prevention: Systematic review. *JMIR MHealth and UHealth, 8*(1), e12516. [CrossRef] [PubMed]

Mercer, D., Douglass, A. B., & Links, P. S. (2009). Meta-analyses of mood stabilizers, antidepressants and antipsychotics in the treatment of borderline personality disorder: Effectiveness for depression and anger symptoms. *Journal of Personality Disorders, 23*(2), 156–174. [CrossRef]

Miguel-Tobal, J., Cano-Vindel, A., Casado-Morales, M., & Spielberger, C. (2001). *Inventario de expresión de la Ira estado-rasgo, S.T.A.X.I.-2./state-trait anger expression inventory*. STAXI-2. TEA Ediciones.

Moore, F., Allott, C., & O'Connor, R. (2023). Impulsivity, aggression, and impulsive aggression in suicidality. *Personality and Individual Differences, 202*, 111971. [CrossRef]

Moynihan, R., Sanders, S., Michaleff, Z. A., Scott, A. M., Clark, J., To, E. J., Jones, M., Kitchener, E., Fox, M., Johansson, M., Lang, E., Duggan, A., Scott, I., & Albarqouni, L. (2021). Impact of COVID-19 pandemic on utilisation of healthcare services: A systematic review. *BMJ Open, 11*(3), e045343. [CrossRef] [PubMed]

Neelam, K., Duddu, V., Anyim, N., Neelam, J., & Lewis, S. (2021). Pandemics and pre-existing mental illness: A systematic review and meta-analysis. *Brain, Behavior, and Immunity—Health, 10*, 100177. [CrossRef]

Nock, M. K., Green, J. G., Hwang, I., McLaughlin, K. A., Sampson, N. A., Zaslavsky, A. M., & Kessler, R. C. (2013). Prevalence, correlates and treatments of lifetime suicidal behavior among adolescents: Results from the national comorbidity survey replication—Adolescente supplement (NCS-A). *JAMA Psychiatry, 70*(3), 300–310. [CrossRef]

Olié, E., Dubois, J., Benramdane, M., Guillaume, S., & Courtet, P. (2021). Psychological state of a sample of patients with mood disorders during the first French COVID-19 lockdown. *Scientific Reports, 11*(1), 23711. [CrossRef]

Oquendo, M. A., Cia, E., Graver, R., Mora, M., Montalvan, V., & Mann, J. (2000). Spanish adaptation of the reasons for living inventory. *Hispanic Journal of Behavioral Sciences, 22*(3), 369–381. [CrossRef]

Ordóñez-Carrasco, J. L., Cuadrado Guirado, I., & Rojas Tejada, A. (2022). Escala de dolor psicológico: Adaptación de la Psychache Scale al español en jóvenes adultos. *Revista de Psiquiatría y Salud Mental, 15*(3), 196–204. [CrossRef]

Ornell, F., Borelli, W. V., Benzano, D., Schuch, J. B., Moura, H. F., Sordi, A. O., Kessler, F. H. P., Scherer, J. N., & von Diemen, L. (2021). The next pandemic: Impact of COVID-19 in mental healthcare assistance in a nationwide epidemiological study. *The Lancet Regional Health—Americas, 4*, 100061. [CrossRef] [PubMed]

Painuly, N., Sharan, P., & Mattoo, S. K. (2007). Antecedents, concomitants and consequences of anger attacks in depression. *Psychiatry Research, 153*(1), 39–45. [CrossRef]

Palmier-Claus, J. E., Ainsworth, J., Machin, M., Barrowclough, C., Dunn, G., Barkus, E., Rogers, A., Wykes, T., Kapur, S., Buchan, I., Salter, E., & Lewis, S. W. (2012). The feasibility and validity of ambulatory self-report of psychotic symptoms using a smartphone software application. *BMC Psychiatry, 12*(1), 172. [CrossRef] [PubMed]

Park, Y. J., Ryu, H., Han, K. S., Kwon, J. H., Kim, H. K., Kang, H. C., Yoon, J. W., Cheon, S. H., & Shin, H. (2010). Anger, anger expression, and suicidal ideation in Korean adolescents. *Archives of Psychiatric Nursing, 24*(3), 168–177. [CrossRef] [PubMed]

Patten, S. B., Kutcher, S., Streiner, D., Gratzer, D., Kurdyak, P., & Yatham, L. (2021). Population mental health and COVID-19: Why do we know so little? *Canadian Journal of Psychiatry, 66*(9), 782–784. [CrossRef]

Patton, J. H., Stanford, M. S., & Barratt, E. S. (1995). Factor structure of the Barratt impulsiveness scale. *Journal of Clinical Psychology, 51*(6), 768–774. [CrossRef]

Paz García-Portilla, M., Alejandra Sáiz, P., Díaz-Mesa, E. M., Fonseca, E., Arrojo, M., Sierra, P., Sarramea, F., Sánchez, E., Manuel Goikolea, J., Balanzá, V., Benabarre, A., & Bobes, J. (2009). Psychometric performance of the Oviedo sleep questionnaire in patients with severe mental disorder. *Revista de Psiquiatría y Salud Mental (English Edition), 2*(4), 169–177. [CrossRef]

Reger, M. A., Stanley, I. H., & Joiner, T. E. (2020). Suicide mortality and coronavirus disease 2019—A perfect storm. *JAMA Psychiatry, 77*(11), 1093–1094. [CrossRef]

Rogers, M. L., Kelliher-Rabon, J., Hagan, C. R., Hirsch, J. K., & Joiner, T. E. (2017). Negative emotions in veterans relate to suicide risk through feelings of perceived burdensomeness and thwarted belongingness. *Journal of Affective Disorders, 208*, 15–21. [CrossRef]

Roster, C. A., Lucianetti, L., & Albaum, G. (2015). Exploring slider vs. categorical response formats in web-based surveys. *Journal of Research Practice*, *11*(1), 1.

Rozek, D. C., Crawford, J. N., LoSavio, S. T., Myers, U. S., Dabovich, P., Warnecke, A., Smith, N. B., & Bryan, C. J. (2021). The protective role of reasons for living on suicidal cognitions for military affiliated individuals with a positive PTSD screen in primary care settings. *Journal of Affective Disorders*, *292*, 424–429. [CrossRef] [PubMed]

Rueda-Jaimes, G. E., Castro-Rueda, V. A., Rangel-Martínez-Villalba, A. M., Moreno-Quijano, C., Martinez-Salazar, G. A., & Camacho, P. A. (2018). Validation of the beck hopelessness scale in patients with suicide risk. *Revista de Psiquiatría y Salud Mental*, *11*(2), 86–93. [CrossRef]

Russell, D. (1996). UCLA loneliness scale (version 3): Reliability, validity and factor structure. *Journal of Personality Assessment*, *66*(42), 3–4. [CrossRef]

Rutherford, C., Costa, D., Mercieca-Bebber, R., Rice, H., Gabb, L., & King, M. (2016). Mode of administration does not cause bias in patient-reported outcome results: A meta-analysis. *Quality of Life Research*, *25*(3), 559–574. [CrossRef] [PubMed]

Santomauro, D. F., Mantilla Herrera, A. M., Shadid, J., Zheng, P., Ashbaugh, C., Pigott, D. M., Abbafati, C., Adolph, C., Amlag, J. O., Aravkin, A. Y., Bang-Jensen, B. L., Bertolacci, G. J., Bloom, S. S., Castellano, R., Castro, E., Chakrabarti, S., Chattopadhyay, J., Cogen, R. M., Collins, J. K., . . . Ferrari, A. J. (2021). Global prevalence and burden of depressive and anxiety disorders in 204 countries and territories in 2020 due to the COVID-19 pandemic. *The Lancet*, *398*(10312), 1700–1712. [CrossRef] [PubMed]

Sanz, J., Perdigón, A. L., & Vázquez, C. (2003). Adaptación española del Inventario para la Depresión de Beck-II (BDI-II): 2. Propiedades psicométricas en población general. *Clínica y Salud*, *14*(3), 249–280.

Sánchez-Teruel, D., Robles-Bello, M. A., & Camacho-Conde, J. A. (2020). Validity of the Spanish version of the herth hope index and the beck hopelessness scale in people who have attempted suicide. *Actas Españolas de Psiquiatría*, *48*(4), 163–168.

Schäfer, S. K., von Boros, L., Schaubruch, L. M., Kunzler, A. M., Lindner, S., Koehler, F., Werner, T., Zappalà, F., Helmreich, I., Wessa, M., Lieb, K., & Tüscher, O. (2024). Digital interventions to promote psychological resilience: A systematic review and meta-analysis. *Npj Digital Medicine*, *7*, 1–12. [CrossRef]

Simeon, D., Stanley, B., Frances, A., Mann, J. J., Winchel, R., & Stanley, M. (1992). Self-mutilation in personality disorders: Psychological and biological correlates. *American Journal of Psychiatry*, *149*, 221–226. [CrossRef]

Spielberger, C. D., Gorsuch, R. L., Lushene, R. E., Vagg, P. R., & Jacobs, G. A. (1983). *Manual for the state-trait anxiety inventory (form Y)*. Consulting Psychologists Press.

Stefansson, J., Nordström, P., & Jokinen, J. (2012). Suicide intent scale in the prediction of suicide. *Journal of Affective Disorders*, *136*(1–2), 167–171. [CrossRef]

Stringer, B., Van Meijel, B., Eikelenbooma, M., Koekkoek, B., Licht, C. M. M., Ad Kerkhof, J. E. M., Penninx, B. W. J. H., & Beekman, A. T. E. (2013). Recurrent suicide attempts in patients with depressive and anxiety disorders: The role of borderline personality traits. *Journal of Affective Disorders*, *151*(1), 23–30. [CrossRef]

Sueki, H. (2022). Relationship between beck hopelessness scale and suicidal ideation: A short-term longitudinal study. *Death Studies*, *46*(2), 467–472. [CrossRef]

Sun, L., Li, H., Zhang, J., & Wu, Q. (2015). Psychological strains and suicide intent: Results from a psychological autopsy study with Chinese rural young suicides. *International Journal of Social Psychiatry*, *61*(7), 677–683. [CrossRef]

Swann, A., Lijffijt, M., O'Brien, B., & Mathew, S. (2020). Impulsivity and suicidal behavior. In *Recent advances in research on impulsivity and impulsive behaviors*. Current Topics in Behavioral Neurosciences. Springer. [CrossRef]

Torous, J., & Roberts, L. W. (2017). The ethical use of mobile health technology in clinical psychiatry. *Journal of Nervous and Mental Disease*, *205*(1), 4–8. [CrossRef]

Troister, T., D'Agata, M. T., & Holden, R. R. (2015). Suicide risk screening: Comparing the beck depression inventory-II, beck hopelessness scale, and psychache scale in undergraduates. *Psychological Assessment*, *27*(4), 1500–1506. [CrossRef]

Troister, T., & Holden, R. R. (2012). A two-year prospective study of psychache and its relationship to suicidality among high-risk undergraduates. *Journal of Clinical Psychology*, *68*(9), 1019–1027. [CrossRef]

Troister, T., & Holden, R. R. (2013). Factorial differentiation among depression, hopelessness, and psychache in statistically predicting suicidality. *Measurement and Evaluation in Counseling and Development*, *46*(1), 50–63. [CrossRef]

Turecki, G., Brent, D. A., Gunnell, D., O'Connor, R. C., Oquendo, M. A., Pirkis, J., & Stanley, B. H. (2019). Suicide and suicide risk. *Nature Reviews Disease Primers*, *5*(1), 1–12. [CrossRef]

Vázquez Morejón, A. J., & Jiménez García-Bóveda, R. (1994). RULS: Escala de soledad UCLA revisada. Fiabilidad y validez de una versión española. *Revista de Psicología de la Salud*, *6*(1), 46–55.

Velarde-Mayol, C., Fragua-Gil, S., & García-de-Cecilia, J. M. (2016). Validación de la escala de soledad de UCLA y perfil social en la población anciana que vive sola. *Medicina de Familia. SEMERGEN*, *42*(3), 177–183. [CrossRef]

Wang, H., Naghavi, M., Allen, C., Barber, R. M., Carter, A., Casey, D. C., Charlson, F. J., Chen, A. Z., Coates, M. M., Coggeshall, M., Dandona, L., Dicker, D. J., Erskine, H. E., Haagsma, J. A., Fitzmaurice, C., Foreman, K., Forouzanfar, M. H., Fraser, M. S., Fullman, N., . . . Zuhlke, L. J. (2016). Global, regional, and national life expectancy, all-cause mortality, and cause-specific mortality for 249 causes of death, 1980–2015: A systematic analysis for the global burden of disease study 2015. *The Lancet, 388*(10053), 1459–1544. [CrossRef] [PubMed]

Wilks, C. R., Morland, L. A., Dillon, K. H., Mackintosh, M. A., Blakey, S. M., Wagner, H. R., & Elbogen, E. B. (2019). Anger, social support, and suicide risk in U.S. military veterans. *Journal of Psychiatric Research, 109*, 139–144. [CrossRef] [PubMed]

Winkler, P., Formanek, T., Mlada, K., Kagstrom, A., Mohrova, Z., Mohr, P., & Csemy, L. (2020). Increase in prevalence of current mental disorders in the context of COVID-19: Analysis of repeated nationwide cross-sectional surveys. *Epidemiology and Psychiatric Sciences, 29*, e173. [CrossRef] [PubMed]

World Health Organization. (2021). *COVID-19 continues to disrupt essential health services in 90% of countries*. Available online: https://www.who.int/news/item/23-04-2021-covid-19-continues-to-disrupt-essential-health-services-in-90-of-countries (accessed on 20 December 2024).

Zalsman, G., Hawton, K., Wasserman, D., van Heeringen, K., Arensman, E., Sarchiapone, M., Carli, V., Höschl, C., Barzilay, R., Balazs, J., Purebl, G., Kahn, J. P., Sáiz, P. A., Lipsicas, C. B., Bobes, J., Cozman, D., Hegerl, U., & Zohar, J. (2016). Suicide prevention strategies revisited: 10-year systematic review. *The Lancet Psychiatry, 3*(7), 646–659. [CrossRef]

Zhang, J., & Jia, C. X. (2007). Validating a short version of the suicide intent scale in China. *Omega: Journal of Death and Dying, 55*(4), 255–265. [CrossRef]

behavioral sciences

MDPI

Article

Regulation Strategies, Contextual Problems, Addictive and Suicidal Behaviors: A Network Perspective with Adolescents

Dalila Eslava [1], Begoña Delgado [2], Miguel Á. Carrasco [3] and Francisco Pablo Holgado-Tello [4,*]

1 Faculty of Health Sciences, Valencian International University, 46002 Valencia, Spain; dalila.eslava@universidadviu.com
2 Department of Developmental and Educational Psychology, Faculty of Psychology, National University of Distance Education, 28040 Madrid, Spain; bdelgado@psi.uned.es
3 Department of Personality, Assessment and Psychological Treatment, Faculty of Psychology, National University of Distance Education, 28040 Madrid, Spain; macarrasco@psi.uned.es
4 Department of Methodology of Behavioural Sciences, Faculty of Psychology, National University of Distance Education, 28040 Madrid, Spain
* Correspondence: pfholgado@psi.uned.es

Abstract: Adolescence is a period marked by challenges, including problems that appear in the adolescent's context. To manage these, adolescents use a series of emotional regulation skills that can be more or less adaptive. Less adaptive regulation is related to problem behaviors such as alcohol abuse, substance addiction, problematic internet use, and/or suicidal behavior. This study employs psychometric networks to analyze the association between these problem behaviors, the existence of contextual problems, and the use of cognitive emotional regulation strategies. We performed this analysis for the total sample: the male sample and the female sample. The total sample consists of 758 participants; 424 females (55.4%) and 341 males (44.6%) between the ages of 12 and 21 years (*M* age = 15.85; *SD* = 2311). The results show that less adaptive regulation strategies are the most central node, exhibiting a positive relationship with problem behaviors and contextual problems. In contrast, adaptive regulation strategies are a less influential node. Finally, problem behaviors are related to each other. Differences emerged between the male sample and the female sample. These findings contribute to improving our understanding of the phenomenon as well as to the construction of preventive interventions.

Keywords: adolescence; emotional regulation; addictions; suicidal behavior; psychometric networks

1. Introduction

Adolescence is a life stage of great strength and potential that extends approximately from the age of 12 to 18, or even 21 [1]. This evolutionary stage is characterized by the need to face, within a relatively short time, various physical, cognitive, psychological, and social challenges and changes [2] that can reveal vulnerabilities and, at times, present difficulties [3]. Appropriate adaptation to these challenges and changes can facilitate the transition to adulthood [2]. However, for some young people these changes can lead to psychosocial maladjustment [4–8] that can have a significant impact on adulthood [9].

Substance use often appears for the first time during adolescence, and some authors point out that, for many adolescents, it can represent a ritual of transition between adolescence and adulthood [10,11]. According to data from the ESTUDES survey (State Survey on Drug Use in Secondary Education) [12], when consulted about their consumption of certain substances within the previous 30 days, 56.6% of Spanish adolescents reported having used alcohol, 21% having used tobacco, and 15.6% having used cannabis. Contact with these substances in adolescence is a concern, not only because of the neurocognitive consequences [13,14] but also because consumption at younger ages often leads to higher rates of consumption in adulthood [15]. Likewise, adolescence is a vulnerable period for problematic internet use [16], which has become a public health concern [17]. Asked about their internet use in the previous 30 days, 23.5% of Spanish adolescents revealed compulsive internet use [18], which can lead to psychological, social, and/or academic difficulties [19].

On the other hand, adolescence is also a vulnerable period in terms of emotional problems, such as suicidal behavior [20]. At this stage, these types of thoughts appear for the first time, along with the first existential crises [21]. The PSICE (Evidence-Based Psychology in Educational Contexts) report estimates that 5.4% of adolescents experience suicidal ideation and that 4.9% have attempted suicide [7]. In fact, suicide is the leading cause of unnatural death among adolescents between 15 and 19 years of age in Spain [22]. Suicidal behavior can be manifested in a variety of ways, from suicidal ideation and planning, through suicidal communication, to suicide attempts and death by suicide [11,23].

These behavioral and emotional problems are interrelated. For example, the prevalence of heavy alcohol use, daily tobacco use, and cannabis use is higher in those adolescents who are prone to compulsive internet use [18]. In addition, substance use is related to suicidal behavior [24], as is problematic internet use [25,26].

These problem behaviors share triggers, risk factors, and maintenance factors [27], one of which is difficulty in emotional regulation [28,29]. Garnefski and Kraaij [30] state that cognitive emotional regulation is the process by which people influence how they experience and express their emotions, and it plays an important role in emotional and behavioral problems. At this stage, adolescents may have to manage demands and challenges [2], and may face problems in their family, social, and/or school contexts [4]. In this sense, it is important to consider the conditions presented by the contexts in which an adolescent develops, especially when such conditions are problematic. To cope with these new challenges, adolescents can count on adaptive regulation skills that allow them to manage their emotions appropriately. However, when these skills are not available, the adolescent may embark on a series of ruminative thoughts, giving rise to intense emotions, as well as less adaptive behaviors to cope with them [31,32]. For example, substance use can be a way to cope with stressful situations [33]. Likewise, suicidal thoughts seem to function as a form of emotional regulation for some individuals [34]. Therefore, assuming that contextual problems are crucial to understanding an adolescent's problem behaviors, the adolescent's emotional regulation plays a key role in determining their impact [35].

It is important to consider gender differences when examining these phenomena. Regarding the prevalence of the aforementioned behaviors, boys have higher rates of cannabis use [12] and compulsive internet use [18], while girls have higher rates of alcohol and tobacco use [12]. Likewise, according to the PSICE study, girls provide a higher proportion of affirmative responses than boys when suicidal behavior is evaluated [7]. However, Espada-Sánchez et al. [25] find that there is a "gender paradox" by which women attempt suicide more frequently, but death by suicide occurs to a greater extent in men. This is partly attributed to the higher prevalence of affective disorders (e.g., depression and anxiety) in girls and the tendency of boys to use more lethal methods of suicide such as hanging or firearms [36]. On the other hand, several authors indicate that boys are more likely than girls to use substances as an emotional regulation strategy [37,38]. However, it seems that girls have greater emotional difficulties [7]. These differences may be due to socially established gender roles, whereby adolescents respond differently to the demands of the adolescent life stage and the problems that arise during it [39]. Therefore, it is important to identify and address these differences when studying these phenomena.

The main aim of this study is to explore the association between problem behaviors (alcohol abuse, substance addiction, problematic internet use, and suicidal behavior), the existence of contextual problems (as a general measure, including indistinctly problems related to the family, school, or relationships with peers), and the use of cognitive emotional regulation strategies (adaptive regulation and less adaptive regulation). This approach is also carried out according to gender. To our knowledge, the existing literature has addressed these relationships in isolation [32,40]. Less adaptive regulation is expected to be positively related to problem behaviors, while more adaptive regulation is expected to be negatively related to problem behaviors. Regarding contextual problems, it is expected that they have a positive relationship with less adaptive regulation strategies, as well as with problem behaviors. Problem behaviors are also expected to have a positive relationship with each other. Regarding the difference between boys and girls, taking into account the differences presented by the literature, it is expected that substance addiction and problematic internet use are more intensely related to emotional regulation strategies in boys, while in girls these relationships pivot on alcohol and tobacco abuse and suicidal behavior. However, this study goes beyond establishing specific hypotheses according to the literature by employing an exploratory perspective based on psychometric networks. Thus, an essential and key objective is to identify which variables are most relevant in the proposed network and how they interact with each other, with the goal of better understanding this complex phenomenon.

2. Materials and Methods

2.1. Participants

The final sample of the study comprised 765 participants, 424 female (55.4%) and 341 male (44.6%), all of them between the ages of 12 and 21 years (*M* age = 15.85; *SD* = 2311). The data were collected in 2023, between January and November. Most of them were high school students (95%), and only 37 participants were university students. The sample was selected from various secondary schools and colleges using non-random and convenience sampling. Given this sampling design, only two regions of Spain were represented: Madrid (79.81%), mainly, and Andalusia.

2.2. Instruments

- Sociodemographic data. An ad hoc questionnaire was administered to collect sociodemographic information (age and sex).
- MULTICAGE CAD-4 [41]. This instrument assesses addictive disorders through eight subscales. For the present study, only the subscales of alcohol abuse/dependence, substance addiction, and internet addiction were used. Respondents answered using "yes" or "no". The subscales have a Cronbach's alpha index above 0.7 [41].
- SENTIA-brief [42]. The Adolescent Suicidal Behavior Assessment Scale was used, specifically the brief 5-item modality. This scale consists of a general factor, suicidal behavior, and three subscales: ideation, communication, and performance/planning. For the present study, the global score was used. The answers follow a five-point Likert scale (1 = "never" and 5 = "many times"). The omega coefficient for the total score is 0.97 [42].
- Cognitive Emotion Regulation Questionnaire (CERQ-short) [43,44]. This is a reduced version of the 18-item CERQ questionnaire. It is composed of two subscales: adaptive regulation (evaluating strategies such as replanning, reevaluating, accepting, and focusing on the positive) and less adaptive regulation (evaluating catastrophizing, rumination, blaming oneself, and blaming others). The answers follow a five-point Likert scale (1 = "almost never" and 5 = "almost always"). In the Spanish version, the Cronbach's alphas of the scales are 0.84 and 0.72, respectively [44].
- Child and Adolescent Assessment System (SENA). This is a global index of contextual problems [45]. It is an instrument for detecting a wide spectrum of emotional and behavioral problems in children and adolescents, as well as areas of vulnerability and psychological resources. The present study uses the "contextual problem index", assessing family-, school- and peer-related aspects. The answers follow a five-point Likert scale (1 = "never or almost never" and 5 = "always or almost always"). A high score on this index is an indicator of a greater severity of mismatch across different contexts and not exclusively in one of them. Direct scores are used.

2.3. Procedure

The study is part of a broader project on adolescents' behavioral problems. It was approved by the ethics committee of the Universidad Nacional de Educacion a Distancia in compliance with the ethical standards established in Law 3/2018 on Data Protection and Guarantee of Digital Rights. Accordingly, it required informed consent to be obtained from both the adolescents and their parents, and participation was voluntary. All data were kept anonymous and confidential. After sampling, data were collected by previously trained researchers in small groups during a 90 min session.

2.4. Data Analysis

The study first conducted a descriptive analysis to obtain the frequencies and other statistics of the problem behaviors for the total sample, as well as for the boys and girls separately. To gain a preliminary understanding of the relationship between the variables, bivariate correlations were performed on the three samples. Two analyses were performed to identify differences between the sample of boys and the sample of girls: the Kolmogorv-Smirnov normality test, followed by the non-parametric Mann-Whitney U test. The SPSS v27 statistical package was used.

To delve deeper into the relationship between the variables, a psychometric network analysis was conducted on the total sample, as well as separately for boys and girls, to explore the relationships between the variables. This analysis graphically represents a model that collects statistically significant relationships; it is composed of nodes (study variables) and edges (relationships between the nodes). In this case, the network was weighted undirected and the pcor method was used, with a $p < 0.05$ significance for the edges. The qgraph and bootnet libraries of R were used. Four measures of centrality were estimated: strength (St), closeness (Clo), intermediation (Bet), and expected influence (EI). The strength of a node refers to the sum of the absolute partial correlation coefficients between one node and all other nodes, i.e., a node with a high strength is a node that influences many other nodes. Proximity refers to how strongly a node is directly related to the rest of the nodes, i.e., a node with high proximity is a node that can predict other nodes well. Intermediation indicates how many of the shortest paths between two nodes pass through the node in question, so if a node has a high brokerage value, this indicates that it is well connected to the rest of the nodes in the network. Finally, expected influence uses the sum of the absolute weights of all the edges of a node, i.e., converting negative edges into positive edges before adding. For this reason, it is presented as a more precise index of centrality [46,47]. However, Bringmann et al. [48] indicate that for the study of psychological variables, proximity and intermediation indices are inadequate to establish the importance of nodes in the network. Their values are unstable in cross-sectional studies, showing wide confidence intervals and, in some cases, incoherence.

Likewise, precision and stability measurements were obtained. The accuracy chart shows the estimated edge value in the sample (red line) and the 95% confidence intervals (gray bars) for those estimates. Finally, the stability graph assesses the consistency of the estimators through resampling procedures, replicating the network with fewer cases. The lines indicate the correlation between the estimates of the indices in the full sample and of those indices when the sample is reduced. If the correlation falls below 0.70, the estimates become unstable, and it is recommended that it should not fall below 0.70 with half of the sample [47,49].

3. Results

We tested whether there were differences between boys and girls on the measured variables. To determine which statistic to use, we first performed the Kolmogorov-Smirnov normality test; as the variables did not follow a normal distribution, we next performed the non-parametric Mann-Whitney U-test and compared the mean ranks between the samples of boys and girls. The results show that there are statistically significant differences between some of the variables. Girls exhibited more problematic internet use ($p < 0.05$) as well as more suicidal behavior ($p < 0.001$) and less adaptive regulation ($p < 0.001$) than boys (means and standard deviations are included in Table 1).

Table 1. Descriptive statistics of the variables and significant differences by gender.

Variables	Sample	Mean	SD	Minimum	Maximum
Alcohol abuse	Total sample	0.52	0.95	0	4
	Boys	0.44	0.86	0	4
	Girls	0.59	1.01	0	4
Substance addiction	Total sample	0.32	0.73	0	4
	Boys	0.32	0.74	0	4
	Girls	0.32	0.71	0	4
Problematic internet * use	Total sample	2.16	1.32	0	4
	Boys	2.04	1.27	0	4
	Girls	2.26	1.35	0	4
Suicidal behavior **	Total sample	1.22	0.55	1	5
	Boys	1.14	0.46	1	5
	Girls	1.29	0.61	1	4.60
Contextual problems	Total sample	5.99	1.00	0.93	15
	Boys	5.95	1.14	0.93	15
	Girls	6.03	0.87	4.05	10.13
Adaptive regulation	Total sample	28.89	8.02	2	50
	Boys	28.15	8.28	10	50
	Girls	28.68	7.80	2	49
Less adaptive regulation **	Total sample	17.86	6.04	1	40
	Boys	16.20	5.64	1	40
	Girls	19.19	6.02	3	34

Note. *SD* = standard deviation. U-test significant difference * $p < 0.05$ and ** $p < 0.01$.

Table 2 shows the bivariate correlations of the three samples.

Table 2. Bivariate Correlations in the total sample (below the diagonal), in the boys' sample (above the diagonal, outside the brackets), and in the girls' sample (above the diagonal, in brackets).

Variables	1	2	3	4	5	6	7
1. Alcohol abuse	1	0.45 ** (0.4 **)	0.12 * (0.22 **)	0.16 ** (0.16 **)	0.00 (0.13 **)	0.02 (0.00)	0.12 * (0.22 **)
2. Substance addiction	0.43 **	1	0.18 ** (0.15 **)	0.23 ** (0.19 **)	0.13 * (0.21 **)	−0.02 (−0.05)	0.19 ** (0.22 **)
3. Problematic internet use	0.18 **	0.16 **	1	0.12 * (0.11 *)	0.14 * (0.32 **)	−0.02 (−0.06)	0.25 ** (0.26 **)
4. Suicidal behavior	0.17 **	0.20 **	0.12 **	1	0.42 ** (0.29 **)	0.00 (−0.07)	0.40 ** (0.32 **)
5. Contextual problems	0.07 *	0.17 **	0.23 **	0.34 **	1	−0.00 (−0.03)	0.35 ** (0.42 **)
6. Adaptive regulation	0.01	−0.04	−0.04	−0.05	−0.02	1	0.34 ** (0.11 **)
7. Less adaptive regulation	0.19 **	0.20 **	0.27 **	0.37 **	0.38 **	0.20 **	1

Note. * $p < 0.05$ and ** $p < 0.01$.

3.1. Psychometric Network Analysis of the Total Sample

Figure 1 shows the results of a psychometric network analysis of the total sample. Panel A shows the estimated network of regulation strategies, contextual problems, and addictive and suicidal behaviors. The network is interconnected. Panel B of Figure 1 presents non-standardized estimates of the centrality measures; according to Isvoranu et al. [50], these are the values that should be reported. The most central node in terms of strength, expected influence, and betweenness is less adaptive regulation strategies (St = 1.04; EI = 1.04; Bet = 6; and Clo = 0.02). Another variable that stands out is the presence of contextual problems (St = 0.77; EI = 0.62; Bet = 0; and Clo = 0.20). The results for the other variables are as follows: suicidal behavior (St = 0.75; EI = 0.53; Bet = 0; and Clo = 0.02), alcohol abuse (St = 0.74; EI = 0.58; Bet = 3; and Clo = 0.02), substance addiction (St = 0.54; EI = 0.54; Bet = 0; and Clo = 0.01), problematic internet use (St = 0.52; EI = 0.36; Bet = 0; and Clo = 0.02), and adaptive regulation (St = 0.45; EI = 0.07; Bet = 0; and Clo = 0.02).

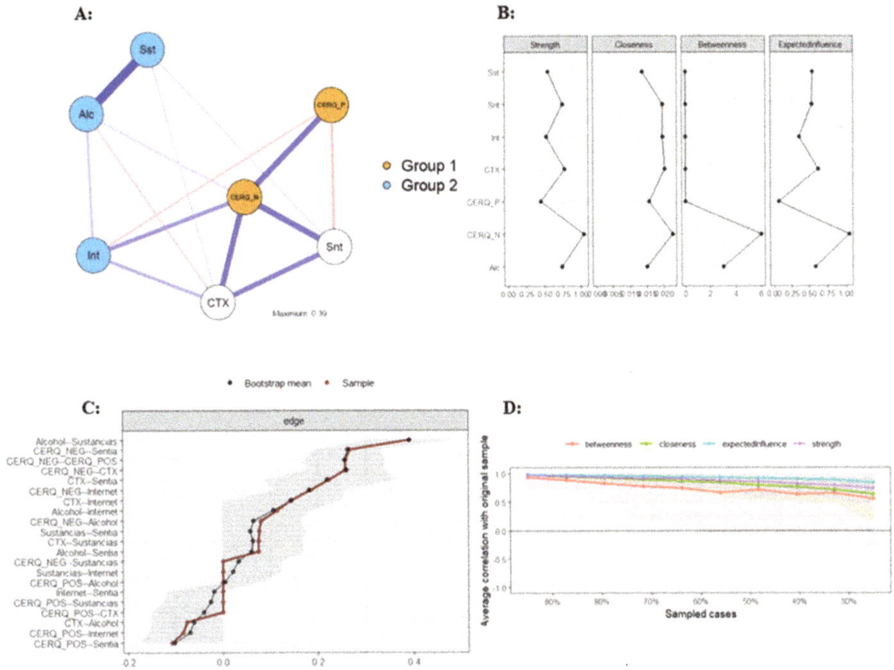

Figure 1. Network analysis of regulation strategies, contextual problems, and addictive and suicidal behaviors in the total sample. Alc/Alcohol = alcohol abuse; Sst/Sustancias = substance addiction; Int/Internet = problematic internet use; Snt/Sentia = suicidal behavior; CTX = contextual problems; CERQ_P/CERQ_POS = adaptative behavior; and CERQ_N/CERQ_NEG = less adaptative behavior. Panel (**A**): Estimated network graph in total sample; Panel (**B**): Non-standardized estimates of the centrality measures in total sample; Panel (**C**): Precision plot of estimated network in total sample; Panel (**D**): Stability indices of the edges in total sample.

In panel C of Figure 1, the precision plot shows that the estimated network demonstrated adequate precision. In most cases, the estimates obtained through resampling (n = 1000) overlap with the original estimates, and none fall outside the confidence interval. Panel D of Figure 1 presents the stability indices of the edges in the estimated network. When the sample size is reduced by 50%, the estimates do not fall below 0.70. These results indicate that the estimated network is stable, and the conclusions drawn from it can be generalized.

3.2. *Psychometric Network Analysis in the Boys' Sample*

Figure 2 presents the psychometric network analysis for the male sample. Panel A shows the estimated network of regulation strategies, contextual problems, and addictive and suicidal behaviors. The network is interconnected. Panel B of Figure 2 presents the non-standardized estimates of the centrality measures. The most central node in terms of strength, standardized influence, and betweenness is less adaptive regulation strategies (St = 1.10; Clo = 0.06; Bet = 5; and EI = 1.10). Another notable variable is suicidal behavior (St = 0.60; Clo = 0.05; Bet = 0; and EI = 0.60). The results for the other variables are as follows: contextual problems (St = 0.54; Clo = 0.04; Bet = 0; and EI = 0.54), alcohol abuse (St = 0.42; Clo = 0.04; Bet = 0; and EI = 0.42), substance addiction (St = 0.42; Clo = NA; Bet = 0; and EI = 0.42), adaptive regulation strategies (St = 0.39; Clo = 0.04; Bet = 0; and EI = 0.39), and problematic internet use (St = 0.21; Clo = 0.03; Bet = 0; and EI = 0.21).

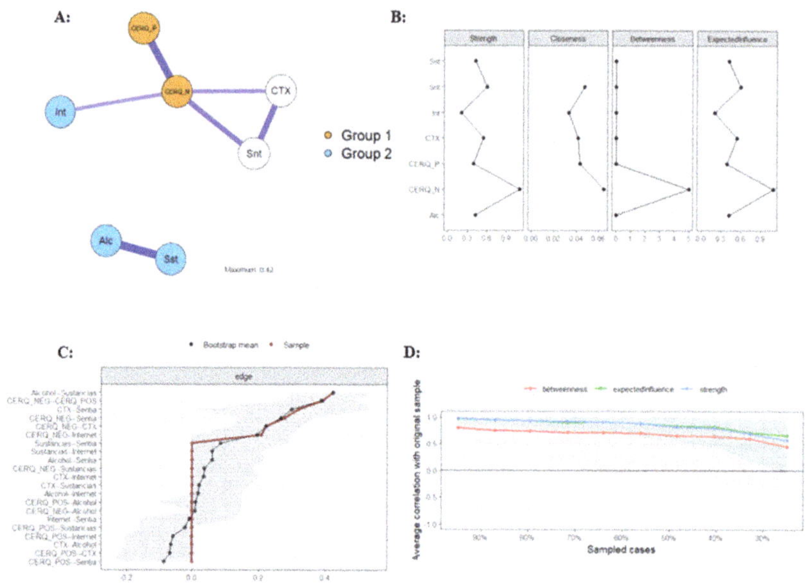

Figure 2. Network analysis of regulation strategies, contextual problems, and addictive and suicidal behaviors in the male sample. Alc/Alcohol = alcohol abuse; Sst/Sustancias = substance addiction; Int/Internet = problematic internet use; Snt/Sentia = suicidal behavior; CTX = contextual problems; CERQ_P/CERQ_POS = adaptative behavior; and CERQ_N/CERQ_NEG = less adaptative behavior. Panel (**A**): Estimated network graph in boys; Panel (**B**): Non-standardized estimates of the centrality measures in boys; Panel (**C**): Precision plot of estimated network in boys; Panel (**D**): Stability indices of the edges in boys.

In panel C of Figure 2, the precision plot indicates that the estimated network does not demonstrate adequate precision in the estimation. There are discrepancies between the sample and the resampling (n = 1000) as most nodes show estimates different from zero, which alters the interpretation of the network. Panel D of Figure 2 presents the stability indices of the edges in the estimated network. In this analysis, the stability of the strength and influence of the variables does not fall below 0.70 when the sample is reduced by 50%, except for strength. The estimation of closeness shows no variance, so the statistical program does not display it. These results suggest that the estimated network is partially stable; therefore, caution should be used when generalizing its results.

3.3. *Psychometric Network Analysis in the Girls' Sample*

Figure 3 presents the psychometric network analysis for the female sample. Panel A shows the estimated network of regulation strategies, contextual problems, and addictive and suicidal behaviors. The network is interconnected. Panel B of Figure 3 presents the non-standardized estimates of the centrality measures. The most central node in terms of strength, standardized influence, and betweenness is less adaptive regulation strategies (St = 0.91; Clo = 0.02; Bet = 5; and EI = 0.92). Another notable variable is the presence of contextual problems (St = 0.82; Clo = 0.02; Bet = 6; and EI = 0.82). The results for the other variables are as follows: alcohol abuse (St = 0.63; Clo = 0.02; Bet = 1; and EI = 0.62), problematic internet use (St = 0.53; Clo = 0.02; Bet = 1; and EI = 0.53), suicidal behavior (St = 0.49; Clo = 0.02; Bet = 0; and EI = 0.29), substance addiction (St = 0.48; Clo = 0.01; Bet = 0; and EI = 0.48), and adaptive regulation strategies (St = 0.27; Clo = 0.01; Bet = 0; and EI = 0.07).

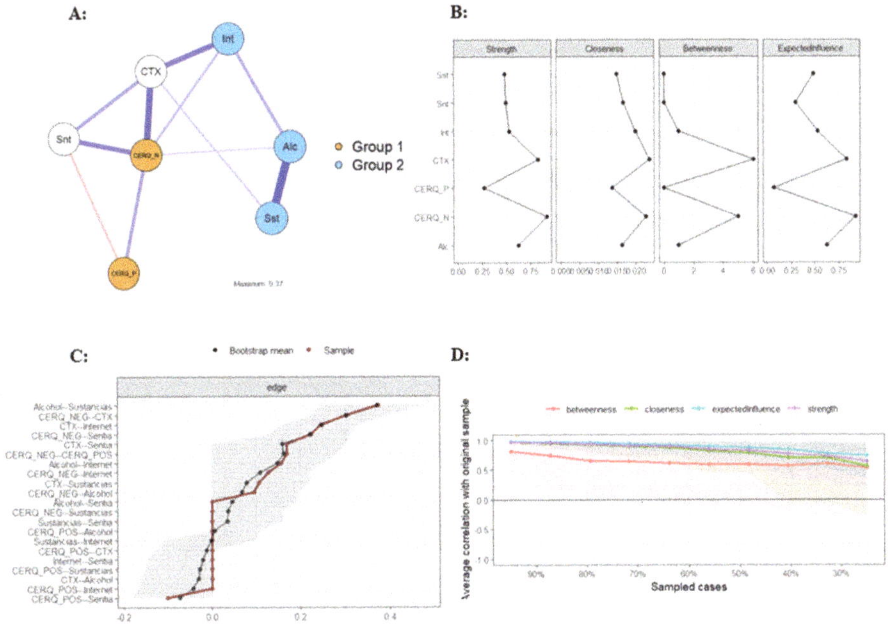

Figure 3. Network analysis of regulation strategies, contextual problems, and addictive and suicidal behaviors in the female sample. Alc/Alcohol = alcohol abuse; Sst/Sustancias = substance addiction; Int/Internet = problematic internet use; Snt/Sentia = suicidal behavior; CTX = contextual problems; CERQ_P/CERQ_POS = adaptative behavior; and CERQ_N/CERQ_NEG = less adaptative behavior. Panel (**A**): Estimated network graph in girls; Panel (**B**): Non-standardized estimates of the centrality measures in girls; Panel (**C**): Precision plot of estimated network in girls; Panel (**D**): Stability indices of the edges in girls.

In panel C of Figure 3, the precision plot shows that the estimated network demonstrated adequate precision in the estimation. Unlike the boys' sample, in most cases the estimates obtained through resampling (n = 1000) overlap with the original estimates, and none fall outside the confidence interval. Panel D of Figure 3 presents the stability indices of the edges in the estimated network. In this analysis, the stability of the strength, closeness, and influence of the variables does not fall below 0.70 when the sample is reduced by 50%, except for strength. These results suggest that the estimated network is partially stable. Therefore, caution should be used when generalizing the conclusions drawn.

4. Discussion

The main objective of this study was to analyze, using psychometric networks, the association between problem behaviors (i.e., alcohol abuse, substance addiction, problematic internet use, and suicidal behavior), the presence of problems within the family, school, or among peers (contextual problems), and the use of cognitive-emotion regulation strategies (adaptive regulation and less adaptive regulation). Additionally, the study aimed to analyze this relationship separately for boys and girls.

The descriptive data for this sample revealed that, compared to boys, girls presented more suicidal behavior, more maladaptive regulation, and more problematic internet use. These preliminary results are in accordance with the previous literature highlighting the higher proportion of affirmative responses among girls when suicidal behavior is evaluated [7,25], even though death by suicide occurs to a greater extent in boys. This gender paradox is partly attributable to the higher prevalence of affective disorders among girls [36] and the stronger tendency to express emotions among girls [51]. Also, in accordance with the existing literature, girls presented a greater amount of regulation strategies such as rumination, catastrophizing, blaming others, and self-blaming, expectantly more prone to exacerbating emotions than mitigating them. Finally, girls presented more problematic internet use than boys. These data deserve more attention. Although some studies have reported lower overall rates of problematic internet use among girls than boys [52,53], girls tend to spend more time on social networking sites. Therefore, gender differences [54] may depend on specific types of online activity (e.g., boys tend to develop more problematic behaviors related to online gaming, while in girls these relate more to social media platforms and online communication) [55,56].

To examine the relationships between the study variables, a psychometric network analysis was conducted using the entire sample, as well as the male and female samples separately. To our knowledge, this is the first study to explore these relationships through a psychometric network structure. Other researchers have applied this type of analysis to understand the relationship between depressive symptoms and substance use [57] or to assess the impact of protective and risk factors on suicidal behavior [58]. However, context-related issues, such as family, school, or peer group problems—which have been identified as risk factors for each of the problem behaviors studied [59]—have not yet been considered using this type of analysis. Network analysis provides a deeper understanding of how the selected problem behaviors, regulation strategies, and contextual issues are interrelated by examining and illustrating the connections between nodes while controlling for the effects of other nodes in the network.

In all three samples, the most central node in the network is less adaptive regulation strategies, which exhibits connections with contextual problems (especially in girls), problematic internet use, suicidal behavior (especially in boys), and—specifically in the female sample—with alcohol consumption. This finding reinforces the idea that inadequate emotion regulation is a key factor in addictive and suicidal behaviors in adolescents. According to the previous literature, less adaptive regulation strategies are associated with higher alcohol consumption [32], cannabis use [60], problematic internet use [61], and suicidal behavior [35]. In summary, our study reinforces the view that maladaptive emotional regulation strategies are a fundamental aspect underlying various behavioral issues. However, as we will discuss further, this relationship differs between boys and girls and across different types of behavioral problems.

Regarding problem behaviors, it is notable that alcohol abuse and substance addiction are positively related in all three of the networks analyzed, reinforcing the findings from the latest national survey that poly-drug use is common among adolescents [12]. This aligns with evidence suggesting that the use of one substance increases the likelihood of starting to use others [62]. In boys, the tendency towards poly-drug use appears as a phenomenon separate from other variables, showing an apparent disconnect from other behavioral problems, poor cognitive-emotional regulation, or contextual issues. This independence from other problems and the lack of connection with personal or contextual variables may be related to the social and cultural acceptance of alcohol and substance use in leisure contexts [63]. It suggests that, for boys, alcohol or substance use might be driven by risk factors not covered in this study, such as the pursuit of sensations or fun.

In contrast, for girls, alcohol and substance use is associated with other variables, and with pathways influenced by problematic internet use, contextual problems, and maladaptive regulation. Specifically, our study indicates that, for girls, substance use is linked to problematic aspects of their social context, and alcohol use is associated with problematic internet use and maladaptive or ineffective emotional regulation. In this regard, Verplaetse et al. [64] noted that alcohol may be more commonly used as a regulation strategy among women than men.

Problematic internet use was found to be related to maladaptive emotional regulation strategies in both girls and boys. Additionally, for girls, compulsive internet use was associated with contextual problems and served as a pathway to alcohol and substance use. This suggests that such behavior may have more complex implications for girls than for boys. According to the national survey, the prevalence of heavy alcohol consumption, daily tobacco use, and cannabis use is higher among adolescents who also exhibit compulsive internet use [18]. However, the meta-analysis by Lanthier-Labonté et al. [65] concludes that this relationship is not very clear, indicating a need for further investigation as well as a clearer conceptualization of problematic internet use [66]. In our study the association between problematic internet use and alcohol use was true only for girls, not for boys.

Lastly, suicidal behavior was found to have a significant positive relationship with less adaptive regulation strategies and contextual problems across all three samples. However, suicidal behavior did not exhibit a significant relationship with other problem behaviors, except for its positive association with substance addiction in the overall sample. Concerning our results, maladaptive cognitive-emotion regulation and contextual problems emerge as fundamental factors in addressing suicidal behavior among adolescents. Nevertheless, it is important to continue exploring the roles these addictive behaviors may play in suicide risk. Some researchers emphasize that internet use plays a significant role in suicidal behavior [25]. Additionally, other studies suggest that the relationship between suicidal behavior and addictive behaviors is more robust when examined in clinical populations, with its relevance in other populations remaining unclear [67].

A notable aspect of the analyzed networks is the greater interconnection between contextual problems, maladaptive cognitive emotion regulation strategies, addictive behaviors, and suicidal behaviors observed among girls. This interconnection aligns with the observance of greater emotional difficulties in girls [7,36]. Interesting, although girls seem to cope with more simultaneous difficulties, as problematic internet use, alcohol use, or substance addiction, our network analyses show that girls are more efficient than boys in avoiding suicidal behavior by using their adaptive cognitive-emotion regulation strategies. Adaptive strategies such as positive reevaluation, or putting things into perspective, are considered by some authors to distinguish the best regulators [68] and are activated by girls specifically in the face of suicidal behavior. Thus, our results suggest that girls may be more efficient in dealing with suicidal behaviors than boys. In contrast, cognitive-emotion regulation and context difficulties are associated with a wider range of behavioral problems in girls than in boys. Therefore, our results suggest that, even when emotion regulation and context difficulties are involved in a wider range of addictive problems in girls than in boys, girls may deal more efficiently with suicidal behaviors than boys. This may be due to girls' earlier maturation rate, in addition to the fact that they have to learn to manage emotions and situations in a more complex way due to a more demanding environment.

Finally, another noteworthy finding across all three networks is the repeated positive association between less adaptive regulation strategies and contextual problems. Context during adolescence, which includes adolescents' family, school, and peers, plays a crucial role in psychosocial development [69]. Adolescents gain new experiences and learning opportunities from their context, providing them with useful tools and skills for life, including cognitive and emotional regulation strategies [70]. It is expected that if an adolescent's context is marked by persistent problems, such as frequent conflicts with their parents, they are more likely to lack adaptive strategies for managing the challenges they may encounter during this period [71]. Similarly, contextual problems were found to be related to substance use and problematic internet use in the total sample and were consistently linked with suicidal behaviors. These results are supported by the previous literature, which identifies family conflicts, peer problems, social isolation, and school issues as risk factors for substance use [6], problematic internet use [72], and suicidal behavior [73]. As mentioned earlier, it is noteworthy that the node of contextual problems is more significant in the female sample compared to the male sample. Additionally, while this node is positively related to substance addiction, problematic internet use, and suicidal behavior in girls, it is only associated with suicidal behavior in boys. This raises the question of why contextual problems have a greater impact on problem behaviors in this demographic. This greater emphasis on context for girls may be due to the fact that they experience a greater number of more challenging psychosocial demands than boys. In addition, Van Droogenbroeck et al. [74] suggest other possible explanations, such as an underestimation of distress by boys or the influence of gender roles, which portray girls as more sensitive to stressors.

The problem behaviors addressed in this study are complex and multifactorial, requiring thorough investigation [11,66,75]. This study aims to contribute information on their management, highlighting the roles of cognitive-emotional regulation and context. However, further research is necessary, especially studies incorporating additional variables of interest and employing analyses that explore relationships in greater detail, such as psychometric networks. It is also crucial to account for gender differences when examining these phenomena. For example, studies have shown that while girls experience more related mental health issues, they are underrepresented in treatment services [76]. Additionally, a "gender paradox" applies to suicidal behavior: rates of suicide attempts are higher in women, but rates of completed suicide are higher in men [25,36,77]. These aspects need to be considered in future research.

This study is not without limitations. First, it is a cross-sectional study, which prevents the establishment of "causal" relationships in the sense of more robust statistical control and temporal dynamics. Thus, while it identifies relationships, these need further exploration as processes are dynamic and, therefore, longitudinal [49]. Second, the variables "substance addiction", "suicidal behavior", and "contextual problems" encompass diverse information. For instance, cannabis use differs from cocaine use, and suicidal ideation is distinct from suicide attempts. Likewise, problems at school differ from those at home. Future studies should consider using more specific variables to examine these phenomena in greater detail. Third, data were collected through self-report questionnaires. Although these instruments generally have good psychometric properties, it would have been useful to include a response inference scale to assess respondent attentiveness. Additionally, incorporating a multi-informant perspective would have been beneficial for this study. Fourth, some of the estimated networks showed only partial stability, which could limit their generalizability. Fifth, regarding psychometric network analysis, a multigroup analysis is needed to determine whether the structure and/or edges vary between boys and girls. While psychometric networks can usefully inform an understanding of the phenomenon under study, caution should be exercised when interpreting the results: as with any cross-sectional and correlational study, the effects observed may be spurious due to the presence of unmeasured variables. Finally, the wide age range of the sample in this study encompasses different developmental stages and processes (e.g., cognitive, emotional, biological, and psychosexual) as well as contextual demands, which were not taken into account in the network analysis. These variables, closely linked to chronological age, may have significant implications and could potentially moderate the findings of the present study. Future research should examine age-related differences in specific developmental processes within the framework of network analysis. Additionally, the ecological and historical context, including the socio-cultural characteristics of the Spanish setting in which the research was conducted, may have influenced the results. These factors should also be taken into account in future studies.

On the other hand, this study also has several strengths. First, it benefits from a substantial sample size, comprising 758 adolescents and young adults. Second, the use of psychometric network analysis is noteworthy. Despite its limitations [78], this approach provides valuable insights into relationships and phenomena [49]. Third, the study is innovative, addressing current issues and providing new data that contribute to the understanding of both substance-related and non-substance-related addictive behaviors, as well as suicidal behavior.

In conclusion, it is crucial to emphasize the need for a collaborative approach between science and practice. To promote psychological well-being, especially during vulnerable periods such as childhood and adolescence, it is essential to implement effective interventions based on scientific research. In this regard, addressing maladaptive regulation strategies and contextual problems appears to be central to improving adolescents' psychological well-being, which will likely lead to the better management of the problematic behaviors discussed.

5. Conclusions

The results of this study highlight that the use of ineffective or maladaptive emotional regulation strategies and the presence of problems in the developmental context are crucial aspects in the prevention of suicidal behaviors in adolescents. The study also warns of relevant gender differences. Specifically, suicidal behaviors could be better managed by girls due to the activation of effective emotional regulation strategies such as putting things into perspective, focusing on the positive, acceptance, and positive reevaluation. This differential effect contributes to understanding why boys commit suicide at a higher rate than girls since it is less likely that they can inhibit the associated negative emotions once the behaviors of suicidal ideation, planning, and attempt have begun. On the other hand, girls and boys may have different motivations for substance and alcohol use. Specifically, in girls these behaviors are related to ineffective emotional regulation and the presence of contextual problems, while in boys these behaviors seem to have independent motivations, and, hypothetically, could be more related to leisure and sensation seeking. Only problematic internet use is related to ineffective emotional regulation in both boys and girls. Consequently, the data obtained are consistent with the gender paradox, presenting a situation of greater vulnerability to contextual problems and addictive behaviors in girls, while suggesting a greater defenselessness in the face of suicidal behaviors in boys.

Author Contributions: Conceptualization, B.D., M.Á.C. and F.P.H.-T.; methodology, D.E. and F.P.H.-T.; software, F.P.H.-T.; formal analysis, D.E. and F.P.H.-T.; investigation, B.D., M.Á.C. and F.P.H.-T.; writing—original draft preparation, D.E., B.D., M.Á.C. and F.P.H.-T.; writing—review and editing, B.D., M.Á.C., F.P.H.-T. and D.E.; visualization, B.D., M.Á.C., F.P.H.-T. and D.E.; supervision, B.D., M.Á.C., F.P.H.-T. and D.E.; project administration, M.Á.C. and F.P.H.-T.; funding acquisition, M.Á.C., B.D. and F.P.H.-T. All authors have read and agreed to the published version of the manuscript.

Funding: This research was funded by The Ministry of Science and Innovation of the Government of Spain, Project Reference: PID2020-114538RB-I00; AEI/10.13039/501100011033.

Institutional Review Board Statement: The study was conducted in accordance with the Declaration of Helsinki and approved by the Institutional Review Board (or Ethics Committee) of the UNED (protocol code 12-PSI-2022, approved 17 June 2022).

Informed Consent Statement: Informed consent was obtained from all subjects involved in the study.

Data Availability Statement: The data will be available in the following repository: https://e-spacio.uned.es/home (accessed on 10 November 2024).

Conflicts of Interest: The authors declare no conflicts of interest.

References

1. Kapur, S. Adolescence: The Stage of Transition. *Horiz. Holist. Educ.* **2015**, *2*, 233–250.
2. Andrews, J.L.; Ahmed, S.; Blakemore, S.J. Navigating The Social Environment in Adolescence: The Role of Social Brain Development. *Biol. Psychiatry* **2020**, *89*, 109–118. [CrossRef] [PubMed]
3. Steinberg, L. *Age of Opportunity: Lessons from the New Science of Adolescence*; Houghton Mifflin Harcourt: Boston, MA, USA, 2015.

4. Al-Halabí, S.; García-Haro, J.M.; Gutiérrez-López, B. Tratamientos psicológicos para la conducta suicida en niños y adolescentes [Psychological treatments for suicidal behavior in children and adolescents]. In *Manual de Tratamientos Psicológicos: Infancia y Adolescencia [Psychological Treatment Manual: Childhood and Adolescence]*; Fonseca-Pedrero, E., Ed.; Pirámide: Madrid, Spain, 2021; pp. 639–667.
5. Schwartz-Mette, R.A.; Lawrence, H.R.; Shankman, J.; Fearey, E.; Harrington, R. Intrapersonal Emotion Regulation Difficulties and Maladaptive Interpersonal Behavior in Adolescence. *Res. Child Adolesc. Psychopathol.* **2021**, *49*, 749–761. [CrossRef] [PubMed]
6. Fernández-Artamendi, S.; López-Núñez, C.; Coloma-Carmona, A.; Carballo, J.L. Tratamientos psicológicos para las conductas adictivas en población infanto-juvenil [Psychological treatments for addictive behaviours in the child and adolescent population]. In *Manual de Tratamientos Psicológicos: Infancia y Adolescencia [Psychological Treatment Manual: Childhood and Adolescence]*; Fonseca-Pedrero, E., Ed.; Pirámide: Madrid, Spain, 2021; pp. 651–698.
7. Fonseca-Pedrero, E.; Calvo, P.; Díez-Gómez, A.; Pérez-Albéniz, A.; Lucas-Molina, B.; Al-Halabí, S. *La Salud Mental de los Adolescentes en Contextos Educativos: Reflexiones Derivadas del Estudio PSICE [Adolescent Mental Health in Educational Settings: Reflections from the PSICE Study]*; Consejo General de la Psicología de España: Madrid, Spain, 2023.
8. Sisk, L.M.; Gee, D.G. Stress and adolescence: Vulnerability and opportunity during a sensitive window of development. *Curr. Opin. Psychol.* **2021**, *44*, 286–292. [CrossRef]
9. Wijbenga, L.; de Winter, A.F.; Almansa, J.; Vollebergh, W.A.; Korevaar, E.L.; Hofstra, J.; Reijneveld, S.A. Multiple health risk behaviors and mental health from a life course perspective: The Dutch TRAILS study. *Prev. Med.* **2021**, *154*, 106870. [CrossRef]
10. Alfonso, J.P.; Huedo-Medina, T.B.; Espada, J.P. Factores de riesgo predictores del patrón de consumo de drogas durante la adolescencia [Risk factors predicting the pattern of drug use during adolescence]. *Ann. Psychol.* **2009**, *25*, 330–338.
11. Al-Halabí, S.; Fonseca-Pedrero, E. Suicidal Behavior Prevention: The Time to Act is Now. *Clin. Salud* **2021**, *32*, 89–92. [CrossRef]
12. Ministerio de Sanidad, Servicios Sociales e Igualdad. Observatorio Español de las Drogas y de las Adicciones. *Encuesta Estatal Sobre Uso de Drogas en Enseñanzas Secundarias (ESTUDES)*. 2023. Available online: https://pnsd.sanidad.gob.es/profesionales/sistemasInformacion/sistemaInformacion/encuestas_ESTUDES.htm (accessed on 10 November 2024).
13. Duperrouzel, J.C.; Granja, K.; Pacheco-Colón, I.; Gonzalez, R. Adverse Effects of Cannabis Use on Neurocognitive Functioning: A Systematic Review of Meta- Analytic Studies. *J. Dual Diagn.* **2020**, *16*, 43–57. [CrossRef]
14. Smith, R.F.; McDonald, C.G.; Bergstrom, H.C.; Ehlinger, D.G.; Brielmaier, J.M. Adolescent nicotine induces persisting changes in development of neural connectivity. *Neurosci. Biobehav. Rev.* **2015**, *55*, 432–443. [CrossRef]
15. Stamates, A.L.; Roberts, R.; Lau-Barraco, C. Alcohol, Cannabis, and Tobacco Polysubstance Use: A Latent Profile Analysis of Age of Onset. *Subst. Abus.* **2021**, *43*, 531–538. [CrossRef]
16. Throuvala, M.A.; Griffiths, M.D.; Rennoldson, M.; Kuss, D.J. School-based prevention for adolescent Internet Addiction: Prevention is the key. A systematic literature review. *Curr. Neuropharmacol.* **2019**, *17*, 507–525. [CrossRef] [PubMed]
17. *Meeting Report 2014: Public Health Implications of Excessive Use of the Internet, Computers, Smartphones and Similar Electronic Devices*; WHO Document Production Services: Geneva, Switzerland, 2014.
18. Observatorio Español de las Drogas y las Adicciones. Informe Sobre Adicciones Comportamentales 2022. *Delegación del Gobierno para el Plan Nacional Sobre Drogas*. Available online: https://pnsd.sanidad.gob.es/profesionales/sistemasInformacion/home.htm (accessed on 10 November 2024).
19. Baloğlu, M.; Şahin, R.; Arpaci, I. A review of recent research in problematic internet use: Gender and cultural differences. *Curr. Opin. Psychol.* **2020**, *36*, 124–129. [CrossRef] [PubMed]
20. Fonseca-Pedrero, E.; Pérez-Albéniz, A.; Al-Halabí, S. Conducta suicida en adolescentes a revisión: Creando esperanza a través de la acción [Suicidal behavior in adolescents under review: Fostering hope through action]. *Papeles Psicól.* **2022**, *43*, 173–184.
21. Glenn, C.R.; Kleiman, E.M.; Kellerman, J.; Pollak, O.; Cha, C.B.; Esposito, E.C.; Porter, A.C.; Wyman, P.A.; Boatman, A.E. Annual Research Review: A meta-analytic review of worldwide suicide rates in adolescents. *J. Child Psychol. Psychiatry* **2019**, *61*, 294–308. [CrossRef]
22. Instituto Nacional de Estadística. Defunciones Según la Causa de Muerte [Deaths by Cause of Death] 2022 [Base de Datos]. Available online: https://www.ine.es/jaxiT3/Tabla.htm?t=7947 (accessed on 10 November 2024).
23. O'Connor, R.C.; Nock, M.K. The psychology of suicidal behaviour. *Lancet Psychiatry* **2014**, *1*, 73–85. [CrossRef]
24. Wang, P.-W.; Yen, C.-F. Adolescent substance use behavior and suicidal behavior for boys and girls: A cross-sectional study by latent analysis approach. *BMC Psychiatry* **2017**, *17*, 392. [CrossRef]
25. Espada-Sánchez, J.P.; Piqueras Rodríguez, J.A.; Soto-Sanz., V.; Morales Sabuco, A. Conducta suicida y autolesiones en la infancia y la adolescencia [Suicidal behaviour and self-harm in childhood and adolescence]. In *Manual de Psicología de la Conducta Suicida [Psychology Manual on Suicidal Behavior]*; Al-Halabí, S., Fonseca-Pedrero, E., Eds.; Pirámide: Madrid, Spain, 2023; pp. 111–142.
26. Zhu, X.; Griffiths, H.; Xiao, Z.; Ribeaud, D.; Eisner, M.; Yang, Y.; Murray, A.L. Trajectories of Screen Time across Adolescence and Their Associations with Adulthood Mental Health and Behavioral Outcomes. *J. Youth Adolesc.* **2023**, *52*, 1433–1447. [CrossRef]
27. Goldston, D.B. Conceptual issues in understanding the relationship between suicidal behavior and substance use during adolescence. *Drug Alcohol Depend.* **2004**, *76*, S79–S91. [CrossRef]
28. González-Roz, A.; Martínez-Loredo, V.; Maalouf, W.; Fernández-Hermida, J.; Al-Halabí, S. Protocol for a Trial Assessing the Efficacy of a Universal School-Based Prevention Program for Addictive Behaviors. *Psicothema* **2023**, *1*, 41–49. [CrossRef]
29. Weiss, N.H.; Kiefer, R.; Goncharenko, S.; Raudales, A.M.; Forkus, S.R.; Schick, M.R.; Contractor, A.A. Emotion regulation and substance use: A meta-analysis. *Drug Alcohol Depend.* **2021**, *230*, 109131. [CrossRef]

30. Garnefski, N.; Kraaij, V. Specificity of relations between adolescents' cognitive emotion regulation strategies and symptoms of depression and anxiety. *Cogn. Emot.* **2016**, *32*, 1401–1408. [CrossRef] [PubMed]
31. Şimşek, O.M.; Koçak, O.; Younis, M.Z. The impact of interpersonal cognitive distortions on satisfaction with life and the mediating role of loneliness. *Sustainability* **2021**, *13*, 9293. [CrossRef]
32. Trujillo, A.; Obando, D.; Trujillo, C.A. Family dynamics and alcohol and marijuana use among adolescents: The mediating role of negative emotional symptoms and sensation seeking. *Addict. Behav.* **2016**, *62*, 99–107. [CrossRef] [PubMed]
33. Wang, Z.; Buu, A.; Lohrmann, D.K.; Shih, P.C.; Lin, H. The role of family conflict in mediating impulsivity to early substance exposure among preteens. *Addict. Behav.* **2021**, *115*, 106779. [CrossRef]
34. Coppersmith, D.D.L.; Millgram, Y.; Kleiman, E.M.; Fortgang, R.G.; Millner, A.J.; Frumkin, M.R.; Bentley, K.H.; Nock, M.K. Suicidal thinking as affect regulation. *J. Psychopathol. Clin. Sci.* **2023**, *132*, 385–395. [CrossRef]
35. Kim, H.S.; Hodgins, D.C.; Kim, B.; Wild, T.C. Transdiagnostic or Disorder Specific? Indicators of Substance and Behavioral Addictions Nominated by People with Lived Experience. *J. Clin. Med.* **2020**, *9*, 334. [CrossRef]
36. Schrijvers, D.L.; Bollen, J.; Sabbe, B.G. The gender paradox in suicidal behavior and its impact on the suicidal process. *J. Affect. Disord.* **2012**, *138*, 19–26. [CrossRef]
37. Turner, S.; Mota, N.; Bolton, J.; Sareen, J. Self-medication with alcohol or drugs for mood and anxiety disorders: A narrative review of the epidemiological literature. *Depress. Anxiety* **2018**, *35*, 851–860. [CrossRef]
38. Vázquez-Reyes, A.; Martín-Rodríguez, A.; Pérez-San-Gregorio, M.; Vázquez-Morejón, A.J. Gender Influence on severe Mental Disorders: Relationship between Behavior Problems and Family Burden. *Clin. Salud* **2021**, *32*, 65–70. [CrossRef]
39. Guo, X.; Lv, B.; Zhou, H.; Liu, C.; Liu, J.; Jiang, K.; Luo, L. Gender Differences in How Family Income and Parental Education Relate to Reading Achievement in China: The Mediating Role of Parental Expectation and Parental Involvement. *Front. Psychol.* **2018**, *9*, 783. [CrossRef]
40. Eslava, D.; Martínez-Vispo, C.; Villanueva-Blasco, V.J.; Errasti, J.M.; Al-Halabí, S. Family Conflict and Suicidal Behaviour in Adolescence: The Mediating Role of the Assertive Interpersonal Schema. *Sustainability* **2023**, *15*, 5149. [CrossRef]
41. Pérez, E.P.; Monje, M.R.; Alonso, F.G.; Girón, M.F.; López, M.P.; Romero, J.C. Validación de un instrumento para la detección de trastornos de control de impulsos y adicciones: El MULTICAGE CAD-4 [Validation of a tool for screening of impulse control disorders and addiction: MULTICAGE CAD-4. *Trastor. Adict.* **2007**, *9*, 269–278. [CrossRef]
42. Díez-Gómez, A.; Sebastián-Enesco, C.; Pérez de Albéniz, A.; Fonseca-Pedrero, E. Evaluación de la conducta suicida en adolescentes: Validación de la escala SENTIA-Breve [Suicidal behavior assessment in adolescents: Validation of the SENTIA-Brief scale]. *Actas Esp. Psiquiatr.* **2021**, *49*, 24–34.
43. Garnefski, N.; Kraaij, V. The Cognitive Emotion Regulation Questionnaire. *Eur. J. Psychol. Assess.* **2007**, *23*, 141–149. [CrossRef]
44. Holgado-Tello, F.P.; Amor, P.J.; Lasa-Aristu, A.; Domínguez-Sánchez, F.J.; Delgado, B. Two new brief versions of the Cognitive Emotion Regulation Questionnaire and its relationships with depression and anxiety. *An. Psicol.* **2018**, *34*, 458–464. [CrossRef]
45. Fernández-Pinto, I.; Santamaría, P.; Sánchez-Sánchez, F.; Carrasco, M.A.; del Barrio, V. *SENA: Sistema de Evaluación de Niños y Adolescentes [SENA: Child and Adolescent Assessment System]*; TEA Ediciones: Madrid, Spain, 2015.
46. Costantini, G.; Epskamp, S.; Borsboom, D.; Perugini, M.; Mõttus, R.; Waldorp, L.J.; Cramer, A.O. State of the art personality research: A tutorial on network analysis of personality data in R. *J. Res. Pers.* **2015**, *54*, 13–29. [CrossRef]
47. Epskamp, S. Network Psychometrics. Doctoral Dissertation, University of Amsterdam, Amsterdam, The Netherlands, April 2017.
48. Bringmann, L.F.; Elmer, T.; Epskamp, S.; Krause, R.W.; Schoch, D.; Wichers, M.; Wigman, J.T.W.; Snippe, E. What do centrality measures measure in psychological networks? *J. Abnorm. Psychol.* **2019**, *128*, 892–903. [CrossRef]
49. Álvarez Díaz, M.; Gallego Acedo, C.; Fernández Alonso, R.; Muñiz, J.; Fonseca Pedrero, E. Análisis de redes: Una alternativa a los enfoques clásicos de evaluación de los sistemas educativos [Network analysis: An alternative to classic approaches for education systems evaluation]. *Psicol. Educ.* **2021**, *28*, 165–173. [CrossRef]
50. Isvoranu, A.; Epskamp, S.; Waldotp, L.J.; Borsboom, D. *Network Psychometrics with R: A Guide for Behavioral and Social Scientists*; Routledge: London, UK, 2022.
51. Chaplin, T.M.; Aldao, A. Gender differences in emotion expression in children: A meta-analytic review. *Psychol. Bull.* **2013**, *139*, 735–765. [CrossRef]
52. Anderson, E.L.; Steen, E.; Stavropoulos, V. Internet use and Problematic Internet Use: A systematic review of longitudinal research trends in adolescence and emergent adulthood. *Int. J. Adolesc. Youth* **2017**, *22*, 430–454. [CrossRef]
53. Kuss, D.J.; Griffiths, M.D. Internet Gaming Addiction: A Systematic Review of Empirical Research. *Int. J. Ment. Health Addict.* **2011**, *10*, 278–296. [CrossRef]
54. Andreassen, C.S.; Pallesen, S.; Griffiths, M.D. The relationship between addictive use of social media, narcissism, and self-esteem: Findings from a large national survey. *Addict. Behav.* **2017**, *64*, 287–293. [CrossRef]
55. Király, O.; Ngygyörgy, K.; Griffiths, M.; Demetrovics, Z. Chapter 4. Problematic online gaming. In *Behavioral Addictions: Criteria, Evidence, and Treatment*; Rosenberg, K.P., Feder, L.C., Eds.; Academic Press: Cambridge, MA, USA, 2014; pp. 61–95.
56. Twenge, J.M.; Joiner, T.E.; Rogers, M.L.; Martin, G.N. Increases in Depressive Symptoms, Suicide-Related Outcomes, and Suicide Rates Among U.S. Adolescents After 2010 and Links to Increased New Media Screen Time. *Clin. Psychol. Sci.* **2017**, *6*, 3–17. [CrossRef]
57. Wasil, A.R.; Venturo-Conerly, K.E.; Shinde, S.; Patel, V.; Jones, P.J. Applying network analysis to understand depression and substance use in Indian adolescents. *J. Affect. Disord.* **2020**, *265*, 278–286. [CrossRef]

58. Fonseca-Pedrero, E.; Al-Halabí, S.; Pérez-Albéniz, A.; Debbané, M. Risk and Protective Factors in Adolescent Suicidal Behaviour: A Network Analysis. *Int. J. Environ. Res. Public Health* **2022**, *19*, 1784. [CrossRef]
59. Fonseca-Pedrero, E. *Manual de Tratamientos Psicológicos: Infancia y Adolescencia [Psychological Treatment Manual: Childhood and Adolescence]*; Pirámide: Madrid, Spain, 2021.
60. McKee, K.; Russell, M.; Mennis, J.; Mason, M.; Neale, M. Emotion regulation dynamics predict substance use in high-risk adolescents. *Addict. Behav.* **2020**, *106*, 106374. [CrossRef]
61. Gioia, F.; Rega, V.; Boursier, V. Problematic internet use and emotional dysregulation among young people: A literature review. *Clin Neuropsychiatry* **2021**, *18*, 41–54.
62. Kandel, D.; Kandel, E. The Gateway Hypothesis of substance abuse: Developmental, biological and societal perspectives. *Acta Paediatr.* **2014**, *104*, 130–137. [CrossRef]
63. Sjödin, L.; Larm, P.; Karlsson, P.; Livingston, M.; Raninen, J. Drinking motives and their associations with alcohol use among adolescents in Sweden. *Nord. Stud. Alcohol Drugs* **2021**, *38*, 256–269. [CrossRef]
64. Verplaetse, T.L.; Cosgrove, K.P.; Tanabe, J.; McKee, S.A. Sex/gender differences in brain function and structure in alcohol use: A narrative review of neuroimaging findings over the last 10 years. *J. Neurosci. Res.* **2020**, *99*, 309–323. [CrossRef]
65. Lanthier-Labonté, S.; Dufour, M.; Milot, D.-M.; Loslier, J. Is problematic Internet use associated with alcohol and cannabis use among youth? A systematic review. *Addict. Behav.* **2020**, *106*, 106331. [CrossRef] [PubMed]
66. Becoña, E. Adicciones comportamentales: Separando el grano de la paja [Behavioral Addictions: Separating the wheat from the chaff]. *Infonova* **2018**, *34*, 11–20.
67. Rodríguez-Cintas, L.; Daigre, C.; Braquehais, M.D.; Palma-Alvarez, R.F.; Grau-López, L.; Ros-Cucurull, E.; Rodríguez-Martos, L.; Abad, A.C.; Roncero, C. Factors associated with lifetime suicidal ideation and suicide attempts in outpatients with substance use disorders. *Psychiatry Res.* **2018**, *262*, 440–445. [CrossRef] [PubMed]
68. Delgado, B.; Amor, P.J.; Domínguez-Sánchez, F.J.; Holgado-Tello, F.P. Relationship between adult attachment and cognitive emotional regulation style in women and men. *Sci. Rep.* **2023**, *13*, 8144. [CrossRef] [PubMed]
69. Lerner, R.M.; Lerner, J.V.P.; Bowers, E.; Geldhof, G.J. Positive youth development and relational-developmental-systems. In *Handbook of Child Psychology and Developmental Science: Theory and Method*; Overton, W.F., Molenaar, P.C.M., Lerner, R.M., Eds.; John Wiley & Sons, Inc.: New York, NY, USA, 2015.
70. Servicio de Información e Investigación Social. *Prevención de las Adicciones. Revisión del Conocimiento Disponible Sobre Efectividad de las Intervenciones [Addiction Prevention. Review of Available Knowledge on Effectiveness of Interventions]*; Eusko Jaurlaritza-Gobierno Vasco: Pais Vasco, Spain, 2023. Available online: https://www.siis.net/es/investigacion/ver-estudio/626/ (accessed on 10 November 2024).
71. Zimmer-Gembeck, M.J.; Rudolph, J.; Kerin, J.; Bohadana-Brown, G. Parent emotional regulation: A meta-analytic review of its association with parenting and child adjustment. *Int. J. Behav. Dev.* **2021**, *46*, 63–82. [CrossRef]
72. Fumero, A.; Marrero, R.J.; de Miguel, A.; Peñate, W. Tratamientos psicológicos para las adicciones comportamentales en población infanto-juvenil [Psychological treatments for behavioural addictions in children and adolescents]. In *Manual de Tratamientos Psicológicos: Infancia y Adolescencia [Psychological Treatment Manual: Childhood and Adolescence]*; Fonseca-Pedrero, E., Ed.; Pirámide: Madrid, Spain, 2021; pp. 699–730.
73. Ati, N.A.L.; Paraswati, M.D.; Windarwati, H.D. What are the risk factors and protective factors of suicidal behavior in adolescents? A systematic review. *J. Child Adolesc. Psychiatr. Nurs.* **2020**, *34*, 7–18. [CrossRef]
74. Van Droogenbroeck, F.; Spruyt, B.; Keppens, G. Gender differences in mental health problems among adolescents and the role of social support: Results from the Belgian health interview surveys 2008 and 2013. *BMC Psychiatry* **2018**, *18*, 6. [CrossRef]
75. Becoña, E.; Cortés, M. *Manual de Adicciones para Psicólogos Especialistas en Psicología Clínica en Formación [Addictions Handbook for Trainee Clinical Psychologists in Clinical Psychology]*; Socidrogalcohol: Barcelona, Spain, 2016.
76. Fernández-Artamendi, S.; López-Núñez, C.; Martínez-Loredo, V. Evaluación de las conductas adictivas en adolescentes [Assessment of addictive behaviours in adolescents]. In *Manual de Conductas Adictivas [Handbook on Addictive Behaviours]*; Secades-Villa, R., García-Fernández, G., Fernández-Artamendi, S., Eds.; Pirámide: Madrid, Spain, 2022.
77. López-Vega, D.J.; Morell García, M.F.; del Río Olvera, F.J. Colectivos vulnerables para la conducta suicida. In *Manual de Psicología de la Conducta Suicida [Psychology Manual on Suicidal Behavior]*; Al-Halabí, S., Fonseca-Pedrero, E., Eds.; Pirámide: Madrid, Spain, 2023; pp. 235–272.
78. Guloksuz, S.; Pries, L.K.; van Os, J. Application of network methods for understanding mental disorders: Pitfalls and promise. *Psychol. Med.* **2017**, *47*, 2743–2752. [CrossRef]

behavioral sciences

MDPI

Review

Suicide Prevention Measures at High-Risk Locations: A Goal-Directed Motivation Perspective

Laura Joyner [1,2,*], Jay-Marie Mackenzie [2], Andy Willis [3], Penny Phillips [3], Bethany Cliffe [2], Ian Marsh [4], Elizabeth Pettersen [5], Keith Hawton [6] and Lisa Marzano [1]

1 Department of Psychology, Middlesex University, London NW4 4BT, UK
2 School of Social Sciences, University of Westminster, London W1W 6UW, UK
3 NSPA Lived Experience Advisory Group, Ewell KT17 2AF, UK
4 Faculty of Medicine, Health and Social Care, Canterbury Christ Church University, Canterbury CT1 1QU, UK
5 Samaritans, Ewell KT17 2AF, UK
6 Centre for Suicide Research, Department of Psychiatry, University of Oxford, Oxford OX3 7JX, UK
* Correspondence: l.joyner@mdx.ac.uk

Abstract

Understanding the effectiveness of suicide prevention measures for high-risk locations can often be challenging as many rely, at least to some degree, on psychological processes (e.g., engaging with help-seeking behaviours). Establishing how these measures may influence decision-making during a suicide attempt could be helpful for understanding how and when they may be most effective at preventing deaths. In the present work, we consider how suicide prevention measures may influence "goal pursuit" as it unfolds. Drawing on findings from across the suicide prevention literature, we apply the descriptive framework outlined in GOAL Architecture to consider how different measures may shape perceptions of "distance", "time", and "rate of progress" and, in turn, could influence levels of motivational drive associated with specific acts (e.g., "accessing means for suicide"). This is discussed in relation to real-time decisions around accessing means for suicide, avoiding intervention by a third party, and engaging in help-seeking behaviours. As well as the psychological processes that could encourage or prevent an individual from disengaging from a suicide attempt, we also consider potential risks and the influence of person-level factors.

Keywords: suicide attempt; suicide prevention; goal pursuit; motivation; means restriction; built environment; surveillance; help-seeking

1. Introduction

Annually, over 720,000 suicides are recorded globally (World Health Organisation, 2025). In the UK, around a third of suicides occur in public places such as railways, carparks, cliffs, and bridges (Office for National Statistics, 2023). Suicide has a lasting impact on families and friends, but suicides that occur in public locations can also create trauma for a wider group of people, including potential witnesses and staff dealing with their aftermath (Giupponi et al., 2019). They can also have substantial financial implications for affected industries, public health organisations, and responders (Holdaway et al., 2012). An additional concern about suicides in public locations is possible media reporting of incidents, which could highlight locations of concern and potentially lead to imitative behaviours (Marzano et al., 2025; World Health Organisation, 2023). Indeed, this explains why over 60% of local authorities in the UK currently implement interventions at high-risk locations, and why in England the National Institute for Health and Care Excellence (2018) recommends that suicide prevention measures are vital at high-risk locations.

Suicide prevention measures at high-risk locations are often categorised into four general approaches: (1) restricting access to means, (2) increasing opportunity and capacity for human intervention, (3) enabling help-seeking, and (4) changing public image of the site (Owens et al., 2015). However, understanding why certain measures have or have not been effective at preventing suicides is not always straightforward. For measures that fully restrict physical access to means for suicide, the explanation of how this can be effective is often clearer than for measures that rely, either to a degree or entirely, on psychological effects (e.g., signage encouraging help-seeking). If the processes underpinning such psychological effects are not considered, this arguably hinders the development of effective intervention design and creates barriers to appropriate evaluation. Exploring the influence of specific factors (e.g., measure placement, design characteristics) in a systematic manner may help to develop understanding around these psychological effects.

In the present paper, we draw from the psychological literature around goal pursuit, motivation, and behaviour with the aim of further understanding how, why, and when measures implemented at high-risk locations may prove effective at preventing suicides. Given the topic under discussion, it is worth noting that the use of formal, academic language to describe behavioural processes may not always align with the sensitivity needed to discuss subjects such as suicide. This is especially the case when key terms may also hold different meanings for wider audiences. To clarify, as we are interested in exploring the potential impact of suicide prevention interventions at high-risk locations on related goal-pursuit processes, the definition of a "goal" being "a cognitive representation of a desired end state that a person is committed to attain" (Milyavskaya & Werner, 2018, p. 5) applies here. For the purpose of this paper, we therefore view a goal to be something that is specific or abstract that an individual wants to approach or avoid in the future that may shape their decisions and ultimately guide their behaviour. The term "motivation" is also used to reflect "a person's willingness to exert physical or mental effort in pursuit of a goal or outcome" (American Psychological Association, n.d.). Our use of this term refers specifically to the amount of motivational drive associated with individual goals (i.e., "motivational value").

While it may seem counterintuitive to view suicide through a lens of "goal attainment", research on goal pursuit has provided the basis of much work on behaviour change, including within health psychology (e.g., Schrooten et al., 2012). When a goal becomes activated, an individual may mobilise resources and identify actions for pursuit. However, both the goal and these underlying processes may occur unconsciously, i.e., without the person being actively aware this is happening (Kopetz et al., 2018). Yet, it is in no way suggested here that decisions and evaluations made when individuals are under mental distress and/or in response to adverse events and circumstances are always conscious.

Throughout this paper, we consider a small selection of specific goals that may or may not be active while an individual is approaching or reaches a high-risk location (i.e., "access area of danger", "avoid intervention by third party", "seek help"), rather than looking at suicidal behaviours more broadly. We believe it is helpful to focus on these specific examples set within what may be a relatively brief moment in time (vs. a person's lifetime) to further our understanding of the psychological effects associated with different types of suicide prevention measures that may be deployed at high-risk locations specifically and to inform ways of quantifying their effectiveness. While this means that the present work does not address the periods leading up to or following an attempt, prior research looking at goal pursuit in the context of self-injurious and other high-risk behaviours suggests that people may be less likely to engage with such behaviours when alternative means to fulfil their needs (e.g., self-regulation of emotions) are provided (Kopetz et al., 2018). While not the main focus of this article, the wider systemic issues that may present barriers for some individuals to fulfil their needs (e.g., accessing help) are therefore worth considering in this context. Examples of this are discussed here in the context of help-seeking (e.g., prior barriers to access).

Before exploring the relationship between specific suicide prevention measures and attempt-related actions in more detail, we look first at existing work from the suicide prevention literature that has addressed issues relating to "goals" and "motivations". Next, we provide some wider background on processes of goal prioritisation and dynamic changes to motivation. We then explore how measures recommended for high-risk locations may influence levels of motivational drive from a goal-directed motivation perspective—specifically, how the use of measures that restrict access to means, that increase the likelihood of third-party intervention, and that encourage help-seeking, may change the path of goal pursuit along the gradients outlined in GOAL Architecture (i.e., rate of progress, distance, time).

1.1. Goal Pursuit & Suicide

Across the suicide prevention literature, the concepts of "goals" and "motivation" have been researched in varying ways. Firstly, a body of work has looked at the motivations associated with suicide attempts, such as hopelessness or burdensomeness (e.g., May et al., 2020; May & Klonsky, 2013). Others have considered suicide risk in the context of goal regulation processes, such as goal re-engagement and disengagement (e.g., O'Connor et al., 2012). Baston (2024) applied a goal system approach to help explain suicidal behaviour. In addition, there is work applying action theory to describe suicidal behaviour as a goal-directed process (e.g., Valach et al., 2006, 2016). While this body of work is useful for developing an understanding of the psychological processes preceding a suicide attempt, less is known about decision-making processes during the attempt itself.

An individual holds multiple goals organised across different levels, some of which may be complementary, potentially even facilitating subsequent or overarching, superordinate goals. From this perspective, an individual who holds an abstract superordinate goal related to "making a suicide attempt" could pursue this goal via several concrete subordinate goals. In turn, these subordinate goals may reflect specific, sequential actions that could contribute towards an attempt (e.g., "access a high-risk area") or support the pursuit of this goal in other ways (e.g., "avoid interventions by other people"). While previous research on suicide prevention and goals has focused more on the superordinate level (e.g., identifying underlying motives), in interviews individuals with lived experience of surviving a suicide attempt have talked about "the steps" involved (Marcinkevičiūtė et al., 2024), suggesting the subordinate level is also relevant.

It is also notable that in both research and guidance, suicide prevention measures for high-risk locations are often categorised in ways that relate to subordinate-level goals—for example, "prevent access to means", "increase opportunity for human intervention", or "encourage help seeking" (e.g., Owens et al., 2015). Exploring the ways in which suicide prevention measures may then influence the "micro-decisions" made by individuals (e.g., approach, retreat, seek out alternate routes, etc.) in relation to these actions could arguably help further our understanding of how and when they prove most effective at preventing suicides, or even identify when they may risk causing harm.

Moreover, the principles of goal-directed behaviour may still apply when individuals are experiencing emotional distress. Kopetz and Orehek (2015) suggest that physical self-harm produces immediate consequences that aid the attainment of emotional regulation goals. For example, previous work found the application of bodily harm (vs. a sham condition) resulted in reduced stress responses in participants who had engaged in non-suicidal self-injury (Reitz et al., 2015). Put simply, rather than a failure of self-regulation, Kopetz and Orehek (2015) propose that behaviours such as self-harm may allow some individuals to achieve an immediate goal of regulating emotional distress. Importantly, however, such self-harming behaviours may also be reduced if alternative means of fulfilling the goal are provided. This body of work not only challenges the idea that emotional distress impairs cognitive control but also illustrates how potentially harmful actions may be pursued in the moment if perceived to be an effective way of addressing immediate needs (especially if safer alternatives are not accessible).

We believe that such an approach is relevant for a number of other reasons. Firstly, viewing goal pursuit as a complex, dynamic process allows for the possibility that individuals hold a broad variety of goals in the lead-up to and during a suicide attempt. Indeed, the goal-directed motivation literature suggests individuals may be unable to pursue all their goals at any one time (and therefore must prioritise specific goals over others). Considering which goals may facilitate an attempt and therefore may be activated (e.g., avoid attention, avoid third-party intervention) and which conflict and therefore may become inhibited (e.g., social or help-seeking goals) may be useful for understanding the effectiveness of specific measures, particularly when used in combination with other interventions.

Moreover, understanding how these measures may themselves shift the prioritisation and pursuit of subordinate-level goals could prove more valuable in understanding their effectiveness than simply focusing on the superordinate (e.g., overarching attempt-related goal). In particular, distinguishing between the expected impact of a suicide prevention measure on the pursuit of a specific action, independent of the reasons behind the presentation, could be a useful step towards understanding their effectiveness across a range of different contexts. This aligns with certain general theories of behaviour—for example, the Theory of Interpersonal Behaviour, where "facilitating conditions" moderates the relationship between "intentions" and "behaviour" (Triandis, 1977). From this perspective, by influencing the situational context, suicide prevention measures have the potential to inform decision-making around goal pursuit in real time, but only to a point (e.g., disengaging from an "access means for suicide goal" at one location does not necessarily mean a person will also disengage from the attempt generally). Such an approach allows us to consider the influence of variations in strength of motivation (i.e., motivational drive) and other person-level factors (e.g., self-efficacy), which, as we discuss throughout the paper, may help those working in suicide prevention distinguish when and how measures relying on psychological effects are most effective.

Goal Prioritisation

Goal prioritisation is a dynamic process allowing us to navigate complex environments via constant decisions around "which goals to prioritise, how much to invest in pursuit of those goals, and when to divert their attention towards other goals" (Ballard et al., 2022, p. 146). While decisions around goal prioritisation may sometimes involve deliberative thinking, research suggests that they can also be made intuitively—for instance, by opting for heuristic strategies when time or cognitive resources are more limited (Alister et al., 2024). Notably, dual-process theories of cognition suggest that such intuitive decisions occur rapidly, are automatic, and at times are made unconsciously (Evans, 2008). This suggests that choices around the prioritisation of which goals to pursue are not always based around effortful decision-making processes based on logic or critical thought. Instead, situational cues may influence choices around whether a person continues to pursue or disengage from a specific goal in ways that do not require effortful deliberation or even conscious thought.

An important factor in goal prioritisation is the goal's motivational value, as in, "the extent to which one is driven to allocate resources to it" (Ballard et al., 2022, p. 146). This drive may firstly be influenced by desire, which is "an affectively charged motivation toward a certain object, person, or activity that is associated with pleasure or relief from displeasure" (Hofmann & Van Dillen, 2012, p. 317). In some instances, desire may correspond with a specific goal and therefore provide varying degrees of motivation towards goal pursuit. In other contexts, desire may conflict with a goal and instead present a temptation to deviate away from said goal, requiring an individual to engage with effortful self-regulation to counter its effect (Hofmann & Van Dillen, 2012). Desire is therefore an important consideration when seeking to understand the pursuit of goals related to suicide attempts, as research suggests suicidal crises may be motivated by strong affective states such as extreme emotional distress (e.g., May et al., 2020; May & Klonsky, 2013). As such, a person may be motivated to pursue a potentially harmful goal (e.g., a suicide attempt) if they associate it with their desires (e.g., a drive to relieve emotional distress and/or feelings of entrapment). If that is the case, the strength of this desire will then also influence how motivated individuals are to pursue such a goal.

While the decision-making processes involved when pursuing a goal may at times be intuitive and even unconscious, they can still inform behaviour (e.g., taking a familiar route). Motivational value may also influence behaviour—for example how much effort an individual is willing to put in, their willingness to persist when faced with obstacles, and specific task-related choices (e.g., if motivated to avoid intervention, a person may turn left if there is a police officer to their right). As illustrated in Figure 1, when an individual is beginning to pursue specific tasks or "steps" leading up to a suicide (e.g., travelling to a location, accessing means, avoiding other people/intervention), the strength of motivation driving those steps may be relatively higher than that for alternative goals (e.g., help-seeking). Moreover, research also suggests that when an individual is highly committed to a "focal goal", alternative goals may be cognitively inhibited (Shah et al., 2002). In other contexts, this automatic and unconscious cognitive process, known as "goal shielding", may be greatly beneficial for helping reduce external distractions that may hinder successful goal attainment. However, given that goal shielding can also be influenced by factors including emotional state (Plessow et al., 2011; Shah et al., 2002), such cognitive processes are likely to also be important considerations for understanding how and when some interventions can prove effective (e.g., help-seeking signage).

The motivational value of any goal also changes over time. On one hand, this may relate to changes to the perceived value of the goal—for instance, how desirable achieving the goal is. However, the motivational value may also be influenced by feasibility—as in, how likely it is the goal will be achieved (Milyavskaya & Werner, 2018). Feasibility may be shaped by a broad range of external factors that may facilitate or, alternatively, threaten goal attainment. For instance, an individual with a goal to have a healthy lunch at work (a subordinate goal relating to a broader, superordinate health goal) may feel less motivated to pursue this specific goal if the store they intended to purchase lunch from is considerably farther away than unhealthier alternatives. Furthermore, while distance alone might not deter an individual from pursuing their healthy lunch goal, if colleagues were then to invite them to lunch at a nearer restaurant, this relative closeness may provide added motivation required to prioritise a different superordinate goal, e.g., one related to social needs. As a result, they may no longer pursue the original goal of visiting the shop for healthy food but instead adjust (e.g., selecting a healthy menu option) or even abandon the healthy eating goal for that day. While it may be distant from the issue of suicide, this example illustrates how the dynamic nature of goals allows us to navigate complex physical and social environments.

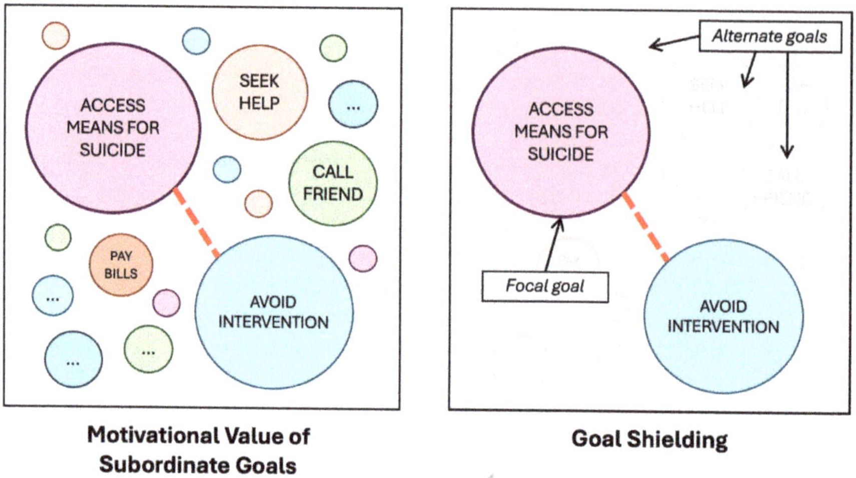

Figure 1. Examples of goal-directed motivation and the goal-shielding process.

In the context of suicide prevention at high-risk locations, it may be that specific preventative measures and other related factors (e.g., the presence of members of the public) at times threaten the perceived feasibility of achieving attempt-related goals in ways that influence their motivational value (Figure 2). If that is the case, then factors within an encountered situation (e.g., means restriction measures, presence of others) may encourage an individual to re-evaluate feasibility and in turn could result in a reduction in the motivational value of the specific goal. At the same time, alternative goals that may previously have been inhibited (e.g., help-seeking) may become more salient, especially if changed conditions make this more feasible or attractive. From this perspective, situational factors could influence the prioritisation of goals in real time in ways that could aid (or, in other cases, potentially undermine) suicide prevention efforts.

Recently, a descriptive framework has been proposed to help quantify these motivational dynamics. The Goal-Orientated Action Linking (GOAL) framework integrates key theories of goal pursuit to help quantify dynamic changes in goal prioritisation (Ballard et al., 2022). Ballard et al. (2022) also note that the framework can be used to better understand the motivational dynamics that occur when pursuing a goal, e.g., across interdependent decisions. This may therefore be particularly relevant when trying to understand the psychological impact of encountering multiple suicide prevention measures at a high-risk location. The framework assumes that the perceived impact of one's actions on goal attainment influences levels of motivation towards achieving one's goal and suggests that motivational value varies and updates in response to three gradients: distance (i.e., proximity), time to deadline, and rate of progress required (i.e., how hard the goal is to achieve). These gradients then provide a basis for quantifying the extent to which an individual may be driven to allocate resources to achieve a particular goal. Throughout this paper, we will therefore consider the potential impact of suicide prevention interventions and other relevant factors on these gradients to understand how they may impact motivation and, in turn, influence behaviour.

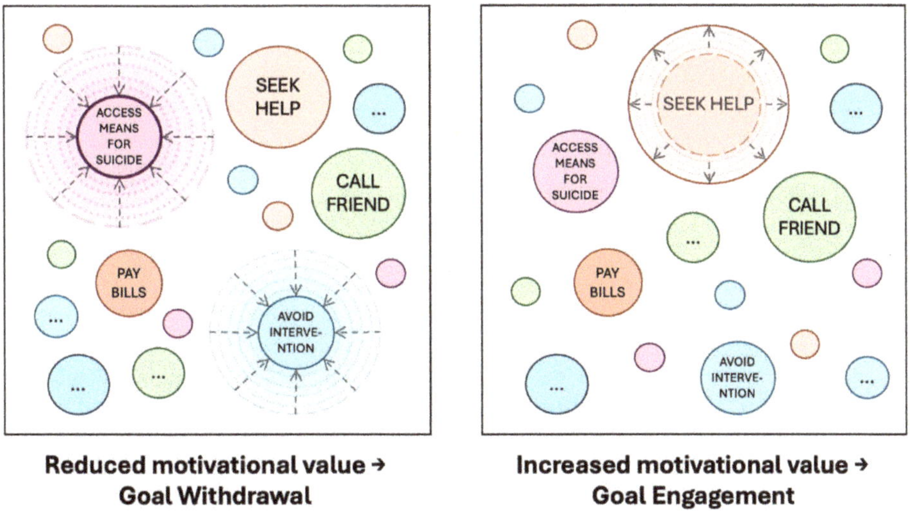

Figure 2. Goal re-prioritisation through changes to motivational value.

2. Restricting Access to Means for Suicide

While arguably not as effective as "full" restriction, research suggests implementing partial restriction to means may help to prevent suicides. These measures do not entirely fully restrict access to an area—for instance, due to barriers or other measures preventing access being lower or not long enough to cover all possible access points (Shin et al., 2024). Despite this, there are examples of partial restriction measures that have contributed to an overall reduction in suicides on railways (e.g., Fredin-Knutzén et al., 2022), at bridges (e.g., Shin et al., 2024), and at high-rise buildings (Mohl et al., 2012), as well as examples where they did not (e.g., Hemmer et al., 2017; Shin et al., 2024). It is therefore important to determine how and why these mitigations work in preventing suicides to better inform intervention design in the future.

As previously discussed, the application of the framework from GOAL Architecture (Ballard et al., 2022) may provide a useful way of interpreting and quantifying the effects of measures that restrict access to means. While certain "full restriction" measures will, of course, present a substantial physical barrier to access, it is sometimes suggested that partial restriction measures act more as a psychological deterrent (e.g., Ross et al., 2020). This is particularly the case where physical access is in no way restricted—for instance, when vehicle (but not pedestrian) access to a high-risk location is restricted (Isaac & Bennett, 2005; Skegg & Herbison, 2009). Yet, research also indicates that not all physical adjustments within an environment will have an impact on suicide rates, suggesting that there are nuances to how and when any psychological deterrent effect occurs. The following section therefore explores how two gradients from GOAL Architecture could be applied to better understand the psychological effects of means restriction measures. First, we discuss how changes to perceived access may influence the effectiveness of some means restriction measures, and how effectiveness may differ across population groups. We then discuss the influence of proximity on motivation to access a high-risk area, both in the context of measures that increase proximity and of measures that cover only some access points.

2.1. Rate-of-Progress Gradient

The Interpersonal–Psychological Theory of Suicide (Van Orden et al., 2010) identifies acquired capability as an important factor for understanding suicide attempts. Experiences such as mental rehearsal, "dry runs", and familiarity (as well as temporary states such as intoxication) may influence perceived capability (Smith & Cukrowicz, 2010). In the context of means restriction, individuals with lived experience of surviving suicide attempts have also indicated that ease of access may be an important decision-making consideration when looking to access a high-risk area (Mackenzie et al., 2025; Marsh et al., 2021; Marzano et al., 2021; Norman et al., 2023; Rosen, 1975). From a goal-pursuit perspective, it is suggested that a "person is motivated to prioritise a goal to the extent that doing so increases their chances of attaining the goal and/or failing to do so decreases their chances" (Ballard et al., 2022, p. 167). As such, a person's beliefs about the likelihood of progressing past full or partial measures (i.e., their outcome expectations) may provide some insight into understanding why and when measures may prove effective at preventing suicides.

Across the goal-pursuit literature, there are different perspectives as to how "rate of progress" may influence motivational value (Ballard et al., 2022). There is the Expectancy Perspective, which suggests that a goal's motivational value will be greater when it is easier to achieve. However, in some contexts, some people may be motivated by challenging goals (the difficulty perspective). Another approach, the achievability perspective, suggests "motivation is the highest when the rate of progress required to reach a desired or undesired state is moderate" (Ballard et al., 2022, p. 151). Depending on the task at hand, there is evidence for all three perspectives. As person-level factors such as individual differences and skill level can also influence the way in which perceived effort impacts motivation (Ballard et al., 2022), considering how the design of measures may increase difficulty–ease of access may also be useful for understanding context-specific effectiveness.

2.1.1. Environmental Changes to Decrease Ease of Access

For some, the potential benefit of applying such a psychological framework to better understand why full means restriction can help prevent suicides may be unclear. Arguably, some measures will simply make the prospect of proceeding past them too physically challenging for most people. For instance, research suggests that barriers above 2.3 m are more effective at preventing suicides on bridges (e.g., Hemmer et al., 2017). Similarly, studies that have investigated the impact of removing restriction measures have found this to be associated with an increase in deaths by suicide at some high-risk locations (Beautrais, 2001; Beautrais et al., 2009). Such examples illustrate how making access to means extremely difficult or at times impossible can help prevent suicides. However, at many high-risk locations, full restrictions to means may not always be possible or even feasible. For example, engineering constraints such as weight restrictions may prevent the installation of new barriers on some bridges. Alternatively, at railway stations that serve different models of trains, variations in door positions may prevent the installation of platform-screen doors. Measures that only partially restrict access to means may therefore be a more viable alternative in some contexts.

While little is known about the psychological mechanisms underpinning any preventative effects of partial restriction measures, researchers have previously suggested that these measures may reduce the perceived ease of access (Fredin-Knutzén et al., 2022; Mohl et al., 2012) or make access more difficult (Mackenzie et al., 2025; Shin et al., 2024). Furthermore, in a previous qualitative study, one individual with lived experience of surviving a suicide attempt indicated that upon encountering a fence that they felt in another context they would be able to climb, the substantial effort to access the high-risk area (e.g., by climbing over) produced doubts that then influenced their decision not to proceed further (Heesen et al., 2024). This might suggest that while an individual's judgements around perceived difficulty may not directly influence any overarching (superordinate) suicide-related goal, they may instead allow a specific attempt-related act (subordinate goal, e.g., access a high-risk area) to be deprioritised in the moment.

Evaluating the literature from this perspective may therefore help provide insights into how, why, and when certain measures prove effective at preventing suicides. Firstly, the height of a barrier provides a clear quantifiable example of how a means restriction measure may impact perceived difficulty. For example, "full" barriers of heights of 5 m (Sinyor & Levitt, 2010), over 3 m (Dwyer et al., 2023; Hemmer et al., 2017; Pelletier, 2007), and over 2.3 m (Hemmer et al., 2017) have previously been associated with complete reductions in suicide rates at bridge locations. Here, the height of these measures alone suggests it is likely difficult for most people to scale them unassisted (although characteristics related to materials and design may play a further role (e.g., Dwyer et al., 2023)).

Moreover, barriers around 1.9 m to 2 m (Bennewith et al., 2007; Hemmer et al., 2017) have been associated with significant, but not total, reductions in suicide rates on bridges (notably, such barriers are below recommended minimums, e.g., 2.5 m, as recommended by Owens et al. (2015)). Learnings around the effectiveness of even lower height barriers may provide important insights into when and how means restrictions measures prove effective at preventing suicides.

Indeed, research suggests that compared to no barriers, lower barriers prevent some (but not all) suicides. For example, installing "half-height platform screen doors" 1.2 m–1.65 m high has previously been associated with a significant, but not complete, reduction in suicide rates on metro platforms (Chung et al., 2016; Okada & Oshima, 2025; Ueda et al., 2015; Xing et al., 2019). In another study, the addition of 1 m-high mid-track fencing (i.e., intermediate fencing between tracks restricting access to high-speed lines) was associated with a reduction in suicides at a railway station (Fredin-Knutzén et al., 2022). An important point to note here is that in both types of environments there previously would have been no physical barrier to entry. This is arguably very different from interventions adding further height to a bridge barrier, for instance, where it is likely that some form of barrier (albeit a smaller one) was already in place. Similarly, previous work suggests that differences in height of as little as 30 cm (i.e., 1.2 m vs. 1.5 m) may influence the level of effectiveness of barriers (Xing et al., 2019). As illustrated in Figure 3, as the height of barriers increases, the perceive ease of access may decrease, which, in turn, may have an additive influence on reducing motivation.

While the extent to which any prevention effects observed with smaller or lower barriers are due to physical factors is unclear, others have suggested barriers of similar heights are not necessarily considered difficult to climb (Ross et al., 2020). As Ross et al. (2020) also suggest, such measures may act as psychological deterrents, at least for some individuals. Indeed, from a goal-pursuit perspective, the presence of partial barriers may influence the perceived ease or difficulty of progressing further (e.g., to reach an area of danger and/or to do so as inconspicuously as possible). If that is the case, then the presence of such measures may prompt individuals to re-evaluate and potentially update their beliefs about the likelihood they will be able (and the effort required) to proceed onwards (i.e., outcome expectations). Where a measure adds a (perhaps unexpected) degree of difficulty, re-evaluation of outcome expectations may, at the very least, prompt hesitation (e.g., Heesen et al., 2024). It may also have the potential to influence the total motivational value of the goal itself (Figure 4). If changes to the perceived rate of progress are substantial enough, for some individuals this could be enough to encourage withdrawal from the goal (at least in the immediate term). This might provide one explanation as to why lower barriers are effective for preventing some, but not all, suicides.

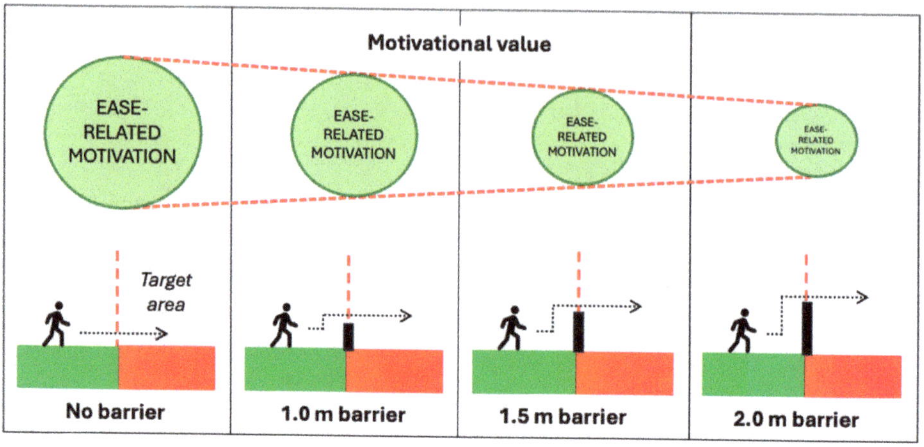

Figure 3. Example of the influence of increasing barrier height on motivational value.

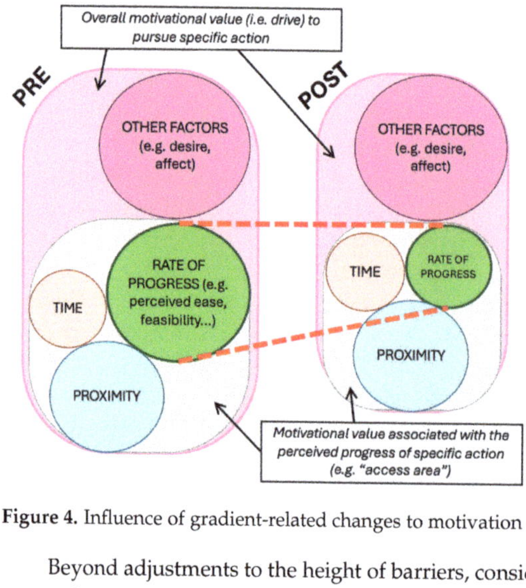

Figure 4. Influence of gradient-related changes to motivation on a goal's total motivational value.

Beyond adjustments to the height of barriers, considering how means restriction measures relate to one another across an ease–difficulty spectrum may be useful for developing a better understanding as to when and why they do (or do not) help prevent suicides. The potential value of this approach perhaps becomes clearer when considering other types of physical adaptations to an environment that have demonstrated some benefits in the context of suicide prevention. For example, research suggests there may be other types of modifications that could also be helpful at preventing suicides by making access more challenging. For example, at bridges, the use of curved barriers (Beautrais et al., 2009; Hemmer et al., 2017; Perron et al., 2013) and rolling bars (Shin et al., 2024) has been associated with reductions in suicides. Such modifications that increase the difficulty of accessing a space in ways other than simply increasing height are also recommended in official guidance (e.g., Owens et al., 2015). However, while factors like changes to height can easily be measured and compared, without formal frameworks to help quantify the psychological impact of other types of changes influencing perceived ease of access, it remains difficult to make formal comparisons. This is where considering the impact of physical adaptations on perceived ease–difficulty of access could be useful for understanding how means restriction measures work, as both physical and psychological deterrents.

Finally, interpreting the influence of a measure in relation to perceived ease–difficulty may also be useful to understand why certain interventions fail to be effective "psychological deterrents" when others appear to prevent at least some deaths. For example, Mohl et al. (2012) found that the placement of a single guard rail bar 18 cm above windowsills reduced suicides from a high-rise hospital building. Yet, while this minimal adjustment to an environment was found to be effective, another study found that the addition of lightweight, 10 cm-tall bird spikes to a 90 cm bridge parapet was not effective at preventing suicides (Shin et al., 2024). On one hand, it may be that the findings observed here are in relation to their impact on barrier height. However, from a goal-pursuit perspective, it could also be that relatively weaker and potentially easier-to-remove mitigations do not present a substantial-enough barrier to impact motivation. Indeed, interviews with individuals with lived experience of surviving a suicide attempt indicate that barriers left in poor condition may be seen as potentially breakable, which in turn can influence the perceived ease of access (Mackenzie et al., 2025). Together, this suggests there may also be a need for measures to influence perceived difficulty in a meaningful way—not just in terms of height, but also in terms of factors such as physical robustness, materials, and surface texture playing a role. For example, industry research has identified some of the strengths and weaknesses of physical attributes for a range of fencing designs, including factors such as ease/difficulty to scale, but also cutting with tools (Stanchak et al., 2015). Distinguishing and quantifying specific design features across an ease–difficulty spectrum may therefore be beneficial to help further develop our understanding of effectiveness of measures across a variety of factors.

2.1.2. Integrating Person-Level Factors

As previously noted, certain means restriction interventions may be effective at preventing some but not all deaths by suicide. This means there is arguably value in understanding for whom the measures are or are not effective, and for determining why this may be the case. From a psychological perspective, it is not just environmental factors that influence behaviour but also person-level factors. This can include factors such as overall motivational desire and affective states, both arguably important factors in understanding suicidal behaviour. However, Social–Cognitive Theory (SCT) suggests that both person-level and environmental-level factors can interact with one another in ways that influence behavioural outcomes (e.g., Schunk & Usher, 2012). Similarly, the Theory of Interpersonal Behaviour suggests the level to which conditions "facilitate" behaviour moderates the relationship between intentions (e.g., affect) and behaviour (Triandis, 1977). Put simply, the extent to which a physical measure is effective in encouraging an individual to disengage from proceeding onwards into a high-risk area is likely to vary in relation to person-level factors.

An example of this is where the level of effectiveness of interventions differs across genders. In one study, a downwards trend in suicides was found only for women after a combination of measures was introduced (including a 1.3 m fence) at a high-risk location (Ross et al., 2020). As previously noted, focus groups with police indicated that the fence itself was not difficult to climb, and the authors therefore suggested the fence may have presented more of a psychological barrier than a physical one. In another study, it was found that only 1 out of 10 people who died after climbing over a half-height platform screen door were women (Xing et al., 2019). While it is of course not possible to rule out differences in physical ability, this suggests there may be potential value in developing a more detailed understanding of the potential impact of person-level factors on intervention effectiveness. For example, understanding when factors such as gender or age influence the effectiveness of certain measures may be useful for informing the development of safer measures in the future.

Additionally, self-efficacy may influence the effectiveness of some means restriction measures if decisions are based on a perceived reality that, despite feeling "true", may not be factually accurate (e.g., about own strength). If beliefs around perceived difficulty and outcome expectations are biased, this could lead an individual to proceed in a situation where others with the same physical ability might refrain. Were an individual to overestimate their ability (e.g., for climbing), their motivation to proceed onwards may not be affected in the way that it might be for others with lower self-efficacy beliefs. This may be particularly important to consider given what is known about who may be at increased risk of suicide. For instance, during a psychotic episode, some individuals may perceive themselves to have special abilities, such as heightened strength (Ritunnano et al., 2022), which could influence their sense of self-efficacy.

Another consideration is where an individual may have challenges around evaluating the likelihood of a negative outcome. For example, individuals at greater risk of experiencing hypomania may perceive the consequences of risk-taking to be less costly (Devlin et al., 2015), which may mean that the requirement to apply additional effort to access a high-risk area may present as less of a psychological deterrent for such individuals compared to others. While research is required to better understand the impact of individual differences on intervention effectiveness via changes to perceived difficulty, together, these examples illustrate the possibility that "psychological deterrent" effects may not produce similar outcomes across the wider population. If it is the case that such effects are influenced by individual differences, adjustments to design standards may be needed to ensure preventative effects occur across all relevant populations. This is particularly important for ensuring both the effective and equitable development and deployment of future suicide prevention initiatives.

Finally, whether the level of effort required to pass means restriction measures is anticipated may be important for understanding their effectiveness as psychological deterrents. For instance, a person may approach an environment having anticipated no substantial barriers to entry and therefore believed the perceived likelihood of being able to proceed to be relatively high. If they were then to unexpectedly encounter, for instance, a fence, this may prompt an individual to re-assess their beliefs around the likelihood of proceeding further. From a goal-directed motivation perspective, if the perceived rate of progress (e.g., level of difficulty) increases enough to change the outcome expectation, then this may lead to a reduction in the motivational value of the related goal. If this reduction were great enough, then an individual may re-evaluate, and potentially disengage from, pursuing the specific act further (at least temporarily). One consideration might therefore be how prepared an individual is to anticipate the level of effort required to proceed into a high-risk area. Where individuals attend a location with an accurate expectation of the effort required to access a high-risk area—for example, due to planning (e.g., Mackenzie et al., 2025; Marsh et al., 2021)—they may be less likely to need to update these beliefs. The influence of accrued knowledge about a location on the context-specific effectiveness of suicide prevention is therefore another potentially important person-level factor to consider.

2.2. Distance Gradient

Another important aspect identified in the framework proposed by GOAL Architecture is the influence of remaining progress (e.g., distance) on motivation. This is because previous work suggests that motivation increases when the target of the goal is closer (Ballard et al., 2022). The influence of distance on motivation operates in two ways. Firstly, when a person is seeking to avoid an undesired state, the motivation to proceed onwards would likely decrease as they get further away from the target. For at least some suicidal individuals, this may mean that increased distance from, for example, a triggering event may gradually reduce motivational drive. Indeed, previous work has identified elevated risk of suicide in the first six months following a cancer diagnosis (Henson et al., 2019) and in the first 30 days following a bereavement (Pitman et al., 2023). In contrast, when a person is approaching a desired goal (e.g., accessing a high-risk area), their motivation to proceed onwards may increase the closer the target becomes (Figure 5). For example, in relation to rail suicides and suicide clusters, several studies have found that most deaths occur in close proximity to the deceased's home address (e.g., Mishara & Bardon, 2016; Norman et al., 2024; Too et al., 2017). Combined, this illustrates the complex, dynamic nature of goals, as well as the potential impact of distance/proximity in the context of suicide prevention.

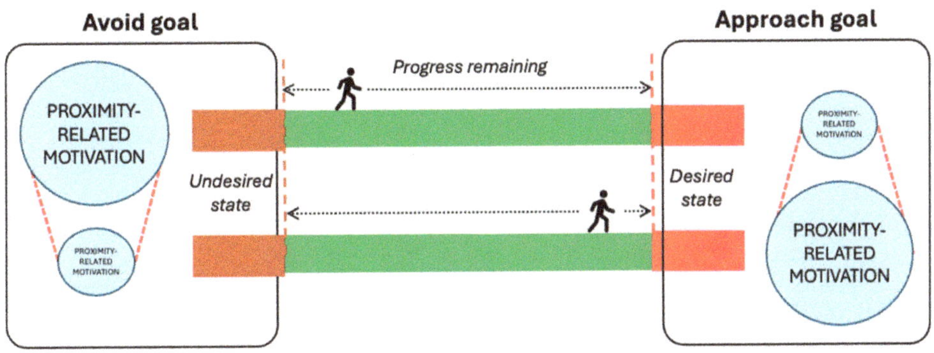

Figure 5. Influence of proximity on motivational value for avoid and approach goals.

In this section, we consider how distance (more specifically, perceived distance remaining) may also influence the effectiveness of means restriction measures. First is the way in which the physical placement of measures may influence their effectiveness. Next, we consider examples where measure design may have not sufficiently increased perceived distance (e.g., through gaps in coverage).

2.2.1. Placement of Intervention

As previously discussed, if a person's goal is to access a specific location (i.e., an approach goal) any "distance-related motivation" may be strongest when there is little further progress remaining. This might suggest that changes that increase the perceived progress required to access means could reduce motivation in ways that could produce a deterrent effect. Indeed, research suggests that introducing restrictions to the quantity of drugs such as paracetamol allowed in a single purchase can help reduce the number (as well as size) of overdoses with these drugs in the population (Hawton et al., 2001). Arguably, such restrictions do not prevent an individual from accessing means but instead increase the amount of effort required to do so (e.g., implementing a need to make multiple purchases across different locations and/or times), which should reduce motivation to proceed onwards. While this, of course, may not result in all suicides by this method being prevented, it provides one potential explanation for the psychological processes associated with this approach.

There is also evidence to suggest that "distance remaining" may be important in the context of high-risk locations. Previous work suggests that proximity to a high-risk area may influence the strength of suicidal thoughts (Marsh et al., 2021) or increase urges (Norman et al., 2023). Individuals have also reported increasing distance (e.g., stepping back) from a high-risk area to self-regulate their behaviour (Marsh et al., 2021). As such, adjustments to perceived proximity (e.g., via changes to physical distance or steps required) may be another relevant (and quantifiable) factor for understanding the effectiveness of suicide prevention measures from a psychological perspective. Indeed, studies suggest that the placement of safety nets placed underneath bridges may be effective at preventing some suicides (Hemmer et al., 2017; Reisch & Michel, 2005; Shin et al., 2025). This is a measure that arguably cannot prevent a person from proceeding beyond the net but does introduce an additional layer to access (i.e., increases progress required) that potentially also creates uncertainty around outcome expectations.

The potential influence of perceived progress on motivation may also help provide insight into why restricting vehicle access to a high-risk location while retaining pedestrian access has previously been associated with reductions in deaths by suicide (Isaac & Bennett, 2005; Skegg & Herbison, 2009). While both sites remained accessible to pedestrians, these temporary road closures meant that the distance required to travel on foot (e.g., vs. from a closer car park) increased during these periods, which were 5 months and 2 years, respectively. For instance, in the study by Skegg and Herbison (2009) a 1.2 km–1.6 km length of road approaching a cliff lookout was closed to vehicles. At both locations, no deaths were recorded during the road closure periods. These findings are particularly notable examples of the dynamic nature of goal value. While in these examples the true physical distance to access a high-risk area did not change, the overall progress required to cover the same ground on foot was greater compared to when a vehicle was used. Arguably, in many cases, the preventative effect observed in these studies would therefore primarily be psychological, as individuals themselves were not prohibited from entering either site (only vehicles). What is not known is whether smaller distances of vehicle restriction would have the same effect. However, from a goal-pursuit perspective, the physical proximity of the placement of such measures would likely be an influencing factor (Figure 6). If the motivational value of approach goals increases as a goal's reference point becomes closer, then this kind of intervention may be more effective the farther away they are positioned. As we discuss in the next section, smaller distances may not be as successful for preventing suicides. However, future research is needed to understand whether the proximity of intervention placements does indeed influence effectiveness for suicide prevention as the goal-directed motivations literature might suggest.

2.2.2. Gaps in Coverage

Another way in which distance may influence the effectiveness of means restriction measures is the proximity of alternative access points. For example, a previous study found that fencing implemented across railways was only associated with a reduction in suicide rates at sites where fencing was over 100 m in length (Clapperton et al., 2023). Specifically, there was a 57% reduction in suicide rates within a 1000 m radius from the midpoint of fences 100 m or greater in length. In contrast, sites with shorter stretches of fencing saw no significant reduction in suicides. This could suggest that some people may have been dissuaded from travelling along the fence to find an access point (i.e., where the fencing ends), but only where the distance required to travel is great enough.

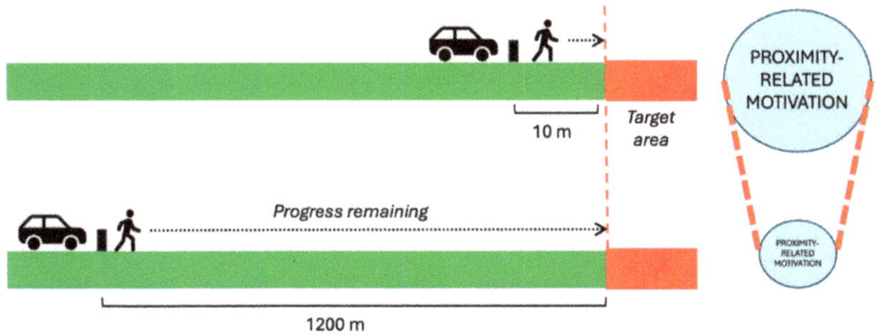

Figure 6. Example of the impact of vehicle restriction measures on perceived proximity and associated motivational value.

Similarly, previous research focusing on bridge sites found barrier-related measures that only covered sections of the bridge (e.g., otherwise leaving gaps for entry elsewhere) were not effective at preventing suicides (Sæheim et al., 2017; Shin et al., 2024). Bridges where barriers have only been added to some (but not all) areas have also observed patterns of localised displacement to other parts of the bridge after installation, albeit with some reduction in suicides (Bennewith et al., 2007). Conversely, removing gaps as part of wider improvements to the design of safety barriers (Beautrais et al., 2009) or through the removal of level crossings (Clapperton et al., 2022) has been associated with a reduction in suicides. Together, these findings suggest that smaller adjustments to perceived progress remaining may not be enough of a deterrent to encourage goal withdrawal, particularly if motivational value (e.g., due to drive) is already relatively high.

3. Increasing Likelihood of Third-Party Intervention

Where an environment is in some way monitored, either formally (e.g., by camera surveillance) or through the presence of other people (e.g., members of the public), it can increase the likelihood that an intervention by a third party may occur. Therefore, while the underlying reasons for a person looking to avoid an intervention may vary (e.g., wanting to avoid police intervention), a common factor is that attention from others may threaten their ability to achieve an "avoid = third-party intervention" goal as well as any associated goals (e.g., "access means"). In this section, we propose that the perceived risk of intervention influences behavioural motivation via changes to the time gradient. In other words, believing that an intervention may occur potentially creates perceived timeframes within which intended actions seem attainable. For example, in a busy environment with overt surveillance (e.g., cameras, patrols) the perceived window of time to "act" without being noticed may potentially be much shorter than in a quiet environment with no visible surveillance. This would have important implications from a goal-pursuit perspective, as motivation can increase when there is a looming deadline, and time available can also influence perceived feasibility, e.g., the likelihood of achieving a goal in the remaining time (Ballard et al., 2022).

Using the existing suicide prevention literature, we first discuss how the presence of other people and surveillance may influence behaviours leading up to a suicide attempt. We then consider the influence of suicide prevention measures on perceived visibility and behaviours. Finally, we discuss how measures can be combined to highlight "atypical behaviours" in ways that indirectly influence means restriction aims.

3.1. Presence of Others and Visibility

Previous work suggests that the presence of other people and potential visibility can be an important factor for some individuals in influencing decisions leading up to or during a suicide attempt. For example, the potential of being seen by other people may influence choice of location (Marsh et al., 2021; Marzano et al., 2019), and as such, they may avoid busy or monitored environments. Additionally, some individuals have indicated that the presence of other people has previously led them to disengage from pursuing an attempt (Marsh et al., 2021). From a goal-pursuit perspective, this might suggest a change to the expected outcome. One reason for this may be the potential negative impact on witnesses (Mackenzie et al., 2025; Marsh et al., 2021; Norman et al., 2023). However, some individuals have reported actively avoiding others or waiting for people to leave as a way of avoiding intervention (Mackenzie et al., 2018). This might suggest that encountering this unexpected development can lead individuals to re-assess the situation in ways that influence outcome expectancies and, in turn, behaviour (indeed, as a participant in one study described, the presence of another person "increases the chance of intervention from zero" (Mackenzie et al., 2025, p. 9)). Notably, re-assessment of beliefs does not necessarily require effortful deliberation and may occur automatically, sometimes even at an unconscious level (Sharot et al., 2023). For instance, if a person were to encounter a barrier to goal attainment, their beliefs about their ability to achieve the goal might change, even if they are not aware of having re-evaluated the situation. This process, known as belief updating, supports dynamic decision making in complex environments and, as such, could influence the perceived likelihood of experiencing an intervention in real time. Simply put, for those seeking to avoid preventive interventions, the presence of others may present a potential barrier to attainment that may lead them to update their beliefs around how likely it is that they will be able to proceed, which in turn may reduce motivation.

Determining how the presence of others might influence motivation may be useful for understanding behaviour. While factors such as proximity of others and ability to avoid them will, of course, be relevant, here we focus on the potential impact on the time gradient—specifically, whether the presence of others increases the salience of a potentially imminent intervention. In creating a perceived timeframe within which an individual must act to avoid intervention, the presence of others may lead some individuals to temporarily disengage from proceeding onwards. Indeed, individuals with lived experience of attempting suicide have reported that being spotted by another person can end a perceived opportunity, and that the presence of others can create a sense of pressure that feels off-putting (Marzano et al., 2019). This might suggest that, at least for some, time pressure produced by the presence of other people may make an action feel less feasible and therefore may act as a short-term deterrent. Yet, another possible outcome in such circumstances is that individuals may act more rapidly, such as refraining from pausing (e.g., Marsh et al., 2021), to avoid intervention.

3.1.1. Lighting-Based Interventions

As we discuss in more detail further on in this section, how an individual responds to a potentially imminent intervention will likely be influenced by other factors (e.g., motivational value, proximity). However, if we assume that any perceived timeframe begins from the moment that an individual is noticed by another person, the anticipation of this may also motivate some individuals to avoid attention. For instance, they may seek out ways to be less visible to others, such as hiding before making an attempt (Mackenzie et al., 2018, 2025; Ryan, 2017). It might therefore be that one way to understand the effectiveness of measures intended to improve visibility within an environment is to consider how they might impact perceived timeframes for potential intervention and, in turn, motivation. For example, previous work suggests that installing blue lights at platform ends may be helpful for preventing suicides (Matsubayashi et al., 2013, 2014), although the extent of the effectiveness of this approach has been contested (Ichikawa et al., 2014). While some suggest this may be due to blue lights producing a "calming effect" on individuals, another pilot intervention at two station platforms in Sweden found that illuminating the ends of platforms with "blue lights" reduced the number of people willing to wait for their train in those areas (National Centre for Suicide Research and Prevention et al., 2022). Such a change in passenger behaviour is arguably difficult to explain through potential "calming effects".

Whether blue light interventions impact motivational drive by influencing expectations about the likelihood of being seen in an environment remains unclear at present. However, the use of lighting as a way to encourage safe behaviour within rail environments has been tested in other ways (Ryan et al., 2022). Within the wider psychological literature, it has been found that the brightness of lighting can be associated with heightened levels of public self-awareness and the self-regulation of behaviour (Steidle & Werth, 2014). In other words, in brightly lit environments, individuals may be more aware of how they are viewed by others and might adapt their behaviour to blend in. From this perspective, a well-lit environment may influence prevention efforts if it increases expectations of being noticed by other people and, in turn, shifts the perceived likelihood of a potentially imminent third-party intervention (e.g., Mackenzie et al., 2025).

Why, then, when thinking about goal-directed motivation might we expect the use of "blue lights" to be any different from standard lighting? Blue-enriched lights (Chellappa et al., 2011) and bright white lights (Vandewalle et al., 2006) are both thought to increase levels of vigilance. It could be the case that by heightening an individual's attention towards situational cues within the environment (e.g., those representing a risk of third-party intervention), blue lights influence perceptions of visibility in a similar way to bright white light. Indeed, research suggests the alerting effects of blue lights are independent of light intensity and instead may be the result of light wavelength (Beaven & Ekström, 2013). As such, a blue light may not need to be as bright as a white light for heightened alertness effects to occur.

Without further research it is not possible to determine the psychological processes that may underpin any potential preventative effect from blue light measures. However, given the ongoing interest in blue lights as a potential suicide prevention measure, whether the properties of blue light (e.g., its shorter wavelengths) make it an appropriate measure for influencing behaviour at high-risk locations is worth considering here. For example, previous work suggests that the influence of blue light on the alerting effect is thought to be mediated by eye colour (Beaven & Ekström, 2013). Specifically, its effects are potentially stronger for those with lighter-coloured irises. There is also evidence to suggest people with blue eyes may be more sensitive to the effects of light generally due to reduced melanin pigment increasing light transmittance (e.g., Nischler et al., 2013; Terman & Terman, 1999). While that is not to say that any influence of blue light on behaviour will necessarily be affected by person-level factors such as eye colour, it does highlight a need for further research outside of suicide prevention to be able to ensure its use would not disadvantage some groups over others (e.g., ethnic groups where darker eyes are a dominant trait) in this context.

3.1.2. Presence of Surveillance Technologies

Given the environmental complexity and scale of some high-risk locations, one potentially useful consideration is whether the proposed "potentially imminent intervention" timeframe can better inform our understanding of how and when surveillance technologies may help prevent suicides. As discussed in the previous section, the perception of being visible to other people may be enough to influence behaviour. Research suggests this may also extend to some surveillance technologies. For example, previous work has found that some suicidal individuals may actively avoid security cameras (Marsh et al., 2021), while others have reported instances of individuals who moved to alternative locations after thinking they could be being watched through CCTV (Mackenzie et al., 2018). This might suggest that the "presence of others" does not need to be physical to be effective at influencing behaviour leading up to a suicide attempt but instead can be inferred in other ways (e.g., through the presence of a surveillance device).

From a psychological perspective, the design of surveillance (and any associated processes) is likely to influence interpretations of intervention timeframes and likelihood in distinct ways (Figure 7). Firstly, if the surveillance is overt, then perceptions of being monitored are likely to be more salient than if covert. Put simply, the more visible and identifiable surveillance devices (e.g., cameras) are, the more aware individuals may be of potentially being under surveillance. As changes in behaviour can occur when an individual believes they are being observed by another person, i.e., "audience effects" (Hamilton & Lind, 2016), it is the perception of being under surveillance, rather than the reality, that is likely to inform outcome expectancies. Indeed, for certain types of technology, anticipated audience effects may not always correspond with actual audience effects (Kaye et al., 2022)—for example, if surveillance cameras are not actually being monitored in real time. This may be why one Australian study found that, after controlling for other factors, the number of cameras visibly installed in and around railway stations was associated with lower rates of suicide (Too et al., 2015). By increasing the salience of being monitored, identifiable devices (e.g., cameras) may indirectly increase the perceived likelihood of experiencing an intervention in ways that could influence motivation to proceed onwards for some individuals.

It could also be the case that the perception of a potential intervention within an uncertain timeframe may be enough to create doubts around proceeding onwards for some individuals. However, without the physical presence of other individuals, the timeline within which a potential intervention may occur is likely to be unclear (but may still be anticipated (e.g., Kaye et al., 2022)). While uncertainty of outcomes may create doubts around how best to proceed, the inability to gauge time remaining and proximity to a person-led response may lead an individual to rely instead on their beliefs, including their prior experiences. As demonstrated in trespass prevention research (da Silva et al., 2006), where overt surveillance technology does not initiate a physical response, its overall effectiveness may wane over time (potentially due to a lack of person-led response becoming known). Therefore, an individual's beliefs about potential consequences may determine whether overt surveillance is an effective psychological deterrent for preventing suicides.

Situational context	Anticipated audience effects	Anticipated vs. actual audience	Perceived timeframe for person-led intervention
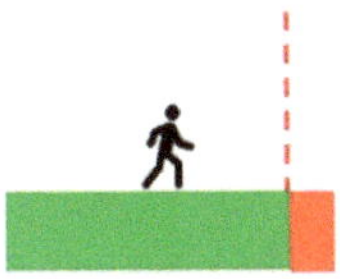 **No surveillance**	Typically lower May vary by person according to beliefs	Varied congruence e.g. if individual believes there may be an audience	Uncertain
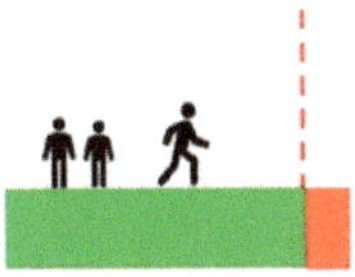 **Other people**	Typically high May vary based on perceived visibility	Typically high congruence	Likely imminent Likely to be influenced by other factors (e.g. proximity)
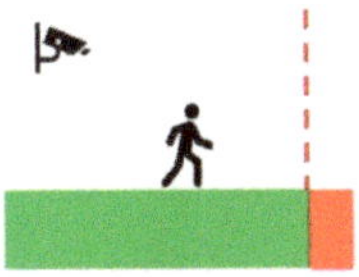 **Overt surveillance**	Medium - high May vary by person according to beliefs (e.g. if the camera feed is monitored in real time), which may also be influenced by prior experiences.	Varied congruence System outputs (e.g. camera feed) may not always be monitored in real-time	Uncertain
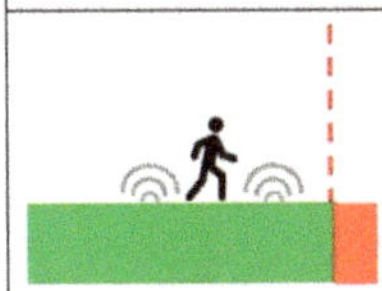 **Covert surveillance**	Typically lower May vary by person according to beliefs	Varied congruence e.g. if individual believes there may be an audience	Uncertain
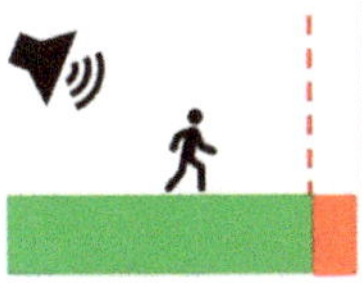 **Automated response**	Typically higher May vary by person according to beliefs and prior experiences.	Varied congruence System may be designed to notify a third party, or could be intended as a standalone measure	Potentially imminent Likely to be influenced by other factors (e.g. prior experiences)

Figure 7. Summary of audience effects and perceived timelines for person-led intervention by surveillance type.

Where surveillance is covert and therefore not visible, it may only influence an individual's behaviour if they anticipate its presence or where its presence becomes known (for example, if a person-led response arrives as a consequence of covert monitoring). Indeed, police officers interviewed in Ross et al.'s (2020) study indicated that after individuals become aware that they had been under surveillance during one suicide attempt at a particular cliff site, they may speed up any future attempts at the same location to avoid similar interventions. As such, perceived timeframes based on prior experiences may influence intervention avoidance behaviour in some circumstances, even without the physical presence of other people. This again illustrates how goal-directed motivation can be influenced by outcome expectancies (i.e., beliefs) rather than simply the information available to individuals in the immediate environment.

3.1.3. Use of Automated Audible and Visual Deterrents

As well as the use of surveillance to promote a person-led response, some systems may produce automated announcements or initiate responsive lighting. While such systems have been trialled in the context of trespass prevention (e.g., da Silva et al., 2006; Kallberg & Silla, 2017), little is known about their effectiveness for suicide prevention. From a cyberpsychology perspective, the activation of these technologies may increase anticipation of a virtual audience due to the synchronous technological response to an individual's behaviour (Kaye et al., 2022). If this also informs the anticipated response (e.g., the expectation that a person will also be notified), it may influence outcome expectancies of a likely intervention. In some cases, any sudden change in perception of an upcoming but uncertain deadline for avoiding intervention may be enough to create doubts about progressing onwards in the immediate moment.

However, concerns have also been raised about the suitability of these approaches for use in suicide prevention due to potential risks (Joyner et al., 2024). If, as we have previously suggested, perceiving a potentially imminent intervention influences motivational value via the time gradient, then there is a chance that this may lead some individuals to act more quickly in an attempt to avoid potential intervention. Indeed, as already noted, the goal-pursuit literature suggests goals become more motivating as the target becomes nearer (Ballard et al., 2022). This would suggest that the rapid presentation of cues signalling a potential intervention within an uncertain timeframe can be associated with a rise in motivational value for some people. Such a process may explain why previous research has shown that audible cues, such as fast train announcements and the sound of trains approaching, may trigger suicidal thoughts in some individuals (Mackenzie et al., 2025; Marzano et al., 2019), potentially even influencing some to speed up when walking towards a platform (Marsh et al., 2021). Others have reported that some individuals move to act quickly when they perceive they may experience an intervention (Ross et al., 2020). Individuals who are highly motivated to either avoid intervention or progress into a high-risk area may therefore be examples of those at particular risk.

In addition to potential intervention, another consideration that may shape an individual's response to an automated surveillance system may be perceptions of associated timeframes. The goal-pursuit literature suggests that the perceived impact of one's actions "are most salient when there is less time available" (Ballard et al., 2022, p. 168). This saliency of timeframes could help to explain, for example, the observed associations between shorter intervals between trains and the number of rail suicides (van Houwelingen et al., 2013). Moreover, the "deadline effect" is associated with a sensitivity to outcome probabilities, which may lead people to prioritise actions with certain outcomes over ones associated with uncertainty (e.g., proceed into a high-risk area vs. remain at the current position and risk potential intervention). The motivational values associated with any distinct but associated goals may therefore be important for understanding the overall drive to act (Figure 8). Although research is needed to determine whether this is the case, it may mean people could be more willing to take risks when an automated deterrent is triggered if their proximity to a high-risk area is relatively low (i.e., distance gradient), if the high-risk area is easy to access (i.e., rate-of-progress gradient), or if they perceive there to be a timebound opportunity in which to act (i.e., time gradient). As such, from a psychological perspective, the conditions around how an individual learns they are under surveillance (whether or not a human-led intervention will be coming in reality) has the potential to produce drastically different outcomes.

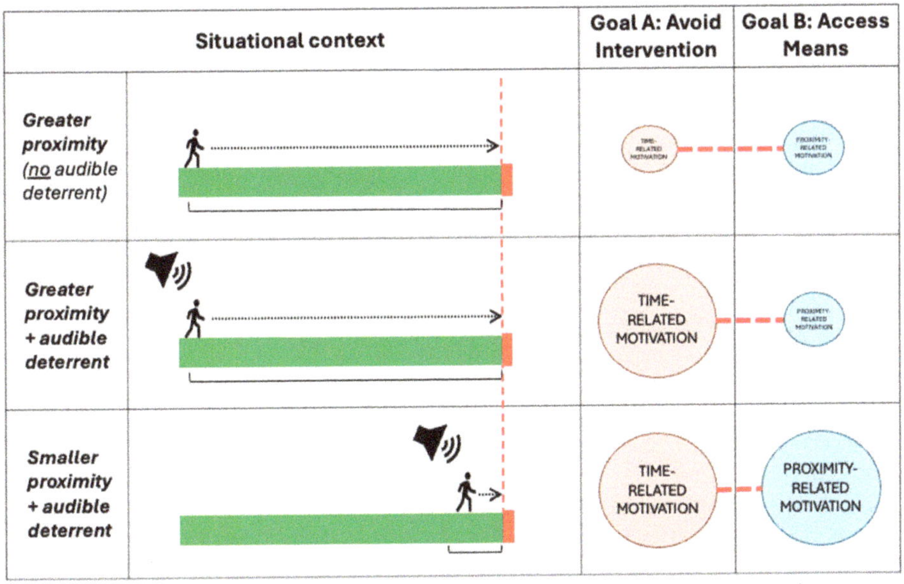

Figure 8. Combined influence of surveillance placement on attempt-related motivation.

A further factor to consider here is the potential influence of individual differences—in particular, the ways in which a person updates their beliefs when presented with new information (e.g., an audible deterrent). While all of us can experience biases when updating our beliefs, some individuals may be more prone than others to experiencing challenges around the integration of new information. One example of this is the relatively common jumping-to-conclusion bias, which relates to a tendency to make hasty decisions based on insufficient information (Kube & Rozenkrantz, 2021) and which has been associated with factors such as cognitive reflection style, openness to the future (Peinado et al., 2024), and psychosis (e.g., Dudley et al., 2016; Rauschenberg et al., 2021). Research also suggests individuals more prone to jumping-to-conclusion bias may be more likely to rely on internal thoughts over contextual information when making these decisions (Özen-Akın & Cinan, 2022). This could mean that some individuals may be more likely than others to associate an audible deterrent with a potentially imminent intervention, without physical evidence that this would be the case (e.g., the presence of other people). While research is again needed to understand whether this would be the case, what is already known about the different ways in which people process information (especially under pressure) suggests that the potential impact of presenting an unexpected intervention (either physically or using technology) will likely differ across the population.

3.2. Drawing Attention to Atypical Behaviours

A final example of how suicide prevention measures may affect ability to avoid intervention is whether the measure can help draw attention to atypical behaviour. Previous work suggests that in the lead-up to a suicide attempt, some people may be motivated to behave in ways that they believe could (but may not actually) reduce attention from other people, e.g., "trying to look normal" (Mackenzie et al., 2018). Therefore, initiating behaviour that may be atypical within an environment (and therefore may draw attention) could create uncertainty for some. As previously discussed, attention from others may increase the salience of a potentially imminent intervention, and therefore anticipation of such attention may be demotivating for some people. This may help explain some of the psychological mechanisms underpinning some interventions.

Firstly, some measures may be designed to make atypical behaviours more prominent to others. An example of this is the use of lengthwise fencing at platform ends in railway stations. This design of fencing notably does not itself block access to the platform end. Instead, a transparent barrier is placed parallel to the platform edge, distinguishing those who stand in the space from others. Research suggests that such a measure may be useful for helping prevent trespassing at some locations, although the observed reduction in suicides was itself not significant (Fredin-Knutzén et al., 2024). It may be the case that when evaluating whether to enter some demarcated spaces, the potential for being noticed becomes more salient and as such presents a deterrent. However, another consideration is whether any time-related impact indirectly influences feasibility in a way that such a measure may be more effective in certain environments. Specifically, for example, in rail and metro environments, coordinating both the timings around avoiding an intervention in addition to the arrival of any train may decrease perceived feasibility of accessing the means for a suicidal act. Therefore, this may increase the likelihood of human-led interventions by drawing attention before a train arrives. Alternatively, the perceived complexity may be demotivating and encourage an individual to move elsewhere. Notably, both outcomes were observed in a study by Fredin-Knutzén et al. (2024). How perceptions of intervention timeframes impact the effectiveness of other measures is therefore a potentially valuable avenue for future research.

Indeed, motivations to avoid interventions may arguably also influence the effectiveness of means restriction measures. Behaviours such as climbing a barrier or standing in a high-risk environment would often be considered atypical and therefore may draw attention. The combination of a barrier both delaying efforts to access high-risk environments and helping draw attention to such efforts can create additional time that can facilitate the arrival of a third-party intervention (e.g., Bennewith et al., 2011). However, where an individual intends to proceed past a means restriction measure into a high-risk area, attention from others may also increase the perceived (not just the actual) likelihood that an intervention could happen. As the GOAL Architecture framework outlines, "rate of progress" is influenced by perceived time remaining (Ballard et al., 2022), and measures that increase the likelihood of a third-party intervention (e.g., surveillance) may impact overall outcome expectancies. Therefore, initiating atypical behaviours may indirectly threaten the perceived feasibility of accessing the area successfully (and the anticipation of which may reduce motivation to proceed).

Both of these perspectives provide examples for why considering how a measure might influence motivation may be helpful for determining any impact of combining different suicide prevention measures. While surveillance itself does not necessarily make it "physically harder" to access a high-risk area, whether it is effective at helping to prevent suicides when combined with means restriction measures is still to be determined. Moreover, measures that inadvertently produce some atypical behaviours (e.g., climbing a barrier) could be more effective if the actions are likely to be observed (e.g., via surveillance), but potentially less effective in a remote, unmonitored area. Understanding whether combined measures lead to an increase in rescues or an overall reduction in attempts may be helpful for determining how and why such measures are effective. Utilising a framework such as GOAL Architecture may be one way of quantifying the environmental changes.

4. Help-Seeking

While a person may proceed towards a high-risk location with the primary intention of accessing an area of danger, they may also hold goals around seeking help, even if these are associated with lower motivational value or are even inhibited. If that is the case, then the psychological mechanisms behind effective engagement with measures related to help-seeking will likely differ. In the following sections, the impact of help-seeking as an alternative goal is discussed before considering how applying the gradients from the GOAL Architecture framework may allow us to better understand willingness to engage in help-seeking behaviours.

4.1. Help-Seeking as an Alternative and/or Additional Goal

For some individuals, help-seeking may be an alternative and/or additional goal (one that is potentially inhibited) that conflicts with (rather than facilitates) the primary goal under pursuit when arriving at a high-risk location. As previously noted, some individuals may disengage from attempt-related goals through dynamic changes to their motivational value. This may present an opportunity for help-seeking goals to be pursued if the situation allows for it, even if the help-seeking goals were not prioritised upon arrival. However, for others, commitment to the pursuit of an attempt-related goal may be so strong that alternative outcomes are inhibited.

4.1.1. Goal Shielding

As previously discussed, when an individual is highly committed to a "focal goal", alternative goals that do not aid the attainment of the focal goal may be cognitively inhibited (Shah et al., 2002). While this "goal shielding" process may be beneficial in other contexts, it is likely to be detrimental if an individual's focal goal is something that may cause harm. Indeed, Kopetz and Orehek (2015) suggest that for risky behaviours, goal shielding can allow alternative concerns to become automatically inhibited and lead to motivated distortion, where any consequences are distorted in line with the goal under pursuit. This may mean that for highly committed individuals, other options (e.g., help-seeking) or potentially even the implication of their actions (e.g., on others) may be inhibited. Simply put, someone who might consider seeking help in other contexts may not when highly motivated to pursue a suicide-related act.

The potential implications of goal-shielding are likely to be particularly relevant for understanding the psychological processes around goal pursuit for those experiencing psychological distress. Indeed, research suggests that people may be more likely to inhibit alternative goals when experiencing greater levels of anxiety (Shah et al., 2002) or when under acute psychosocial stress (Plessow et al., 2011). Similarly, affective states high in motivational intensity (e.g., fear) may narrow cognitive scope in ways that can hinder the processing of peripheral information (see Harmon-Jones et al., 2012). As these processes allow attentional resources to be allocated to a focal goal, they may therefore be particularly relevant when considering the effectiveness of help-seeking-related measures, such as signage encouraging help-seeking from a helpline, for example.

4.1.1.1. "Bursting the Bubble"

Interviews with people with lived experience of surviving a suicide attempt suggest that in some cases external stimuli can potentially disrupt these focused states—for example, a child screaming (Geerling et al., 2019; Marsh et al., 2021) or haptic cues from digital devices (Heesen et al., 2024). From a psychological perspective, novel sensory changes within an environment may sometimes hinder behavioural performance, such as the introduction of auditory (SanMiguel et al., 2010) or tactile (Parmentier et al., 2011b) novel stimuli. Research suggests distraction may be more likely to occur when the stimulus is unexpected rather than predictable (Parmentier et al., 2011a). This might suggest that distraction from focused states may be more likely to occur when the stimulus is not anticipated during goal pursuit. Such a process may be one explanation for the "bursting the bubble" effect and may provide some insights into the conditions needed to help an individual disengage from an attempt-related goal.

Furthermore, given the previously noted concerns that unexpected stimuli (e.g., audible deterrents) may impact behaviour in opposing ways, it is important to highlight how "distracting" stimuli may not always produce the same outcomes. Indeed, while novel stimuli may distract in some contexts, they can facilitate goal pursuit in others—for example, when they inform individuals about the timing of a target's arrival (see Schomaker & Meeter, 2015). This may suggest that, in some contexts, novel stimuli may provide information that can help an individual pursue their intended goal (e.g., audible deterrents alerting to a potentially imminent intervention). Recent research also indicates that the relevance of stimuli to primary and secondary tasks may influence whether it is perceived as distracting (Mandal et al., 2024), and therefore, unexpected stimuli may affect behaviour in some but not all situations.

With this in mind, it may be that some "unexpected stimuli" identified in previous interviews (e.g., baby crying, haptic alert) increase the salience of alternative social goals in ways that are sometimes (but potentially not always) helpful in the context of suicide prevention. For example, research suggests photographs of family may create feelings that conflict with any attempt-related goal, which could encourage some individuals to disengage from an attempt (Owens et al., 2019; Stevenson, 2016). However, depending on the circumstances surrounding an attempt, reminders of specific people may not be helpful (e.g., Lin et al., 2009). Moreover, while sounds of babies crying may disrupt focused states for some (Geerling et al., 2019; Marsh et al., 2021), for others it may exacerbate an existing situation, such as for women with perinatal mental health problems (Gair, 2008; Geerling et al., 2019). Therefore, while approaches to help "burst the bubble" may be a useful strategy for helping prevent suicides, the design of any such interventions would still need to be carefully considered.

4.2. Contextualising Help-Seeking at a High-Risk Location

There is no single reason why an individual may wish to seek help while at a high-risk location. For example, they may have disengaged from an attempt-related goal in ways that allow help-seeking-related goals to become salient. Others may approach a high-risk location with the intention of leaving outcomes up to fate (Marsh et al., 2021), which for some might mean they may be open to engaging in help-seeking if the right opportunity were to present itself. Alternatively, it has been suggested that in some instances suicide attempts may have a communicative function—for example, to signal distress or a desire to seek help (May et al., 2020). Moreover, while potentially less common, these "communication motivations" have also been associated with reduced intent and increased probability of intervention (May & Klonsky, 2013). As such, underlying reasons for pursuing a suicide attempt may also influence willingness to engage with help-seeking opportunities. However, regardless of whether an individual has gone to a location to seek help, or if they happen to be at the location when they become motivated to seek help, it may be beneficial to consider what is known about help-seeking behaviours in relation to gradients identified in GOAL Architecture.

Measures that enable help-seeking at high-risk locations may be implemented in a variety of ways. In some cases, there might be people based at the location—for example, staff who have completed gatekeeper training who may be able to facilitate referral to appropriate support (Burnette et al., 2015). Other measures may encourage or mediate help-seeking without the physical presence of a person—for example, installing signage offering support and identifying routes to access help (e.g., helpline signage placed at the location) or placing technology to mediate communication between an individual and remote support (e.g., crisis phones). From a proximity perspective, it may be the case that the location is relatively closer and/or easier to reach than other locations associated with potential support.

If that were the case, then the distance-related motivational value of pursuing help-seeking should be greatest for locations that are most accessible to reach. Indeed, evidence from the wider suicide prevention literature supports this idea. For example, Tadmon and Bearman (2023) found that the suicide risk of individuals was greater the further away they were from accessing mental health care. Similarly, a recent study found men may be at increased risk of dying by suicide as travel time to getting care from the nearest general or psychiatric hospital increases (Barry et al., 2023). Previous work also found that living distance from school was positively associated with increased suicidal ideation in male students (Armstrong & Manion, 2006), suggesting the influence of "distance" is not only associated with formal sources of help. While distance to support is often likely to be reflective of wider systemic issues and other potential co-founders (e.g., distance from hospital in relation to rurality), the general concept of "proximity" to help may also be useful for developing effective ways to tackle these wider issues. For example, a study found providing veterans located in rural areas with a video-enabled tablet helped to increase their levels of engagement with mental health care (e.g., psychotherapy sessions) and was associated with a reduction in suicide behaviours (Gujral et al., 2022). However, these examples illustrate why it may be beneficial to consider the role of distance as a factor potentially informing choice of help-seeking location, as well as to understand the most effective ways to engage those who may be motivated to seek help.

Furthermore, understanding the wider societal context in relation to the time gradient may be a potentially important consideration both for those who are or become motivated to seek help, and those for whom a waning motivation to pursue a suicide attempt may present an opportunity for prevention efforts encouraging help-seeking. Indeed, delays and long wait times for support may lead some individuals to perceive that they may never receive help, which research suggests may be a consideration leading up to an attempt (Punton et al., 2022). This ties into the importance of wider availability and accessibility of mental health support beyond the high-risk location. Others have found long wait lists can also present a barrier for accessing formal support (e.g., Heinig et al., 2021; Wilson & Marshall, 2010), demonstrating the importance of facilitating provision of help when requested. Arguably, some of the factors relating to why someone may be, or become, motivated to seek help while at a high-risk location will be beyond the control of those who oversee the site. However, the dynamic nature of goal pursuit highlights the potential need to encourage engagement with help-seeking goals as, if disengaged from these, potentially harmful alternatives may instead be prioritised.

Effectiveness of Help-Seeking Measures from a Goal-Pursuit Perspective

If, as proposed by GOAL Architecture (Ballard et al., 2022), motivation to pursue help-seeking actions is influenced by time, proximity, and perceived ease, then it may also be valuable to consider how help-seeking measures relate to these gradients, both for evaluation purposes and for supporting the development of effective initiatives. Openly providing individuals with relevant information may be one example that could be beneficial for increasing associated motivational value. For example, advertising phone numbers for helplines may remove the need to research or ask for such information, arguably reducing the progress required to access help (i.e., distance gradient), which in turn may increase the motivational value of help-seeking goals. Furthermore, effective messaging may help destigmatise help-seeking (i.e., rate-of-progress gradient) and potentially encourage individuals in ways that may influence motivation to act (e.g., Duthie et al., 2024). Such measures do appear to influence help-seeking behaviour. Research from the rail industry suggests that running advertising campaigns with local suicide prevention helplines has been associated with increased rates of calls (Gabree et al., 2019). Another study found that over the course of 16 months, signage placed at platform ends at a railway station in Denmark encouraged at least 13 people to call a suicide prevention helpline (Erlangsen et al., 2023). As these examples illustrate, evaluating help-seeking measures using outcomes related to the targeted goal (e.g., number of calls made) may be useful for understanding their effectiveness.

In turn, considering the design elements of help-seeking measures in line with gradients outlined in GOAL Architecture may help optimise their effectiveness. For example, by removing some of the additional barriers individuals may encounter contacting a helpline (e.g., finding a phone or mobile signal, memorising and entering numbers), it may be that the addition of crisis telephones or call help points may reduce some of the potential difficulties around making a call. Such resources do appear to be used for help-seeking (Erlangsen et al., 2023) even if their overall effectiveness for suicide prevention is somewhat mixed (see Pirkis et al., 2015). However, previous work has identified the importance of being able to discretely engage in help-seeking behaviours at public locations (Mackenzie et al., 2025). As such, whether overtly labelled help points could increase perceived likelihood of being noticed by passers-by may be another important design consideration. In contrast to other types of suicide prevention measures, ensuring that interventions to support help-seeking quickly facilitate accessible and/or nearby support may be some of the ways in which they could help encourage help-seeking behaviours.

A further consideration is whether it is possible for some measures that enable help-seeking to be developed in ways that also challenge beliefs related to attempt-related goals in an appropriate manner. Indeed, research by Owens et al. (2019) suggests that during a person-led intervention, caring gestures and (permitted) touch may be useful for tackling feelings of isolation. Others have suggested that offering practical support to confront and address specific stressors may be helpful for some people to regain some sense of control (Player et al., 2015). While signposting to support may also be useful for improving perceived proximity and/or rate of progress towards addressing stressors, considering ways in which this could be tailored to specific needs may be especially important from a goal-pursuit perspective. Indeed, previous research with farmers suggest that they may not always feel that support available to the general public will be useful, especially if they anticipate that these those manning these services may not have a good understanding of their specific needs (Hagen et al., 2022). The ability to signpost to tailored support where possible—for example, by making staff aware of official databases of support organisations that can be filtered by specific need (e.g., publicly accessible websites such as Hub of Hope (https://hubofhope.co.uk/) and Find a Helpline (https://findahelpline.com/))—could be one way of helping to reduce steps to access relevant support. While these approaches will not work for everyone, understanding how existing help-seeking measures (e.g., communications) may help to facilitate or challenge specific goals may be a useful step for understanding when they may be most effective.

Finally, identifying potential barriers to attaining help-seeking goals is likely to be important for developing effective measures. An individual may be willing to pursue a help-seeking goal but may not be able to access the offered support. For example, they may encounter a sign encouraging them to approach members of staff for help but find themselves unable to locate anyone (Marsh et al., 2021). By increasing the effort required to find help, this may reduce motivation via the rate-of-progress gradient. Alternatively, help may not arrive within an anticipated timeframe, creating uncertainty around waiting times that could be demotivating and risk reinforcing feelings of hopelessness for some individuals (Punton et al., 2022). Ensuring offers of help are fulfilled may arguably be important for these measures to be effective. Furthermore, concerns about the consequences of engaging in help-seeking—for example, due to prior negative experiences (Holt et al., 2024) or uncertainty of what might happen (Marsh et al., 2021)—may also influence motivation to engage in help-seeking behaviour generally. For others, uncertainty around potential costs that might arise after accessing support may amplify existing financial concerns (Hagen et al., 2022). Clear and transparent communication where appropriate may therefore be helpful for ensuring accurate outcome expectations. Together, these examples illustrate the importance of carefully designed processes around help-seeking measures at high-risk locations to ensure their effectiveness.

5. Discussion

In this article, we have sought to explore the potential ways suicide prevention measures implemented at high-risk locations could influence levels of goal-directed motivation based on the principles outlined in GOAL Architecture (Ballard et al., 2022). Specifically, by identifying how they may impact perceptions of distance, time remaining, and rate of progress, we have considered how these measures could impact motivational drive associated with attempt-related actions, in terms of both prevention and potential risks. We began by exploring the ways in which measures that only partially restrict access to means of suicide may shift the motivational value associated with related goals. First, we discussed the potential role of half-height barriers and other physical adaptations (e.g., spinning bars) in reducing perceived ease of access (while not making access impossible). We then proposed that previously observed psychological deterrent effects may be in part due to the impact of partial measures on perceived rate of progress, which in turn may influence motivational drive to proceed past them. We also described how person-level factors, including self-efficacy and appraisals of risks, may influence the strength of any psychological deterrent effect of measures that partially restrict access to means, which could in turn impact the effectiveness of the measures for certain groups of people. The impact of measure design on perceived distance to suicide means was also discussed in the context of measure placement and proximity of alternative access points.

Next, we proposed that perceptions of being monitored may create a timeframe within which an individual believes they can act, which may in turn influence levels of motivation to avoid a third-party intervention. We firstly considered how the presence of others may influence expectancies of a potentially imminent intervention, and discussed the role that lighting-based interventions (e.g., blue lights) may play in informing perceived visibility. We then explored the impact that different types of surveillance technologies (e.g., covert,

overt) may have on perceptions of monitoring and timeframes for third-party intervention. The potential implications of this for the use of automated systems (e.g., that emit an audible deterrent upon activation) as a suicide prevention measure was also discussed. Moreover, the ability of some measures to help draw attention to atypical behaviours, potentially influencing perceived feasibility (via changes to rate of progress), were considered.

Finally, we looked at help-seeking as an alternative and/or additional goal that for some may exist alongside a primary goal (e.g., "accessing means of suicide") and could at times be inhibited (e.g., due to goal-shielding processes). The implications of goal-shielding on the effectiveness of measures to enable help-seeking was discussed, as well as the potential role of external stimuli for disrupting these states of focused goal pursuit (e.g., "bursting the bubble"). We also applied the gradients identified by the GOAL Architecture framework (Ballard et al., 2022) to contextualise the role of help-seeking measures at high-risk locations and consider how the framework may be applied to aid the evaluation and development of these measures.

Many suicide prevention measures implemented at high-risk locations will to some extent be reliant on psychological mechanisms for their effectiveness, whether they encourage disengagement from an attempt-related goal or promote engagement with actions like help-seeking. Alternatively, others may indirectly influence goal pursuit (e.g., by increasing perceptions of a potentially imminent third-party intervention). Through examining the existing literature on suicide prevention at high-risk locations with a goal-pursuit lens, we have sought to identify potential psychological mechanisms that may help explain these effects. We hope that our formulation adds to previous research that has considered suicidal and self-injurious behaviours in the context of goal-directed processes (e.g., Kopetz et al., 2018; Valach et al., 2006, 2016). However, we have also discussed the potential influence of encountering suicide prevention measures on the pursuit of subordinate-level goals in a way that allowed us to not only consider the extent to which a measure may be effective at preventing suicides but also to identify possibilities for increased harm.

Limitations and Opportunities

There are, of course, limitations to the approach taken here. By integrating theories of goal pursuit, GOAL Architecture provides a descriptive framework to quantify the influence of changes to goal attainability on motivation (Ballard et al., 2022). Considering how goal dynamics may play out in relation to gradients of distance, time remaining, and rate of progress can be a useful exercise for identifying future areas of investigation, as we have attempted to do here. However, alternative approaches may also provide useful insights in this area, such as situated or embodied cognition. Future work may therefore approach this issue from different perspectives.

Moreover, the extent to which suicide prevention measures have the potential to adjust attempt-related motivational drive should not be overestimated. Firstly, the characteristics of any corresponding, higher-level goals (e.g., approach vs. avoid) will also determine whether motivation increases or declines as goal pursuit unfolds. As discussed here in the context of means restriction measures and proximity, the effectiveness of a measure may be somewhat dependent on the types of higher-level goals involved. Overall levels of desire are likely to play a central role in determining whether any measure is likely to influence behaviour.

From this perspective, the psychological effects of encountering a suicide prevention measure would be additive and therefore determined by existing motivational states. As such, it is not our intention to dismiss the importance of other sources of motivation potentially driving an attempt, but rather to consider how suicide prevention measures may further influence attempt-related decisions and behaviour. For example, the model proposed in the Theory of Interpersonal Behaviour identifies "facilitating conditions" as a moderator between two factors ("habits" and "intentions"; i.e., attitudes, social factors, and affect) and behaviour (Triandis, 1977). In previous studies, "facilitating conditions" has been represented by factors such as time constraints (Kupfer et al., 2019), perceived difficulty/ease of an act, and walking distance (Osei et al., 2024). Therefore, the framework proposed in GOAL Architecture may be a useful way of identifying ways of quantifying the influence of suicide prevention measures so that any effects may be appropriately accounted for in other models of behaviour.

Moreover, we have focused on three recommended categories of suicide prevention measures for high-risk locations and how they may impact judgements and behaviour relating to specific attempt-related goals within these environments. This adds to previous work that has considered the potential role of suicide prevention measures at high-risk locations at different stages of the suicidal process (Mackenzie et al., 2025) and in relation to events leading up to an attempt (Burkhardt et al., 2014). By focusing on a relatively small number of subordinate goals (i.e., accessing means, avoiding third-party intervention, help-seeking), we do not address the periods leading up to and after an attempt, or the wider dynamic network of goals (including higher-level goals related to the attempt and conflicting goals). Such a granular approach, we believe, may be a necessary step in furthering our understanding of how, why, and when certain measures are (or are not) effective at preventing suicides in these environments.

This is particularly important when thinking about the range of factors that may influence suicidal behaviour and, in particular, suicide attempts. Focusing on any impact on goal pursuit as it unfurls may be useful for understanding the role prevention measures play within high-risk environments at specific points in time, as well as acknowledging their limits. For example, while an individual may disengage from an "access means" goal at a specific location (e.g., subordinate goal), it does not mean the overall motivation to pursue a suicide attempt has reduced or ceased. While for some individuals, disengagement from accessing means at one location may be enough to protect them in the immediate (but not necessarily longer) term, for others there may be a risk of displacement. Alternatively, an individual may engage in help-seeking behaviours but then encounter barriers to accessing help (e.g., busy phone lines). From this perspective, being motivated to engage in behaviours will not necessarily result in goal attainment. These kinds of considerations are arguably important when designing safe environments and effective processes and therefore warrant further attention; however, they are not long-term solutions when it comes to helping an individual.

We hope that our detailed consideration of the psychological processes associated with suicidal behaviour at high-risk locations will prompt further thinking about the complex interplay of factors that may influence suicidal behaviour and its prevention in these and other situations. As others have previously noted (e.g., Kopetz et al., 2018), examining complex behaviours through a goal-pursuit lens can help us develop a deeper understanding of them. It may also therefore be beneficial for those designing suicide prevention measures more generally to consider how principles of goal pursuit and goal prioritisation could be applied in a similar manner—for example, to understand different types of experiences, such as feelings of ambivalence or distress presentations. Applying frameworks like GOAL Architecture (Ballard et al., 2022) to explore concepts of dynamic goal prioritisation at various stages of the suicidal process may be one approach that could prove useful for identifying areas of opportunity for suicide prevention.

Author Contributions: Conceptualisation, L.J., J.-M.M., A.W., P.P., B.C., I.M., E.P., K.H. and L.M.; writing—original draft preparation, L.J.; writing—review and editing, J.-M.M., A.W., P.P., B.C., I.M., E.P., K.H. and L.M.; visualisation, L.J.; funding acquisition, L.M., J.-M.M., I.M. and E.P. All authors have read and agreed to the published version of the manuscript.

Funding: This project is funded by the NIHR Public Health Research programme (NIHR151521). The views expressed are those of the authors and not necessarily those of the NIHR or the Department of Health and Social Care.

Institutional Review Board Statement: Not applicable.

Informed Consent Statement: Not applicable.

Data Availability Statement: No new data were created or analysed in this study. Data sharing is not applicable to this article.

Acknowledgments: We would firstly like to thank the group of NSPA (National Suicide Prevention Alliance) Lived Experience Influencers who formed an advisory group that continues to provide invaluable feedback across this project. We are also grateful for the advice and support from our colleagues from the wider project team (consisting of Peter Craig, Anthony Purvis, Robin Pharoah, Alex Dark, Manuela Deidda, Philip Worrall, Giorgio Ciminata, Carlisle George, and Amina Mahmood) and steering group (consisting of Rachel Aldred, Amy Chandler, Frank De Vocht, Keith Hawton, Fiona Malpass, Emma McIntosh, and Hilary Norman). For the purpose of open access, the authors have applied a Creative Commons Attribution (CC BY) licence to any Author Accepted Manuscript version arising from this submission.

Conflicts of Interest: The authors declare no conflicts of interest. The funders had no role in the design of the study; in the collection, analyses, or interpretation of data; in the writing of the manuscript; or in the decision to publish the results.

References

Alister, M., Herbert, S. L., Sewell, D. K., Neal, A., & Ballard, T. (2024). The impact of cognitive resource constraints on goal prioritization. *Cognitive Psychology*, *148*, 101618. [CrossRef] [PubMed]

American Psychological Association. (n.d.). Motivation. In *APA dictionary of psychology*. American Psychological Association. Available online: https://dictionary.apa.org/motivation (accessed on 22 April 2025).

Armstrong, L. L., & Manion, I. G. (2006). Suicidal ideation in young males living in rural communities: Distance from school as a risk factor, youth engagement as a protective factor. *Vulnerable Children and Youth Studies*, *1*(1), 102–113. [CrossRef]

Ballard, T., Neal, A., Farrell, S., Lloyd, E., Lim, J., & Heathcote, A. (2022). A general architecture for modeling the dynamics of goal-directed motivation and decision-making. *Psychological Review*, *129*(1), 146–174. [CrossRef] [PubMed]

Barry, R., Rehm, J., de Oliveira, C., Gozdyra, P., Chen, S., & Kurdyak, P. (2023). The relationship between rurality, travel time to care and death by suicide. *BMC Psychiatry*, *23*(1), 345. [CrossRef] [PubMed]

Baston, R. (2024). What underlies death/suicide implicit association test measures and how it contributes to suicidal action. *Philosophical Psychology*, *37*(5), 993–1016. [CrossRef]

Beautrais, A. L. (2001). Effectiveness of barriers at suicide jumping sites: A case study. *Australian & New Zealand Journal of Psychiatry*, *35*(5), 557–562. [CrossRef]

Beautrais, A. L., Gibb, S. J., Fergusson, D. M., Horwood, L. J., & Larkin, G. L. (2009). Removing bridge barriers stimulates suicides: An unfortunate natural experiment. *Australian & New Zealand Journal of Psychiatry*, *43*(6), 495–497. [CrossRef] [PubMed]

Beaven, C. M., & Ekström, J. (2013). A comparison of blue light and caffeine effects on cognitive function and alertness in humans. *PLoS ONE*, *8*(10), e76707. [CrossRef] [PubMed]

Bennewith, O., Nowers, M., & Gunnell, D. (2007). Effect of barriers on the Clifton suspension bridge, England, on local patterns of suicide: Implications for prevention. *The British Journal of Psychiatry*, *190*(3), 266–267. [CrossRef] [PubMed]

Bennewith, O., Nowers, M., & Gunnell, D. (2011). Suicidal behaviour and suicide from the Clifton Suspension Bridge, Bristol and surrounding area in the UK: 1994–2003. *European Journal of Public Health*, *21*(2), 204–208. [CrossRef] [PubMed]

Burkhardt, J.-M., Rådbo, H., Silla, A., & Paran, F. (2014). A model of suicide and trespassing processes to support the analysis and decision related to preventing railway suicides and trespassing accidents at railways. In *Transport research arena (TRA) 2014 proceedings*. Transportation Research Board.

Burnette, C., Ramchand, R., & Ayer, L. (2015). Gatekeeper training for suicide prevention. *Rand Health Quarterly*, *5*(1), 16. [PubMed]

Chellappa, S. L., Steiner, R., Blattner, P., Oelhafen, P., Götz, T., & Cajochen, C. (2011). Non-visual effects of light on melatonin, alertness and cognitive performance: Can blue-enriched light keep us alert? *PLoS ONE*, *6*(1), e16429. [CrossRef] [PubMed]

Chung, Y. W., Kang, S. J., Matsubayashi, T., Sawada, Y., & Ueda, M. (2016). The effectiveness of platform screen doors for the prevention of subway suicides in South Korea. *Journal of Affective Disorders*, *194*, 80–83. [CrossRef] [PubMed]

Clapperton, A., Dwyer, J., Spittal, M., & Pirkis, J. (2023). The effectiveness of installing trackside fencing in preventing railway suicides: A pre-post study design in Victoria, Australia. *Injury Prevention*, *29*(6), 525–527. [CrossRef] [PubMed]

Clapperton, A., Dwyer, J., Spittal, M. J., Roberts, L., & Pirkis, J. (2022). Preventing railway suicides through level crossing removal: A multiple-arm pre-post study design in Victoria, Australia. *Social Psychiatry and Psychiatric Epidemiology*, *57*(11), 2261–2266. [CrossRef] [PubMed]

da Silva, M., Baron, W., & Carroll, A. A. (2006). *Highway-railroad grade crossing safety research: Railroad infrastructure trespassing detection systems research in Pittsford, New York* (Report No. DOT-VNTSC-FRA-05-07). U.S. Department of Transportation Federal Railroad Administration. Available online: https://rosap.ntl.bts.gov/view/dot/8901 (accessed on 1 May 2024).

Devlin, H. C., Johnson, S. L., & Gruber, J. (2015). Feeling good and taking a chance? Associations of hypomania risk with cognitive and behavioral risk taking. *Cognitive Therapy and Research*, *39*(4), 473–479. [CrossRef]

Dudley, R., Taylor, P., Wickham, S., & Hutton, P. (2016). Psychosis, delusions and the "jumping to conclusions" reasoning bias: A systematic review and meta-analysis. *Schizophrenia Bulletin*, *42*(3), 652–665. [CrossRef] [PubMed]

Duthie, G., Reavley, N., Wright, J., & Morgan, A. (2024). The impact of media-based mental health campaigns on male help-seeking: A systematic review. *Health Promotion International*, *39*(4), daae104. [CrossRef] [PubMed]

Dwyer, J., Spittal, M. J., Scurrah, K., Pirkis, J., Bugeja, L., & Clapperton, A. (2023). Structural intervention at one bridge decreases the overall jumping suicide rate in Victoria, Australia. *Epidemiology and Psychiatric Sciences*, *32*, e58. [CrossRef] [PubMed]

Erlangsen, A., la Cour, N., Larsen, C. Ø., Karlsen, S. S., Witting, S., Ranning, A., Wang, A. G., Ørnebjerg, K., Schou, B., & Nordentoft, M. (2023). Efforts to prevent railway suicides in Denmark. *Crisis*, *44*(2), 169–172. [CrossRef] [PubMed]

Evans, J. S. B. T. (2008). Dual-processing accounts of reasoning, judgment, and social cognition. *Annual Review of Psychology*, *59*, 255–278. [CrossRef] [PubMed]

Fredin-Knutzén, J., Hadlaczky, G., Andersson, A.-L., & Sokolowski, M. (2022). A pilot study evaluating the effectiveness of preventing railway suicides by mid-track fencing, which restrict easy access to high-speed train tracks. *Journal of Safety Research*, *83*, 232–237. [CrossRef] [PubMed]

Fredin-Knutzén, J., Hadlaczky, G., Wigren, A., & Sokolowski, M. (2024). A pilot study evaluating the preventive effects of platform-end lengthwise fencing on trespassing, person struck by train and traffic delays. *Journal of Safety Research*, *88*, 78–84. [CrossRef] [PubMed]

Gabree, S. H., Hiltunen, D., & Ranalli, E. (2019). *Railroad implemented countermeasures to prevent suicide: Review of public information* (Report No. DOT/FRA/ORD-19/04). U.S. Department of Transportation Federal Railroad Administration. Available online: https://rosap.ntl.bts.gov/view/dot/39205 (accessed on 1 May 2024).

Gair, S. (2008). The psychic disequilibrium of adoption: Stories exploring links between adoption and suicidal thoughts and actions. *Australian E-Journal for the Advancement of Mental Health*, *7*(3), 207–216. [CrossRef]

Geerling, I., Roberts, R. M., & Sved Williams, A. (2019). Impact of infant crying on mothers with a diagnosis of borderline personality disorder: A qualitative study. *Infant Mental Health Journal: Infancy and Early Childhood*, *40*(3), 405–421. [CrossRef] [PubMed]

Giupponi, G., Thoma, H., Lamis, D., Forte, A., Pompili, M., & Kapfhammer, H. P. (2019). Posttraumatic stress reactions of underground drivers after suicides by jumping to arriving trains; feasibility of an early stepped care outpatient intervention. *Journal of Trauma & Dissociation*, *20*(5), 495–510. [CrossRef] [PubMed]

Gujral, K., Van Campen, J., Jacobs, J., Kimerling, R., Blonigen, D., & Zulman, D. M. (2022). Mental health service use, suicide behavior, and emergency department visits among rural us veterans who received video-enabled tablets during the COVID-19 pandemic. *JAMA Network Open*, *5*(4), e226250. [CrossRef] [PubMed]

Hagen, B. N. M., Sawatzky, A., Harper, S. L., O'Sullivan, T. L., & Jones-Bitton, A. (2022). "Farmers aren't into the emotions and things, right?": A qualitative exploration of motivations and barriers for mental health help-seeking among Canadian farmers. *Journal of Agromedicine*, *27*(2), 113–123. [CrossRef] [PubMed]

Hamilton, A. F. d. C., & Lind, F. (2016). Audience effects: What can they tell us about social neuroscience, theory of mind and autism? *Culture and Brain*, *4*(2), 159–177. [CrossRef] [PubMed]

Harmon-Jones, E., Gable, P., & Price, T. F. (2012). The influence of affective states varying in motivational intensity on cognitive scope. *Frontiers in Integrative Neuroscience*, *6*, 73. [CrossRef] [PubMed]

Hawton, K., Townsend, E., Deeks, J., Appleby, L., Gunnell, D., Bennewith, O., & Cooper, J. (2001). Effects of legislation restricting pack sizes of paracetamol and salicylate on self poisoning in the United Kingdom: Before and after study. *BMJ*, *322*(7296), 1203. [CrossRef] [PubMed]

Heesen, K., Mérelle, S., van den Brand, I., van Bergen, D., Baden, D., Slotema, K., Gilissen, R., & van Veen, S. (2024). The forever decision: A qualitative study among survivors of a suicide attempt. *eClinicalMedicine*, *69*, 102449. [CrossRef] [PubMed]

Heinig, I., Wittchen, H.-U., & Knappe, S. (2021). Help-seeking behavior and treatment barriers in anxiety disorders: Results from a representative German community survey. *Community Mental Health Journal*, *57*(8), 1505–1517. [CrossRef] [PubMed]

Hemmer, A., Meier, P., & Reisch, T. (2017). Comparing different suicide prevention measures at bridges and buildings: Lessons we have learned from a national survey in Switzerland. *PLoS ONE*, *12*(1), e0169625. [CrossRef] [PubMed]

Henson, K. E., Brock, R., Charnock, J., Wickramasinghe, B., Will, O., & Pitman, A. (2019). Risk of suicide after cancer diagnosis in England. *JAMA Psychiatry*, *76*(1), 51–60. [CrossRef] [PubMed]

Hofmann, W., & Van Dillen, L. (2012). Desire: The new hot spot in self-control research. *Current Directions in Psychological Science*, *21*(5), 317–322. [CrossRef]

Holdaway, S., Evans, E., & Webb, S. (2012). *Improving suicide prevention measures on the rail network in Great Britain. Literature review* (No. T845). Rail Safety Standards and Board.

Holt, N. R., Botelho, E., Wolford-Clevenger, C., & Clark, K. A. (2024). Previous mental health care and help-seeking experiences: Perspectives from sexual and gender minority survivors of near-fatal suicide attempts. *Psychological Services*, *21*(1), 24–33. [CrossRef] [PubMed]

Ichikawa, M., Inada, H., & Kumeji, M. (2014). Reconsidering the effects of blue-light installation for prevention of railway suicides. *Journal of Affective Disorders*, *152–154*, 183–185. [CrossRef] [PubMed]

Isaac, M., & Bennett, J. (2005). Prevention of suicide by jumping: The impact of restriction of access at Beachy Head, Sussex during the foot and mouth crisis 2001. *Public Health Medicine*, *6*(1), 19–22.

Joyner, L., Cliffe, B., Mackenzie, J. M., Pettersen, E., Marsh, I., Phillips, P., & Marzano, L. (2024). *The use of smart surveillance technologies for suicide prevention in public spaces: A professional stakeholder survey from the United Kingdom*. Research Square. [CrossRef]

Kallberg, V.-P., & Silla, A. (2017). Prevention of railway trespassing by automatic sound warning—A pilot study. *Traffic Injury Prevention*, *18*(3), 330–335. [CrossRef] [PubMed]

Kaye, L. K., Rousaki, A., Joyner, L. C., Barrett, L. A. F., & Orchard, L. J. (2022). The online behaviour taxonomy: A conceptual framework to understand behaviour in computer-mediated communication. *Computers in Human Behavior*, *137*, 107443. [CrossRef]

Kopetz, C., & Orehek, E. (2015). When the end justifies the means: Self-defeating behaviors as "rational" and "successful" self-regulation. *Current Directions in Psychological Science*, *24*(5), 386–391. [CrossRef]

Kopetz, C., Woerner, J. I., & Briskin, J. L. (2018). Another look at impulsivity: Could impulsive behavior be strategic? *Social and Personality Psychology Compass*, *12*(5), e12385. [CrossRef] [PubMed]

Kube, T., & Rozenkrantz, L. (2021). When beliefs face reality: An integrative review of belief updating in mental health and illness. *Perspectives on Psychological Science*, *16*(2), 247–274. [CrossRef] [PubMed]

Kupfer, T. R., Wyles, K. J., Watson, F., La Ragione, R. M., Chambers, M. A., & Macdonald, A. S. (2019). Determinants of hand hygiene behaviour based on the theory of interpersonal behaviour. *Journal of Infection Prevention*, *20*(5), 232–237. [CrossRef]

Lin, Y. Y., Huang, X.-Y., Chen, C.-Y., & Shao, W.-C. (2009). The lived experiences of brokered brides who have attempted suicide in Taiwan. *Journal of Clinical Nursing*, *18*(24), 3409–3420. [CrossRef] [PubMed]

Mackenzie, J. M., Borrill, J., Hawkins, E., Fields, B., Kruger, I., Noonan, I., & Marzano, L. (2018). Behaviours preceding suicides at railway and underground locations: A multimethodological qualitative approach. *BMJ Open*, *8*(4), e021076. [CrossRef] [PubMed]

Mackenzie, J. M., Marsh, I., Fields, B., Kruger, I., Katsampa, D., Crivatu, I., & Marzano, L. (2025). Preventing suicides on the railways: Learning from lived and living experiences. *BMC Public Health*, *25*(1), 1625. [CrossRef] [PubMed]

Mandal, A., Liesefeld, A. M., & Liesefeld, H. R. (2024). The surprising robustness of visual search against concurrent auditory distraction. *Journal of Experimental Psychology: Human Perception and Performance*, *50*(1), 99–118. [CrossRef] [PubMed]

Marcinkevičiūtė, M., Vilutytė, L., & Gailienė, D. (2024). Experience of pre-suicidal suffering: Insights from suicide attempt survivors. *International Journal of Qualitative Studies on Health and Well-Being*, *19*(1), 2370894. [CrossRef] [PubMed]

Marsh, I., Marzano, L., Mosse, D., & Mackenzie, J. M. (2021). First-person accounts of the processes and planning involved in a suicide attempt on the railway. *BJPsych Open*, *7*(1), e39. [CrossRef] [PubMed]

Marzano, L., Katsampa, D., Mackenzie, J. M., Kruger, I., El-Gharbawi, N., Ffolkes-St-Helene, D., Mohiddin, H., & Fields, B. (2021). Patterns and motivations for method choices in suicidal thoughts and behaviour: Qualitative content analysis of a large online survey. *BJPsych Open*, *7*(2), e60. [CrossRef] [PubMed]

Marzano, L., Mackenzie, J. M., Kruger, I., Borrill, J., & Fields, B. (2019). Factors deterring and prompting the decision to attempt suicide on the railway networks: Findings from 353 online surveys and 34 semi-structured interviews. *The British Journal of Psychiatry, 215*(4), 582–587. [CrossRef] [PubMed]

Marzano, L., Spence, R., Marsh, I., Barbin, A., & Kruger, I. (2025). How does news coverage of suicide affect suicidal behaviour at a high-frequency location? A 7-year time series analysis. *BMJ Public Health, 3*(1). [CrossRef] [PubMed]

Matsubayashi, T., Sawada, Y., & Ueda, M. (2013). Does the installation of blue lights on train platforms prevent suicide? A before-and-after observational study from Japan. *Journal of Affective Disorders, 147*(1), 385–388. [CrossRef] [PubMed]

Matsubayashi, T., Sawada, Y., & Ueda, M. (2014). Does the installation of blue lights on train platforms shift suicide to another station?: Evidence from Japan. *Journal of Affective Disorders, 169*, 57–60. [CrossRef] [PubMed]

May, A. M., & Klonsky, E. D. (2013). Assessing motivations for suicide attempts: Development and psychometric properties of the inventory of motivations for suicide attempts. *Suicide & Life-Threatening Behavior, 43*(5), 532–546. [CrossRef]

May, A. M., Pachkowski, M. C., & Klonsky, E. D. (2020). Motivations for suicide: Converging evidence from clinical and community samples. *Journal of Psychiatric Research, 123*, 171–177. [CrossRef] [PubMed]

Milyavskaya, M., & Werner, K. M. (2018). Goal pursuit: Current state of affairs and directions for future research. *Canadian Psychology/Psychologie Canadienne, 59*(2), 163–175. [CrossRef]

Mishara, B. L., & Bardon, C. (2016). Systematic review of research on railway and urban transit system suicides. *Journal of Affective Disorders, 193*, 215–226. [CrossRef] [PubMed]

Mohl, A., Stulz, N., Martin, A., Eigenmann, F., Hepp, U., Hüsler, J., & Beer, J. H. (2012). The "Suicide Guard Rail": A minimal structural intervention in hospitals reduces suicide jumps. *BMC Research Notes, 5*(1), 408. [CrossRef] [PubMed]

National Centre for Suicide Research and Prevention (NASP), Region Stockholm & Karolinska Institutet. (2022). Pilot study of blue LED-lights in high risk environments. In *"Suicide prevention traffic administration/NASP" report* (pp. 25–33). Available online: https://restrail.eu/toolbox/IMG/pdf/pilot_study_of_blue_led-lights_in_high_risk_environments-stockholm-v.1.0.pdf (accessed on 14 March 2025).

National Institute for Health and Care Excellence. (2018). *Preventing suicide in community and custodial settings* (NICE Guideline NG105). Available online: https://www.nice.org.uk/guidance/ng105 (accessed on 13 May 2025).

Nischler, C., Michael, R., Wintersteller, C., Marvan, P., van Rijn, L. J., Coppens, J. E., van den Berg, T. J. T. P., Emesz, M., & Grabner, G. (2013). Iris color and visual functions. *Graefe's Archive for Clinical and Experimental Ophthalmology, 251*(1), 195–202. [CrossRef] [PubMed]

Norman, H., Marzano, L., Fields, B., Brown, S., MacDonald Hart, S., & Kruger, I. (2024). Characteristics and circumstances of rail suicides in England 2019–2021: A cluster analysis and autopsy study. *Journal of Affective Disorders, 354*, 397–407. [CrossRef] [PubMed]

Norman, H., Marzano, L., Winter, R., Crivatu, I., Mackenzie, J. M., & Marsh, I. (2023). Factors prompting and deterring suicides on the roads. *BJPsych Open, 9*(3), e81. [CrossRef] [PubMed]

O'Connor, R. C., O'Carroll, R. E., Ryan, C., & Smyth, R. (2012). Self-regulation of unattainable goals in suicide attempters: A two year prospective study. *Journal of Affective Disorders, 142*(1), 248–255. [CrossRef] [PubMed]

Office for National Statistics. (2023, December 19). *Suicides in England and Wales: 2022 registrations. Statistical bulletin.* Available online: https://www.ons.gov.uk/peoplepopulationandcommunity/birthsdeathsandmarriages/deaths/bulletins/suicidesintheunitedkingdom/2022registrations (accessed on 3 June 2024).

Okada, A., & Oshima, T. (2025). Assessing the potential of half-height platform screen doors to prevent personal injury accidents: Evidence from the Tokyo metropolitan area railway network. *IATSS Research, 49*(1), 81–92. [CrossRef]

Osei, K. K., Obiri-Yeboah, A. A., Adu-Gyamfi, Lord, & Ackaah, W. (2024). Road crossing behavior and preferences among pedestrians: From the lens of the theory of interpersonal behavior. *Traffic Injury Prevention, 25*(1), 91–100. [CrossRef] [PubMed]

Owens, C., Derges, J., & Abraham, C. (2019). Intervening to prevent a suicide in a public place: A qualitative study of effective interventions by lay people. *BMJ Open, 9*(11), e032319. [CrossRef] [PubMed]

Owens, C., Hardwick, R., Charles, N., & Watkinson, G. (2015). *Preventing suicides in public places: A practice resource* (No. 2015497). Public Health England. Available online: https://assets.publishing.service.gov.uk/media/5c2f6f8b40f0b66cf8298a70/Preventing_suicides_in_public_places.pdf (accessed on 24 June 2024).

Özen-Akın, G., & Cinan, S. (2022). People with jumping to conclusions bias tend to make context-independent decisions rather than context-dependent decisions. *Consciousness and Cognition, 98*, 103279. [CrossRef] [PubMed]

Parmentier, F. B. R., Elsley, J. V., Andrés, P., & Barceló, F. (2011a). Why are auditory novels distracting? Contrasting the roles of novelty, violation of expectation and stimulus change. *Cognition, 119*(3), 374–380. [CrossRef] [PubMed]

Parmentier, F. B. R., Ljungberg, J. K., Elsley, J. V., & Lindkvist, M. (2011b). A behavioral study of distraction by vibrotactile novelty. *Journal of Experimental Psychology: Human Perception and Performance, 37*(4), 1134–1139. [CrossRef] [PubMed]

Peinado, V., Valiente, C., Contreras, A., Trucharte, A., & Vázquez, C. (2024). Unravelling the jumping to conclusions bias in daily life and health-related decision-making scenarios. *Personality and Individual Differences, 230*, 112782. [CrossRef]

Pelletier, A. R. (2007). Preventing suicide by jumping: The effect of a bridge safety fence. *Injury Prevention, 13*(1), 57–59. [CrossRef] [PubMed]

Perron, S., Burrows, S., Fournier, M., Perron, P.-A., & Ouellet, F. (2013). Installation of a bridge barrier as a suicide prevention strategy in Montréal, Québec, Canada. *American Journal of Public Health, 103*(7), 1235–1239. [CrossRef] [PubMed]

Pirkis, J., Too, L. S., Spittal, M. J., Krysinska, K., Robinson, J., & Cheung, Y. T. D. (2015). Interventions to reduce suicides at suicide hotspots: A systematic review and meta-analysis. *The Lancet Psychiatry, 2*(11), 994–1001. [CrossRef] [PubMed]

Pitman, A., Logeswaran, Y., McDonald, K., Cerel, J., Lewis, G., & Erlangsen, A. (2023). Investigating risk of self-harm and suicide on anniversaries after bereavement by suicide and other causes: A Danish population-based self-controlled case series study. *Epidemiology and Psychiatric Sciences, 32*, e53. [CrossRef] [PubMed]

Player, M. J., Proudfoot, J., Fogarty, A., Whittle, E., Spurrier, M., Shand, F., Christensen, H., Hadzi-Pavlovic, D., & Wilhelm, K. (2015). What interrupts suicide attempts in men: A qualitative study. *PLoS ONE, 10*(6), e0128180. [CrossRef] [PubMed]

Plessow, F., Fischer, R., Kirschbaum, C., & Goschke, T. (2011). Inflexibly focused under stress: Acute psychosocial stress increases shielding of action goals at the expense of reduced cognitive flexibility with increasing time lag to the stressor. *Journal of Cognitive Neuroscience, 23*(11), 3218–3227. [CrossRef] [PubMed]

Punton, G., Dodd, A. L., & McNeill, A. (2022). 'You're on the waiting list': An interpretive phenomenological analysis of young adults' experiences of waiting lists within mental health services in the UK. *PLoS ONE, 17*(3), e0265542. [CrossRef] [PubMed]

Rauschenberg, C., Reininghaus, U., ten Have, M., de Graaf, R., van Dorsselaer, S., Simons, C. J. P., Gunther, N., Henquet, C., Pries, L. K., Guloksuz, S., Bak, M., & van Os, J. (2021). The jumping to conclusions reasoning bias as a cognitive factor contributing to psychosis progression and persistence: Findings from NEMESIS-2. *Psychological Medicine, 51*(10), 1696–1703. [CrossRef] [PubMed]

Reisch, T., & Michel, K. (2005). Securing a suicide hot spot: Effects of a safety net at the bern muenster terrace. *Suicide and Life-Threatening Behavior, 35*(4), 460–467. [CrossRef] [PubMed]

Reitz, S., Kluetsch, R., Niedtfeld, I., Knorz, T., Lis, S., Paret, C., Kirsch, P., Meyer-Lindenberg, A., Treede, R. D., Baumgärtner, U., Bohus, M., & Schmahl, C. (2015). Incision and stress regulation in borderline personality disorder: Neurobiological mechanisms of self-injurious behaviour. *The British Journal of Psychiatry, 207*(2), 165–172. [CrossRef] [PubMed]

Ritunnano, R., Kleinman, J., Oshodi, D. W., Michail, M., Nelson, B., Humpston, C. S., & Broome, M. R. (2022). Subjective experience and meaning of delusions in psychosis: A systematic review and qualitative evidence synthesis. *The Lancet Psychiatry, 9*(6), 458–476. [CrossRef] [PubMed]

Rosen, D. H. (1975). Suicide survivors. *Western Journal of Medicine, 122*(4), 289–294. [PubMed]

Ross, V., Koo, Y. W., & Kõlves, K. (2020). A suicide prevention initiative at a jumping site: A mixed-methods evaluation. *EClinicalMedicine, 19*, 100265. [CrossRef] [PubMed]

Ryan, B. (2017). What do we know about rail suicide incidents? An analysis of 257 fatalities on the rail network in Great Britain. *Proceedings of the Institution of Mechanical Engineers, Part F: Journal of Rail and Rapid Transit, 231*(10), 1150–1173. [CrossRef]

Ryan, B., Hallewell, M., Hughes, N., Coad, N., Eliseu, J., Lira, M., Grant, A., Parrott, N., & Thompson, K. (2022). Field testing two innovative lighting interventions to influence waiting behaviours and movements on stairways in train stations. *Lighting Research & Technology, 54*(3), 237–259.

SanMiguel, I., Linden, D., & Escera, C. (2010). Attention capture by novel sounds: Distraction versus facilitation. *European Journal of Cognitive Psychology, 22*(4), 481–515. [CrossRef]

Sæheim, A., Hestetun, I., Mork, E., Nrugham, L., & Mehlum, L. (2017). A 12-year national study of suicide by jumping from bridges in Norway. *Archives of Suicide Research, 21*(4), 568–576. [CrossRef] [PubMed]

Schomaker, J., & Meeter, M. (2015). Short- and long-lasting consequences of novelty, deviance and surprise on brain and cognition. *Neuroscience & Biobehavioral Reviews, 55*, 268–279. [CrossRef]

Schrooten, M. G., Vlaeyen, J. W. S., & Morley, S. (2012). Psychological interventions for chronic pain: Reviewed within the context of goal pursuit. *Pain Management, 2*(2), 141–150. [CrossRef] [PubMed]

Schunk, D. H., & Usher, E. L. (2012). Social cognitive theory and motivation. In *The Oxford handbook of human motivation* (pp. 13–27). Oxford University Press. [CrossRef]

Shah, J. Y., Friedman, R., & Kruglanski, A. W. (2002). Forgetting all else: On the antecedents and consequences of goal shielding. *Journal of Personality and Social Psychology, 83*(6), 1261–1280. [CrossRef] [PubMed]

Sharot, T., Rollwage, M., Sunstein, C. R., & Fleming, S. M. (2023). Why and when beliefs change. *Perspectives on Psychological Science, 18*(1), 142–151. [CrossRef] [PubMed]

Shin, S., Pirkis, J., Clapperton, A., & Spittal, M. (2025). Change in suicides during and after the installation of barriers at the Golden Gate Bridge. *Injury Prevention*. [CrossRef] [PubMed]

Shin, S., Pirkis, J., Clapperton, A., Spittal, M., & Too, L. S. (2024). Effectiveness of partial restriction of access to means in jumping suicide: Lessons from four bridges in three countries. *Epidemiology and Psychiatric Sciences, 33*, e38. [CrossRef] [PubMed]

Sinyor, M., & Levitt, A. J. (2010). Effect of a barrier at Bloor Street Viaduct on suicide rates in Toronto: Natural experiment. *BMJ, 341*, c2884. [CrossRef] [PubMed]

Skegg, K., & Herbison, P. (2009). Effect of restricting access to a suicide jumping site. *Australian & New Zealand Journal of Psychiatry, 43*(6), 498–502. [CrossRef] [PubMed]

Smith, P. N., & Cukrowicz, K. C. (2010). Capable of suicide: A functional model of the acquired capability component of the interpersonal-psychological theory of suicide. *Suicide & Life-Threatening Behavior, 40*(3), 266–275. [CrossRef]

Stanchak, K., Foderaro, F., & da Silva, M. (2015). *High-security fencing for rail right-of-way applications: Current use and best practices* (Technical Report No. DOT-VNTSC-FRA-14-08). U.S. Department of Transportation Federal Railroad Administration. Available online: https://railroads.dot.gov/elibrary/high-security-fencing-rail-right-way-applications-current-use-and-best-practices (accessed on 27 March 2025).

Steidle, A., & Werth, L. (2014). In the spotlight: Brightness increases self-awareness and reflective self-regulation. *Light, Lighting, and Human Behaviour, 39*, 40–50. [CrossRef]

Stevenson, O. (2016). Suicidal journeys: Attempted suicide as geographies of intended death. *Social & Cultural Geography, 17*(2), 189–206. [CrossRef]

Tadmon, D., & Bearman, P. S. (2023). Differential spatial-social accessibility to mental health care and suicide. *Proceedings of the National Academy of Sciences, 120*(19), e2301304120. [CrossRef] [PubMed]

Terman, J. S., & Terman, M. (1999). Photopic and scotopic light detection in patients with seasonal affective disorder and control subjects. *Biological Psychiatry, 46*(12), 1642–1648. [CrossRef] [PubMed]

Too, L. S., Pirkis, J., Milner, A., Bugeja, L., & Spittal, M. J. (2017). Railway suicide clusters: How common are they and what predicts them? *Injury Prevention, 23*(5), 328–333. [CrossRef] [PubMed]

Too, L. S., Spittal, M. J., Bugeja, L., Milner, A., Stevenson, M., & McClure, R. (2015). An investigation of neighborhood-level social, economic and physical factors for railway suicide in Victoria, Australia. *Journal of Affective Disorders, 183*, 142–148. [CrossRef] [PubMed]

Triandis, H. C. (1977). *Interpersonal behavior*. Brooks/Cole.

Ueda, M., Sawada, Y., & Matsubayashi, T. (2015). The effectiveness of installing physical barriers for preventing railway suicides and accidents: Evidence from Japan. *Journal of Affective Disorders, 178*, 1–4. [CrossRef] [PubMed]

Valach, L., Michel, K., & Young, R. A. (2016). Suicide as a distorted goal-directed process: Wanting to die, killing, and being killed. *The Journal of Nervous and Mental Disease, 204*(11), 812. [CrossRef] [PubMed]

Valach, L., Michel, K., Young, R. A., & Dey, P. (2006). Suicide attempts as social goal-directed systems of joint careers, projects, and actions. *Suicide and Life-Threatening Behavior, 36*(6), 651–660. [CrossRef] [PubMed]

Vandewalle, G., Balteau, E., Phillips, C., Degueldre, C., Moreau, V., Sterpenich, V., Albouy, G., Darsaud, A., Desseilles, M., & Dang-Vu, T. T. (2006). Daytime light exposure dynamically enhances brain responses. *Current Biology, 16*(16), 1616–1621. [CrossRef] [PubMed]

van Houwelingen, C., Baumert, J., Kerkhof, A., Beersma, D., & Ladwig, K.-H. (2013). Train suicide mortality and availability of trains: A tale of two countries. *Psychiatry Research, 209*(3), 466–470. [CrossRef] [PubMed]

Van Orden, K. A., Witte, T. K., Cukrowicz, K. C., Braithwaite, S. R., Selby, E. A., & Joiner, T. E., Jr. (2010). The interpersonal theory of suicide. *Psychological Review, 117*(2), 575–600. [CrossRef] [PubMed]

Wilson, A., & Marshall, A. (2010). The support needs and experiences of suicidally bereaved family and friends. *Death Studies, 34*(7), 625–640. [CrossRef] [PubMed]

World Health Organisation. (2023). *Preventing suicide: A resource for media professionals, update 2023*. Available online: https://iris.who.int/bitstream/handle/10665/372691/9789240076846-eng.pdf?sequence=1#page=13.12 (accessed on 13 May 2025).

World Health Organisation. (2025, March 25). *Suicide 2021*. Available online: https://www.who.int/news-room/fact-sheets/detail/suicide (accessed on 13 May 2025).

Xing, Y., Lu, J., & Chen, S. (2019). Evaluating the effectiveness of platform screen doors for preventing metro suicides in China. *Journal of Affective Disorders, 253*, 63–68. [CrossRef] [PubMed]

behavioral sciences

MDPI

Review

The Sociology of Suicide After COVID-19: Assessment of the Spanish Case

Enrique Fernández-Vilas [1,*], Juan R. Coca [1], Juan José Labora González [2] and Marcos Iglesias Carrera [3]

[1] Department of Sociology and Social Work, University of Valladolid, José Tudela 12D, 42004 Soria, Spain; juanr.coca@uva.es
[2] Department of Political Science and Sociology, University of Santiago de Compostela, Ángel Jorge Echeverri, 15782 Santiago de Compostela, Spain; juan.labora@usc.es
[3] School of Labor Relations, University of Salamanca, San Torcuato 43, 49014 Zamora, Spain; marcosiglesias@usal.es
* Correspondence: enrique.fvilas@uva.es

Abstract: The phenomenon of suicide has become a significant global concern, claiming over 800,000 lives annually and resulting in millions of suicide attempts worldwide. In the aftermath of the COVID-19 pandemic, these troubling statistics have worsened, with notable increases in suicidal behavior, especially among vulnerable populations such as the youth, the elderly, and those in socioeconomically disadvantaged groups. This paper aims to explore the impact of the COVID-19 pandemic on suicide rates in Spain, using a theoretical ex post facto analysis. Spain has witnessed an alarming rise in suicide rates, particularly among young people, and a disturbing trend of increased suicidal ideation and self-harm behaviors. While some studies report no significant change in suicide rates during the pandemic, others point to the exacerbating effects of social isolation, economic instability, and public health measures. This study provides an in-depth examination of the psychosocial consequences of the pandemic on mental health in Spain, emphasizing the urgency of the need to address pre-existing inequalities and implement effective suicide prevention measures. Furthermore, it highlights the importance of gender-sensitive strategies and the need for systemic reforms to ensure better mental healthcare access for all segments of society. To achieve this goal, this paper uses a narrative literature review combined with a theoretical ex post facto analysis to assess the influence of the COVID-19 pandemic on suicide patterns in Spain.

Keywords: suicide; COVID-19; mental health; suicide prevention; gender differences; socioeconomic inequalities; post-pandemic mental health; public health

1. Introduction

The social phenomenon of suicide claims the lives of more than 800,000 individuals globally each year. In addition, it has been estimated that around 16 million suicide attempts are estimated to occur worldwide each year (Clua-García et al., 2021). That is, more than 2000 people die by suicide and almost 45,000 attempt suicide every day. Adult males have been found to be at higher risk of suicide, while young women are more likely to attempt suicide. Nearly one-third of all suicide attempts worldwide are made by young people, making it the second leading cause of death among 15–29 year olds and 15–19-year-old females (Mental Health and Substance Use, 2021).

The most common ways of committing suicide include the use of pesticides, hanging, or firearms, although jumping from high places and overdose are also common (Mental Health and Substance Use, 2021). However, there are significant differences in the choice of method between different countries and genders, with 71% of women opting for poisoning compared to 50% of men (Clua-García et al., 2021). The lethality of these methods varies considerably by region.

In the aftermath of the COVID-19 pandemic, suicide rates and mental health disorders have shown varying trends globally. While some studies found no significant changes in suicide rates during the pandemic (Pathirathna et al., 2022), others reported an increase in suicidal ideation and suicide attempts (Schnitzer et al., 2023). Prolonged social isolation and economic uncertainty have contributed to the deterioration of human well-being and have promoted this phenomenon (Sher, 2020). One of the most affected age groups was children and young people, whose members experienced disruptions to their education and social life. Also, the older age group of the elderly suffered a higher degree of isolation and lost more people they were close to due to death (Yan et al., 2023).

On the other hand, the pandemic led to an increase in gender inequality within suicide rates, with higher rates of suicidal ideation and suicide attempts seen in young women, while men continued to have higher rates of completed suicide due to the use of more lethal methods (Da Cunha Varella et al., 2024).

In Spain, recent studies have shown an increase in the incidence of disorders such as anxiety, depression, and post-traumatic stress disorder during periods of confinement and social restrictions (González-Sanguino et al., 2020). This deterioration in the mental health of the Spanish population has been reflected in an increase in suicide rates. According to data from the Instituto Nacional de Estadística [Spanish Institute of Statistics], 3941 suicides were recorded in 2020 (Instituto Nacional de Estadística, 2021), which represents an increase from the 3671 cases reported in 2019 (Instituto Nacional de Estadística, 2020). This increase is particularly worrying in certain demographic groups. For example, an increase in suicide rates among young people and adolescents during the pandemic has been observed. In 2020, 14 children under the age of 15 died by suicide in Spain, doubling the previous year's figure (Paricio del Castillo et al., 2024). In addition, the pandemic has exacerbated pre-existing social inequalities, whose impact on groups in situations of socioeconomic vulnerability is clear, contributing to the increase in suicidal behavior (De la Torre Luque et al., 2024).

The aim of this paper is to study the phenomenon of suicide in Spain by means of a theoretical ex post facto analysis. This analysis refers to the examination of suicide trends after the occurrence of the COVID-19 pandemic, without manipulating the variables and instead interpreting the observed consequences. This method is particularly useful in sociology when retrospective interpretation is required.

2. Background: COVID-19 and the "New Normal"

In late 2019, several cases of an atypical form of pneumonia in the Wuhan region (China) put health authorities on alert, with the academic community initially referring to these cases as 2019-nCov (2019-novel coronavirus) (Huang et al., 2020). Shortly afterward, and given its taxonomy, the International Committee on Taxonomy of Viruses (ICTV) labelled the causative agent of this disease Sars-CoV-2 (Coronaviridae Study Group of the International Committee on Taxonomy of Viruses, 2020).

More than four years after the onset of the pandemic, over 650 million people have been infected and more than 6.8 million have died from the infection, as reflected in data from Johns Hopkins University (2023), which created an interactive map to monitor real-time disease data.

In addition to the physical deterioration caused by the disease, the distancing and confinement measures implemented led to major stress for the entire population (Manchia et al., 2022). Therefore, it is worth highlighting the relevance of the social study of the psyche in at-risk societies. Great concern exists regarding mental health, at least in relation to the phenomenon of suicide in the Western world. Since the COVID-19 pandemic, with increasing diagnoses of anxiety and depression across the world, concern for the most vulnerable populations, such as children, the elderly, low-income individuals, and those with pre-existing mental health conditions, has been evident in the literature. These groups have experienced heightened levels of stress due to factors like isolation, economic instability, and disrupted healthcare access. Research highlights the need for targeted interventions and support systems to address the unique challenges faced by these populations in coping with the long-term psychological impacts of the pandemic (Holmes et al., 2020; Pappa et al., 2020). Evidence indicates that individuals from lower social classes may have limited access to primary and secondary mental healthcare, leading to a higher likelihood of them seeking help through crisis services. Additionally, patients in lower social classes may not receive the full benefits of mental health interventions, which may be less effective for them (Barnett et al., 2023).

During the months of COVID-19's greatest impact, there was an increase in the symptoms of other disorders, which have also continued until the present, such as eating disorders (Ji et al., 2024), attention deficit disorder and hyperactivity (Lopes et al., 2022), the appearance of new symptoms and diagnoses after overcoming COVID-19 (Fair Health, 2022), and issues such as insomnia and an ongoing fear of death, among others. But of greatest concern is the rising suicide rates seen since the pandemic. These rates were already high in many countries such as Spain, where the number one cause of unnatural death is now suicide. During 2019, 309 individuals aged 15 to 29 died by suicide in Spain. This same year, 307 people from this same age range died in traffic accidents, making suicide the leading cause of death among this age group.

In 2021, a suicide occurred every two and a half hours in Spain, leading to a total of 4003 suicides during the year (Instituto Nacional de Estadística, 2023). In 2022, suicide remained the leading cause of unnatural death in Spain (Ministerio de Sanidad, 2024). A total of 4097 people died by suicide in Spain during this year, an increase of 2.3% from 2021. Furthermore, the number of suicides increased for individuals under the age of 20 in particular (84 compared to 75 in 2021). Therefore, we can conclude that between 2018 and 2022, there has been an increase in suicide rates in Spain (Instituto Nacional de Estadística, 2023).

Infectious disease outbreaks have been associated with the appearance of mental health disorders in healthcare workers (medical and nursing staff in healthcare systems, social workers in elderly care centers, etc.), who are exposed to great stress given the nature of their work (Aymerich et al., 2022). These workers have faced emergency situations, sick patients, and the possibility of contracting illnesses. This has most likely had a major impact on their mental health, since it has been shown that these workers are at greater risk of developing mental disorders such as depression, generalized anxiety, and post-traumatic stress disorder (Nicolini, 2020). It has also been shown that this is more common in women than in men. Specifically, care and healthcare workers may have developed additional problems during the pandemic, as individuals experiencing significant health-related anxiety are prone to mistakenly perceiving benign physical symptoms as signs of infection (Pearman et al., 2020). This misinterpretation heightens their anxiety, impacts their capacity for logical decision-making, and alters their behavior. This anxiety about their health may simultaneously lead to maladaptive behaviors such as excessive handwashing, social withdrawal, and shopping anxiety (Asmundson & Taylor, 2020).

The uncertainty created by the pandemic has also affected other sectors and social groups, making them particularly vulnerable, such as staff at nursing homes, day centers, survivors, families, and adolescents. This vulnerability includes anxiety and stress associated with the risk of infection, the death of loved ones, uncertainty, social isolation measures, the physical and emotional fatigue of health workers, massive job losses, financial insecurity, poverty, and misinformation and information overload. Contrary to what was suggested during some periods of the pandemic, the literature has shown that the impacts of COVID-19 are correlated with belonging to certain social classes (Bajos et al., 2021; Holst et al., 2021; Lee & Singh, 2021; Soria & Horgos, 2020).

Studying the sociology of health has allowed people to gather evidence on the social processes to be considered in relation to all diseases, as various studies have mentioned (Cockerham, 2021, 2022; Nettleton, 2021). From this perspective, at-risk societies (Beck, 2009) have been subject to a growing concern for their health, mental health, and safety, as reflected in a diverse range of works (e.g., Nettleton, 2021, among others).

The COVID-19 pandemic has underscored and exacerbated pre-existing inequalities across the world, disproportionately affecting various segments of the population in terms of economics, healthcare access, gender, and education (Sohn et al., 2022; Wu & Qian, 2022). Within the Spanish context, these pandemic-amplified inequalities can be linked to an increased vulnerability among certain groups to mental health issues, including the risk of suicide.

The psychosocial impact of the pandemic, characterized by social isolation, job loss, economic uncertainty, and health-related stress, has contributed to a rise in anxiety, depression, and other mental disorders, which are known risk factors for suicide. In Spain, as in many parts of the world, there has been a growing concern for the population's mental health during and after the pandemic, reflecting the importance of addressing these structural inequalities and their effects on the populace (Husain et al., 2021; Vadivel et al., 2021).

Suicide, as an extreme indicator of psychological distress, can be understood within this context as a manifestation of inadequate support for some social groups. Inequality in the access to healthcare may have limited the availability of mental health resources for those in need, while gender and educational inequalities might have exacerbated existing vulnerabilities, especially among women and the youth, who have been particularly impacted by the psychosocial effects of the pandemic (Shidhaye, 2023).

3. Materials and Methods

The primary objective of this paper is to compile a comprehensive review of the information available to enhance our understanding of the current situation in terms of suicidal behavior. For this, a thorough search of databases and journals including PubMed, Scopus, and Web of Science was conducted. We used adapted keywords, including "suicide behavior", "suicide in Spain", "social stigma", "suicide and gender", "vulnerability", "covid and suicide", "sociodemographic disparities", and others. We also carefully screened out irrelevant studies and selected relevant articles, the references of which were further scrutinized to enhance the scholarly value of this discussion. We also accessed resources and datasets from organizations such as the World Health Organization and, principally, the Spanish Statistical Office Database.

The secondary objective of this article is to explain the variations and trends seen in suicide rates in Spain during and after the COVID-19 pandemic, with a particular focus on how factors such as gender, age, and socioeconomic status influence suicidal behavior.

The present study is based on a narrative literature review (NLR) and official statistical data. The literature search included approximately 300 documents published between 2020 and 2024 in English and Spanish that focus on the relationship between suicide and the COVID-19 pandemic (see Figure 1). After screening for relevance, 96 sources were selected for the final analysis. In parallel, statistical data were obtained from official sources, including the World Health Organization (WHO), the Spanish National Institute of Statistics (INE), and the Ministry of Health (Spain). Both data streams were combined in an integrated narrative analysis.

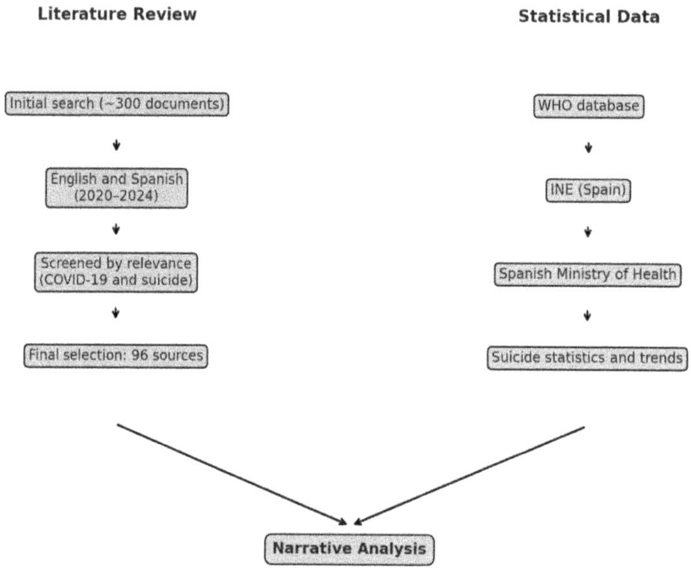

Figure 1. Overview of the methodological process, which included combining the NLR with statistical data from official sources. Source: self-made.

This review includes studies on the incidence of suicide and suicidal behavior and utilizes a theoretical ex post facto approach to assess the effects of confinement and other restrictive measures on mental health. This study employed an NLR approach due to the broad and conceptual nature of the research objective, aiming to identify sociological patterns and contextual interpretations rather than evaluate clinical effectiveness or effect sizes. This method allows for flexible exploration of heterogeneous data sources relevant to the social determinants of suicide in the Spanish context.

4. Results and Analysis: Suicide in Spain During COVID-19

Suicidal behavior in Spain is a serious social and public health concern. Included in the goals proposed in the WHO Mental Health Action Plan for the period 2013–2020 was the aim to reduce suicide rates by 10% by 2020 (Mental Health and Substance Use, 2013). However, figures show that this target has not been met. In fact, in 2020, 3941 deaths by suicide were recorded, a rate of 8.4 per 100,000 members of the population, making it the leading cause of unnatural death in this region.

4.1. Findings from Official Data

Between 2018 and 2022, Spain recorded a sustained increase in the number of deaths by suicide within its population. During this period, the figures increased by approximately 20%, from 3539 cases in 2018 to a total of 4227 in 2022. This worrying rise reflects an alarming trend that has substantially affected the population (Instituto Nacional de Estadística, 2024). In 2023, a slight decrease in the total number of deaths by suicide was observed, as they fell to 4116. However, this overall decline was not evenly distributed across different age groups. While some segments of the population experienced a reduction, others showed an increase in cases (Ministerio de Sanidad, 2024).

Specifically, in young people aged 15–29 and adults aged 30–44 there was an increase in deaths by suicide compared to the previous year. In the 15–29 age group, there were 13 additional cases, while in the 30–44 age group, the increase was by 30 cases.

In this vein, the statistic that suicide is the leading cause of unnatural death among 15–29 year olds in Spain highlights the fact that this an emerging mental health crisis (Instituto Nacional de Estadística, 2023). This trend is a clear indicator that existing prevention strategies and support networks are insufficient to address the complexities and diverse underlying causes of death by suicide in children and youths.

The ANAR Foundation in Spain estimates that there was a 244% increase in suicide attempts and suicidal ideation and a 241% increase in self-harming behaviors among young Spaniards in 2020 (ANAR Foundation, 2021) compared to previous years, although empirical evidence has not verified these high numbers. Despite this, there has been an undeniable increase in suicidal ideation (Instituto Nacional de Estadística, 2024) and its materialization in the young population highlights the real impact that global events such as the COVID-19 pandemic have had on child and youth mental health.

In this sense, the COVID-19 crisis has significantly impacted Spanish society, not only due to its direct health consequences—such as its successive waves of infections and elevated mortality, especially during 2020—but also as a result of the restrictive public health measures implemented to contain the spread of the virus. In the field of suicide prevention, the scenario has become increasingly worrisome. Data from recent years indicate a progressive rise in deaths by suicide since 2018. Rather than interrupting this pattern, the pandemic appears to have reinforced it, with sharper increases in certain segments of the population. Specifically, 3941 individuals died by suicide in 2020, a 3.6% rise compared to 2019 and a 5.5% increase from 2018. This upward trend continued in 2021, with 4003 deaths, which was a slight increase from the previous year and still significantly above pre-pandemic levels (De la Torre Luque, 2023).

Following the height of the pandemic, an increase in the total number of deaths by suicide was observed from 2020 to 2021 (see Figure 2). This increase may be indicative of worsening mental health conditions in the general population, which could be related to the prolonged effects of the COVID-19 pandemic. These would range from socioeconomic stress to social isolation and continued uncertainty about the future.

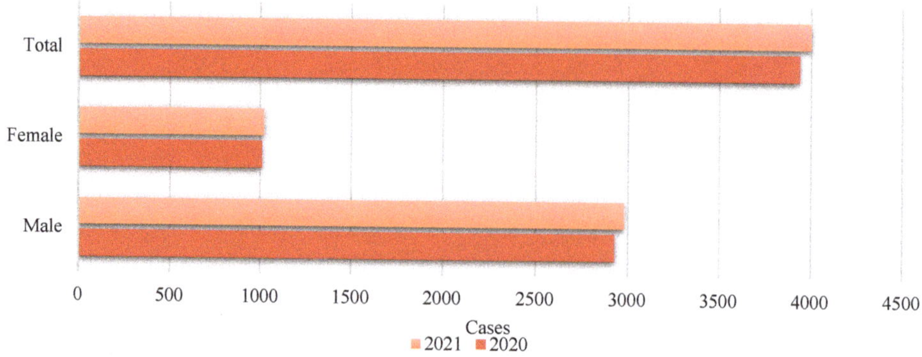

Figure 2. Deaths by suicide in Spain according to sex. Evolution from 2020 to 2021. Source: self-made. Instituto Nacional de Estadística (2023).

From a gender perspective, the difference in the number of cases between men and women is substantial, with men accounting for a higher proportion of deaths by suicide. This is consistent with the sociological and biomedical literature, which indicates that while women tend to have higher rates of suicide attempts, men have higher rates of completed suicide (Freeman et al., 2017; Mościcki, 1994). The exception to this dynamic is in the youth age group (10–17 years) where, in 2021, age-adjusted mortality (standardized rate) reached 1.49 per 100,000 persons. This portion of the population presented the greatest equity in terms of gender distribution, with a proportion of 55.4% of the deaths in this group registered in males and 44.6% in females[1].

Also, the increase in total deaths by suicide and in each of the gender categories points to 2021 being a particularly paradigmatic year. This may be linked to the late stages of the pandemic and the cumulative consequences of long periods of stress and disruption (Kim, 2022; Pathirathna et al., 2022).

These microdata also show that the highest incidence of suicide in absolute terms is found in the 45–54 age group. In 2020, this age group had one of the highest incidences of suicide in Spain, with a rate of 11.0 per 100,000 inhabitants. This population faces various socioeconomic and mental health pressures that contribute to this phenomenon. Historically, factors such as work stress, financial pressure, family responsibilities, and the onset of health problems, among other factors, are particularly relevant at this stage of life, as the literature has shown (Favril et al., 2022; Meltzer et al., 2011).

In addition, some of the studies on risk and protective factors for suicide in older people indicate that social isolation and perceived loneliness are common risk factors in older age (Ahmed & Patil, 2024; Hong et al., 2023; Motillon-Toudic et al., 2022; Solomonov et al., 2023; among others). Although this study focuses on other specific age groups, some middle-aged adults also face similar problems related to social isolation.

Younger age groups experience fewer deaths by suicide (see Figure 3), but the presence of these deaths at younger ages is still worrying for the Spanish case, indicating the need for prevention policies focused on youth mental health and the early detection of suicide risks. A gradual decline in incidence is observed with increasing age, especially after 65 years of age. This may be related to factors such as retirement, which may alleviate certain types of work and economic stress, but may also reflect a survival effect, where more resilient individuals or those with better social support survive longer.

Across all age groups in our dataset, men have higher suicide rates than women, which is consistent with trends observed globally. This is often related to cultural factors such as gender roles and the stigma associated with seeking help for mental health problems among men (Möller-Leimkühler, 2003; Schrijvers et al., 2012).

Thus, in line with historic global trends, there are more deaths by suicide among men than among women recorded every year (see Figure 4). Although the numbers for both genders seem to follow a parallel trend, there are variations in the gap between the two. The gap seems to remain the same or even increase slightly over time, indicating that suicide risk factors are affecting men to a greater extent or that men are less likely to seek or receive help for mental health problems (Houle et al., 2008; Keohane & Richardson, 2018; Shi et al., 2021).

The gender gap is widest in the middle ages of life, suggesting that men in these groups may be subject to additional risk factors or have fewer mental health support networks compared to women (see Canetto & Cleary, 2012).

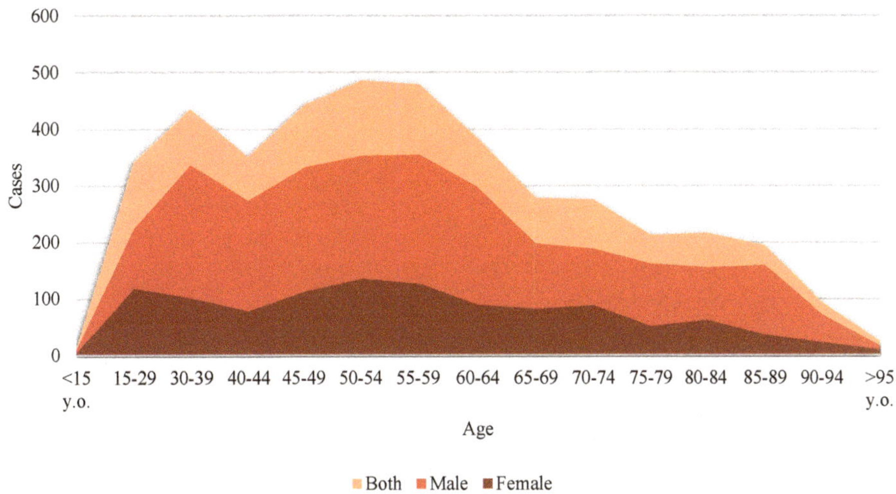

Figure 3. Deaths by suicide in Spain (2022) in terms of age and sex. Source: self-made. Instituto Nacional de Estadística (2023).

These trends underline the importance of considering social determinants of health and gender-specific risk factors when designing suicide prevention policies. The steady increase in cases could be indicative of deeper structural problems in society, such as unemployment, economic crises, and changes in family structure, which may contribute to social isolation and hopelessness; as the literature, particularly the sociological literature, has been warning us (Chandler, 2020; Mueller et al., 2021) from as early as Durkheim (1897/1951).

The data shown above could be related to substantial economic events, such as, for example, the 2008 financial crisis (Great Recession), which had a notable impact on Spain. The consequences of such events may include increased unemployment, economic insecurity, and job insecurity, which are known risk factors for mental health deterioration and suicide, as discussed in a multitude of papers from those years (see Chang et al., 2013; Coope et al., 2014; Corcoran et al., 2015; Harper & Bruckner, 2017; Haw et al., 2015). Using global risk theory, this increase can be interpreted as a manifestation of society's inability to mitigate emerging psychosocial risks and provide effective safety nets. These patterns may reflect gender and age dynamics in Spanish society, where different expectations, roles, and stresses associated with each life stage and gender may contribute to mental health and suicidal behavior (see Bacigalupe et al., 2020; Toribio-Caballero et al., 2022).

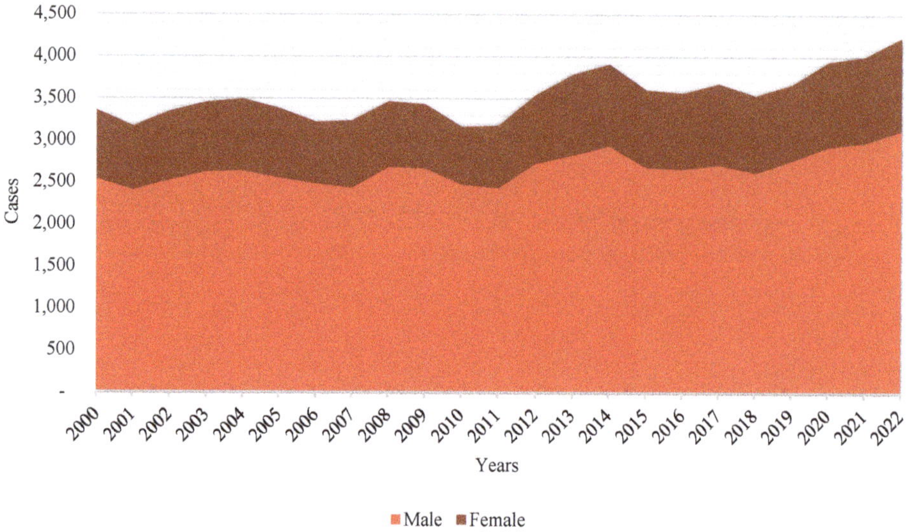

Figure 4. Evolution of deaths by suicide in Spain in 21st century according to sex. Source: self-made. Instituto Nacional de Estadística (2023).

4.2. *Sociological and Theoretical Insights*

The COVID-19 pandemic has demonstrated not only a capacity to affect physical health globally, but also a capacity to substantially exacerbate mental health problems, especially among those already vulnerable due to pre-existing mental disorders or poor structural conditions. In addition, the pandemic has led to a range of psychological stressors, intensifying symptoms in people with mental disorders and leading to the emergence of new clinical conditions. Social isolation, stigmatization, and information overload, a term already known as 'infodemia' (Caceres et al., 2022; Patwa et al., 2021; Bin Naeem & Kamel Boulos, 2021), have contributed significantly to the deterioration of mental health (Fiorillo & Gorwood, 2020). Indeed, previous research has indicated how social isolation may causally influence suicidal tendencies and how, conversely, social support may offer a protective effect, making it critical in efforts to prevent suicide (Bornheimer et al., 2020; Bränström et al., 2020).

Could this combination of factors be considered a 'perfect storm' for the deterioration of mental health (Reger et al., 2020)? Some of the research that has tracked the evolution of mental health since before and during the pandemic has identified increases in the frequency of depression and suicidal thoughts (Daly et al., 2022; Niedzwiedz et al., 2021; Pierce et al., 2020; Winkler et al., 2020). However, other studies have found no significant variations compared to mental health levels before the pandemic (Kwong et al., 2021). The first cohort study conducted in Spain (Ayuso-Mateos et al., 2023) found notable changes in the prevalence of depression when comparing the periods before and after the start of the first wave of the pandemic. However, no significant increase in the rates of suicidal ideation was identified in the period analyzed relative to pre-pandemic levels.

Studies focused on public health during this period have highlighted the particular vulnerability of people with mental disorders, underscoring the urgency of adapting and strengthening support systems for this population in times of crisis (Shinn & Viron, 2020). The need to investigate the interaction between COVID-19 and mental health has become imperative, particularly in terms of identifying and mitigating risk factors; improving the detection and treatment of symptoms of anxiety, depression, and stress; and assessing the impact of the pandemic on the prevalence of infections among those with and without mental disorders. This approach will not only address people's immediate needs during health crises, but also improve the resilience and emotional well-being of people with mental disorders in the longer term.

The Spanish case is not unique in having this upward trend in recent decades (Hedegaard & Warner, 2021; Kwon et al., 2009; Martini et al., 2019; Radhakrishnan & Andrade, 2012; Tanaka & Okamoto, 2021). The analysis of deaths by suicide in this paper highlights the urgent need for suicide prevention measures. Suicide is a global public health problem affecting, to a greater or lesser extent, people of all ages, genders, and regions. Although the age-adjusted rate of deaths by suicide is currently displaying a global downward trend, not all countries are experiencing this decline. If the current trend continues, the global SDG and WHO targets to reduce deaths by suicide by one-third by 2030 will not be met.

The Live Life: implementation guide for suicide prevention in countries (World Health Organization, 2021) proposes four evidence-based interventions to prevent suicide. These interventions include limiting access to means of suicide, such as highly dangerous pesticides and firearms; collaborating with the media to ensure responsible coverage of suicide; promoting social–emotional skills in adolescents; and the early identification, assessment, management, and follow-up of people displaying suicidal behavior. While the WHO guidance provides a seemingly robust framework, its success depends on local adaptation and implementation, as well as continued commitment to address this problem from multiple angles. The literature has argued that some of the main problems with this approach involve addressing different social gaps (see Breet et al., 2021; Chen et al., 2024; Kasal et al., 2023; Krishnamoorthy et al., 2024; Minian et al., 2024; Werdin & Wyss, 2024).

5. Discussion: Suicide and the Pandemic—A Perfect Storm?

Many countries lack the resources to implement these interventions effectively. This includes funding, infrastructure, and trained personnel. It is important to increase access to mental healthcare in low-income and rural communities (World Health Organization, 2023c). The stigma associated with mental health and suicide can prevent people from seeking help. Some institutions believe that more work is needed to raise awareness and educate in order to change cultural and social perceptions (Centers for Disease Control and Prevention, 2022a). Others point out that the lack of accurate and detailed data on suicide and suicide attempts makes it difficult to plan and implement prevention strategies. Therefore, continued research is essential to better understand the risk factors involved and develop more effective interventions (Mayo Clinic, 2023). In turn, other related institutions believe that interventions must be culturally sensitive and take into account individual differences, such as age, gender, sexual orientation, and ethnicity, to be truly effective (American Psychiatric Association, 2021). One way or another, the social character of both the phenomenon and potential interventions seems to be evident. In this sense, there is a need to address the root causes of suicide, including socioeconomic conditions, trauma, substance abuse, and mental illness. Primary prevention therefore involves working on these underlying factors before suicide or suicidal behaviors manifest (National Institutes of Health, 2023). The initial identification and management of those at risk is only the first step. Continued follow-up and support is needed to ensure long-term recovery and prevent relapse (Substance Abuse and Mental Health Services Administration, 2023).

Encouraging community involvement in suicide prevention can be an effective way to reach people at risk and build support networks. This also includes general awareness-raising (Centers for Disease Control and Prevention, 2022b). Harnessing technology and digital media for suicide prevention and mental health promotion, especially among young people, is an effective strategy that has not yet been fully exploited (World Health Organization, 2023a). As shown in recent years, it is imperative to intensify, strengthen, and accelerate suicide prevention efforts to prevent further loss of life due to this public health problem (World Health Organization, 2023b). The implementation of primary and secondary prevention strategies, along with the recognition and treatment of underlying mental health conditions, is critical (Centers for Disease Control and Prevention, 2022b). This includes not only making improvements in the therapies available and early diagnosis, but also a significant increase in funding for research and prevention programs (National Institutes of Health, 2023). Adequate resource allocation is essential to develop effective and accessible interventions that can reach those at risk before they face crisis (Substance Abuse and Mental Health Services Administration, 2023).

The COVID-19 pandemic has shown that with concerted efforts and effective health planning, it is possible to address major public health challenges. However, suicide, often described as an 'orphan disease' due to the lack of attention and resources allocated to it, requires a similar commitment (Merayo-Cano et al., 2023). The data reinforce the need for targeted mental health interventions, especially post-pandemic, where psychological sequelae may continue to manifest. The implementation of suicide prevention and support programs should be gender-sensitive, recognizing the different needs and behaviors of men and women (Holmes et al., 2020). In addition, it has been proven necessary to examine and address the underlying causes of crisis-related increases in deaths by suicide, such as economic instability and social isolation, in order to develop more effective public policies (Pierce et al., 2020). Longitudinal studies are recommended to understand how risk trajectories change over time and to adjust interventions to make them more effective (Hawton et al., 2021).

Other lines of research have included investigating the relationship between public health interventions implemented during the pandemic and suicide rates, thus providing insights into managing future public health crises without exacerbating mental health problems (Reger et al., 2020). Prevention strategies must be designed to address the specific needs of the most vulnerable age groups, such as middle-aged adults, and must be gender-sensitive if they are to create the desired impact (Wetherall & O'Connor, 2023). It is therefore particularly important to continue researching this topic to better understand the underlying factors contributing to these trends, such as the impact of economic crises, unemployment, social isolation, and other stressors related to the pandemic and its aftermath (O'Connor et al., 2021). This will enable the development of more effective approaches to mitigating adverse effects on mental health during and after crisis situations (Kawohl & Nordt, 2020).

Although this study is based on a theoretical ex post facto analysis, it is important to acknowledge the relative scarcity of formal theoretical frameworks in the literature on the relationship between COVID-19 and suicide. Most of the available studies are descriptive or epidemiological in nature, focusing on trends and risk factors without grounding their analysis in sociological or psychological theory (Gunnell et al., 2020). This theoretical gap limits our ability to fully understand the underlying mechanisms by which large-scale social disruptions contribute to mental health crises and suicidal behavior.

In other fields, researchers have successfully used established theories to analyze the effects of COVID-19 on social outcomes. For example, Agnew's General Strain Theory

(Agnew, 1992) and Felson and Cohen's Routine Activities Theory (Cohen & Felson, 1979) have been used to explain changes in crime rates during the pandemic. Although these theories originate in criminology, they offer a compelling illustration of how structured theoretical models can help make sense of social strain, routine disruption, and institutional breakdowns during periods of crisis. In this sense, COVID-19 should be understood not merely as a health emergency but as a disruptive social event[2] comparable to natural disasters, wars, or economic collapses (van Bavel et al., 2020), which alter key patterns of social organization and lead to cascading consequences, including suicide, depression, and social isolation. We therefore encourage the production of more theoretically driven research to better understand how such disruptions create vulnerability, particularly among marginalized groups.

Additionally, future research would benefit from developing and testing causal models that link social disruptions like pandemics to mental health outcomes. While the current study does not propose such a model, we recognize the potential value of structural or multilevel approaches that integrate social, economic, and psychological variables. Quantitative methods, such as time series analyses, could be particularly helpful in assessing how suicide rates evolve before, during, and after crises like COVID-19. Such tools have already shown value in criminological research (Abrams, 2021) and could offer similar insights for suicide studies.

The development of these theoretical and methodological approaches would not only strengthen our understanding of the Spanish situation regarding suicides but also allow for comparisons across societies similarly affected by global health crises.

Finally, one of the main strengths of this study is its comprehensive and sociologically grounded approach, which integrates statistical data with a theoretical framework. However, its limitations include its reliance on secondary data and the absence of primary empirical data, which may constrain the depth of this causal analysis. Additionally, as a narrative review, this study is subject to selection bias in terms of the choices made regarding the inclusion of certain studies; therefore, it is necessary to continue investigating the phenomenon using quantitative sociological analyses, which continue to provide empirical evidence.

6. Conclusions

The study of the evolution of deaths by suicide in Spain during and after the COVID-19 pandemic reveals a series of concerning trends that demand deep reflection on the current situation and the public policies necessary to address this social and public health issue. Despite efforts to reduce suicide rates in recent years, the data reveal a continuous rise in cases, particularly among vulnerable groups such as young people and those in socioeconomically disadvantaged conditions. This trend is not isolated but rather part of a broader pattern that spans across different societies in post-pandemic contexts, highlighting the urgent need to rethink prevention approaches.

The COVID-19 pandemic has accelerated and amplified a range of pre-existing risk factors affecting mental health, such as economic instability, social isolation, and overwhelmed healthcare systems. These factors, which have disproportionately affected various segments of the population, have directly contributed to an increase in psychological disorders and suicidal behavior. In particular, social isolation, mobility restrictions, and economic uncertainty have had devastating effects on the mental health of the most vulnerable sectors, creating a breeding ground conducive to suicide. The disparity in their effects based on age, gender, and social class underscores the importance of addressing suicide not only as an individual health issue but also as a phenomenon deeply influenced by social and economic structures.

A broader cultural transformation of how societies conceptualize and address suicide and mental health disorders is required. Destigmatizing these issues is fundamental to encouraging individuals to seek help without fear of rejection or discrimination. Mental health education should be an integral part of educational and social policies, ensuring that people can identify and manage mental health risks from childhood through to adulthood. Raising awareness about suicide and supporting those with suicidal thoughts must be a priority in political, social, and educational agendas in order to create a culture of prevention that empowers individuals to take action before it is too late. From a theoretical standpoint, these findings reinforce the sociological interpretation of suicide as a phenomenon deeply rooted in structural inequalities. In conclusion, the increase in deaths by suicide in Spain during the COVID-19 pandemic highlights the urgent need for multidimensional prevention strategies that take into account structural and psychosocial factors. These findings suggest that suicide cannot be addressed solely through individual interventions, but that it must be situated within a broader sociological framework that considers economic instability, social isolation, and access to mental healthcare. These results reinforce the need to translate sociological insights into actionable policies within both public health and clinical practice.

Author Contributions: Conceptualization, E.F.-V. and J.R.C.; methodology, E.F.-V. and J.R.C.; software, E.F.-V.; validation, E.F.-V. and J.R.C.; formal analysis, E.F.-V., J.J.L.G. and J.R.C.; investigation, E.F.-V., J.J.L.G. and J.R.C.; resources, E.F.-V.; data curation, E.F.-V.; writing—original draft preparation, E.F.-V. and M.I.C.; writing—review and editing, E.F.-V. and M.I.C.; visualization, E.F.-V.; supervision, J.R.C. and M.I.C.; project administration, J.R.C. and J.J.L.G.; funding acquisition, E.F.-V. and J.R.C. All authors have read and agreed to the published version of the manuscript.

Funding: This research was funded by University of Valladolid and The Bank of Santander (Spain), Grant number: 2024-3608.

Institutional Review Board Statement: Not applicable.

Informed Consent Statement: Not applicable.

Data Availability Statement: Available from the Spanish Statistical Office Database (www.ine.es).

Acknowledgments: The authors would like to express their sincere gratitude to the reviewers and the editor for their valuable comments, constructive suggestions, and careful reading of the manuscript. Their input greatly contributed to improving the quality and clarity of this work.

Conflicts of Interest: The authors declare no conflicts of interest. The funders had no role in the design of the study; in the collection, analyses, or interpretation of data; in the writing of the manuscript; or in the decision to publish the results.

Notes

1 The magnitude of the gender gap remains relatively constant from one year to the next (2020–2021), suggesting that gender-associated risk factors, such as social norms about the expression of distress and access to lethal means, may not have changed significantly between these two years. For example, according to data from the US Center for Disease Control and Prevention (CDC), in 2021, the suicide rate among men was approximately four times that of women, with 22.8 deaths per 100,000 men versus 5.7 per 100,000 women. Between 2020 and 2021, an increase in suicide rates was observed for both genders. For men, the rate increased from 21.9 to 22.8 per 100,000, while for women, it rose from 5.5 to 5.7 per 100,000. This increase may be related to several factors, including the late phases of the pandemic and the cumulative consequences of long periods of stress (Centers for Disease Control and Prevention, 2024; Substance Abuse and Mental Health Services Administration, 2023).

2 Cf. The Concept of Total Social Fact, by Mauss (1925/1990), for a sociological approach.

References

Abrams, D. S. (2021). COVID and crime: An early empirical look. *Journal of Public Economics*, *194*, 104344. [CrossRef] [PubMed]

Agnew, R. (1992). Foundation for a general strain theory of crime and delinquency. *Criminology*, *30*(1), 47–88. [CrossRef]

Ahmed, A., & Patil, P. S. (2024). Navigating the Shadows: A Comprehensive Review of Suicide in the Geriatric Population. *Cureus*, *16*(1), e53352. [CrossRef] [PubMed]

American Psychiatric Association. (2021). *Diversity and mental health*. Available online: https://www.psychiatry.org/patients-families (accessed on 15 February 2025).

ANAR Foundation. (2021). *Informe anual 2020: El teléfono/chat ANAR en tiempos de COVID-19*. Available online: https://lc.cx/wz4n72 (accessed on 15 February 2025).

Asmundson, G. J. G., & Taylor, S. (2020). How health anxiety influences responses to viral outbreaks like COVID-19: What all decision-makers, health authorities, and health care professionals need to know. *Jornal Anxiety Disord*, *71*, 102211. [CrossRef]

Aymerich, C., Pedruzo, B., Pérez, J. L., Laborda, M., Herrero, J., Blanco, J., Mancebo, G., Andrés, L., Estévez, O., Fernandez, M., Salazar de Pablo, G., Catalan, A., & González-Torres, M. A. (2022). COVID-19 pandemic effects on health worker's mental health: Systematic review and meta-analysis. *European Psychiatry*, *65*(1), e10. [CrossRef]

Ayuso-Mateos, J. L., Morillo, D., Haro, J. M., Olaya, B., Lara, E., & Miret, M. (2023). Changes on depression and suicidal ideation under severe lockdown restrictions during the first wave of the COVID-19 pandemic in Spain: A longitudinal study in the general population. *Epidemiology and Psychiatric Sciences*, *32*, e55. [CrossRef]

Bacigalupe, A., Cabezas, A., Bueno, M. B., & Martín, U. (2020). Gender as a determinant of mental health and its medicalization. SESPAS Report 2020. *Gaceta Sanitaria*, *34*(Suppl. S1), 61–67. [CrossRef]

Bajos, N., Jusot, F., Pailhé, A., Spire, A., Martin, C., Meyer, L., Lydié, N., Franck, J. E., Zins, M., Carrat, F., & SAPRIS Study Group. (2021). When lockdown policies amplify social inequalities in COVID-19 infections: Evidence from a cross-sectional population-based survey in France. *BMC Public Health-Springer Nature*, *21*, 705. [CrossRef]

Barnett, P., Oshinowo, I., Cooper, C., Taylor, C., Smith, S., & Pilling, S. (2023). The association between social class and the impact of treatment for mental health problems: A systematic review and narrative synthesis. *Social Psychiatry and Psychiatric Epidemiology*, *58*(4), 581–603. [CrossRef]

Beck, U. (2009). *World at risk*. Polity.

Bin Naeem, S., & Kamel Boulos, M. N. (2021). COVID-19 misinformation online and health literacy: A brief overview. *International Journal of Environmental Research and Public Health*, *18*(15), 8091. [CrossRef]

Bornheimer, L. A., Li, J., Im, V., Taylor, M., & Himle, J. A. (2020). The role of social isolation in the relationships between psychosis and suicidal ideation. *Clinical Social Work Journal*, *48*, 54–62. [CrossRef]

Bränström, R., van der Star, A., & Pachankis, J. E. (2020). Untethered lives: Barriers to societal integration as predictors of the sexual orientation disparity in suicidality. *Social Psychiatry and Psychiatric Epidemiology*, *55*(1), 89–99. [CrossRef] [PubMed]

Breet, E., Matooane, M., Tomlinson, M., & Bantjes, J. (2021). Systematic review and narrative synthesis of suicide prevention in high-schools and universities: A research agenda for evidence based practice. *BMC Public Health*, *21*(1), 1116. [CrossRef] [PubMed]

Caceres, M. M., Sosa, J. P., Lawrence, J. A., Sestacovschi, C., Tidd-Johnson, A., Rasool, M. H. U., Gadamidi, V. K., Ozair, S., Pandav, K., Cuevas-Lou, C., Parrish, M., Rodriguez, I., & Fernandez, J. P. (2022). The impact of misinformation on the COVID-19 pandemic. *AIMS Public Health*, *9*(2), 262–277. [CrossRef]

Canetto, S. S., & Cleary, A. (2012). Men, masculinities and suicidal behaviour. Social *Science & Medicine (1982)*, *74*(4), 461–465. [CrossRef]

Centers for Disease Control and Prevention. (2022a). *Mental health*. Available online: https://www.cdc.gov/mental-health/about/?CDC_AAref_Val= (accessed on 15 February 2025).

Centers for Disease Control and Prevention. (2022b). *Suicide prevention*. Available online: https://www.cdc.gov/suicide/risk-factors/?CDC_AAref_Val= (accessed on 17 February 2025).

Centers for Disease Control and Prevention. (2024). *Web-based Injury Statistics Query and Reporting System (WISQARS)*. Available online: https://www.cdc.gov/injury/wisqars/index.html (accessed on 14 February 2025).

Chandler, A. (2020). Socioeconomic inequalities of suicide: Sociological and psychological intersections. *European Journal of Social Theory*, *23*(1), 33–51. [CrossRef]

Chang, S. S., Stuckler, D., Yip, P., & Gunnell, D. (2013). Impact of 2008 global economic crisis on suicide: Time trend study in 54 countries. *BMJ (Clinical Research ed.)*, *347*, f5239. [CrossRef]

Chen, J. I., Roth, B., Dobscha, S. K., & Lowery, J. C. (2024). Implementation strategies in suicide prevention: A scoping review. *Implementation Science: IS*, *19*(1), 20. [CrossRef]

Clua-García, R., Casanova-Garrigós, G., & Moreno-Poyato, A. R. (2021). Suicide care from the nursing perspective: A meta-synthesis of qualitative studies. *Journal of Advanced Nursing*, *77*(7), 2995–3007. [CrossRef]

Cockerham, W. C. (2021). *Sociology of mental disorder*. Routledge.

Cockerham, W. C. (2022). *Medical sociology*. Routledge.

Cohen, L. E., & Felson, M. (1979). Social change and crime rate trends: A routine activity approach. *American Sociological Review, 44*(4), 588–608. [CrossRef]

Coope, C., Gunnell, D., Hollingworth, W., Hawton, K., Kapur, N., Fearn, V., Wells, C., & Metcalfe, C. (2014). Suicide and the 2008 economic recession: Who is most at risk? Trends in suicide rates in England and Wales 2001–2011. Social *Science & Medicine (1982), 117*, 76–85. [CrossRef]

Corcoran, P., Griffin, E., Arensman, E., Fitzgerald, A. P., & Perry, I. J. (2015). Impact of the economic recession and subsequent austerity on suicide and self-harm in Ireland: An interrupted time series analysis. *International Journal of Epidemiology, 44*(3), 969–977. [CrossRef] [PubMed]

Coronaviridae Study Group of the International Committee on Taxonomy of Viruses. (2020). The species Severe acute respiratory syndrome-related coronavirus: Classifying 2019-nCoV and naming it SARS-CoV-2. *Nature Microbiology, 5*(4), 536–544. [CrossRef] [PubMed]

Da Cunha Varella, A. P., Griffin, E., Khashan, A., & Kabir, Z. (2024). Suicide rates before and during the COVID-19 pandemic: A systematic review and meta-analysis. *Social Psychiatry and Psychiatric Epidemiology, 59*(11), 1897–1905. [CrossRef]

Daly, M., Sutin, A. R., & Robinson, E. (2022). Longitudinal changes in mental health and the COVID-19 pandemic: Evidence from the UK Household Longitudinal Study. *Psychological Medicine, 52*(13), 2549–2558. [CrossRef]

De la Torre Luque, A. (2023). *Evolución del suicidio en España en este milenio (2000–2021)*. Universidad Complutense de Madrid.

De la Torre Luque, A., Perez-Diez, I., Pemau, A., Martinez-Ales, G., Borges, G., Perez-Sola, V., & Ayuso-Mateos, J. L. (2024). Suicide mortality in Spain during the COVID-19 pandemic: Longitudinal analysis of sociodemographic factors. *European Neuropsychopharmacology, 82*, 29–34. [CrossRef]

Durkheim, E. (1951). *Suicide: A study in sociology*. Free Press. (originally in French 1897).

Fair Health. (2022). *Patients diagnosed with post-COVID conditions. An analysis of private healthcare claimsusing the OfficialICD-10 diagnostic code*. Fair Health Inc.

Favril, L., Yu, R., Uyar, A., Sharpe, M., & Fazel, S. (2022). Risk factors for suicide in adults: Systematic review and meta-analysis of psychological autopsy studies. *Evidence-Based Mental Health, 25*(4), 148–155. [CrossRef]

Fiorillo, A., & Gorwood, P. (2020). The consequences of the COVID-19 pandemic on mental health and implications for clinical practice. *European Psychiatry, 63*(1), e32. [CrossRef]

Freeman, A., Mergl, R., Kohls, E., Székely, A., Gusmao, R., Arensman, E., Koburger, N., Hegerl, U., & Rummel-Kluge, C. (2017). A cross-national study on gender differences in suicide intent. *BMC Psychiatry, 17*, 1–11. [CrossRef]

González-Sanguino, C., Ausín, B., Castellanos, M. Á., Saiz, J., López-Gómez, A., Ugidos, C., & Muñoz, M. (2020). Mental health consequences during the initial stage of the 2020 Coronavirus pandemic (COVID-19) in Spain. *Brain, behavior, and Immunity, 87*, 172–176. [CrossRef]

Gunnell, D., Appleby, L., Arensman, E., Hawton, K., John, A., Kapur, N., Khan, M., O'Connor, R. C., Pirkis, J., & COVID-19 Suicide Prevention Research Collaboration. (2020). Suicide risk and prevention during the COVID-19 pandemic. *The Lancet Psychiatry, 7*(6), 468–471. [CrossRef] [PubMed]

Harper, S., & Bruckner, T. A. (2017). Did the Great Recession increase suicides in the USA? Evidence from an interrupted time-series analysis. *Annals of Epidemiology, 27*(7), 409–414. [CrossRef] [PubMed]

Haw, C., Hawton, K., Gunnell, D., & Platt, S. (2015). Economic recession and suicidal behaviour: Possible mechanisms and ameliorating factors. *The International Journal of Social Psychiatry, 61*(1), 73–81. [CrossRef]

Hawton, K., Lascelles, K., Pitman, A., Gilbert, S., Bale, E., & Muniz, J. (2021). Self-harm and the COVID-19 pandemic: A study of factors contributing to self-harm during lockdown restrictions. *Journal of Affective Disorders, 295*, 441–449. [CrossRef]

Hedegaard, H., & Warner, M. (2021). *Suicide mortality in the United States, 1999–2019*. Department of Health and Human Services, Centers for Disease Control and Prevention, National Center for Health Statistics.

Holmes, E. A., O'Connor, R. C., Perry, V. H., Tracey, I., Wessely, S., Arseneault, L., Ballard, C., Christensen, H., Silver, R. C., Everall, I., & Ford, T. (2020). Multidisciplinary research priorities for the COVID-19 pandemic: A call for action for mental health science. *The Lancet Psychiatry, 7*(6), 547–560. [CrossRef]

Holst, H., Fessler, A., & Niehoff, S. (2021). COVID-19, social class and work experience in Germany: Inequalities in work-related health and economic risks. *European Societies, 23*(Suppl. S1), S495–S512. [CrossRef]

Hong, R., Cheng, W. H., Cheng, L. J., Lau, Y., & Lau, S. T. (2023). Global prevalence of social isolation among community-dwelling older adults: A systematic review and meta-analysis. *Archives of Gerontology and Geriatrics, 107*, 104904.

Houle, J., Mishara, B. L., & Chagnon, F. (2008). An empirical test of a mediation model of the impact of the traditional male gender role on suicidal behavior in men. *Journal of Affective Disorders, 107*(1–3), 37–43. [CrossRef]

Huang, C., Wang, Y., Li, X., Ren, L., Zhao, J., Hu, Y., Zhang, L., Fan, G., Xu, J., Gu, X., & Cheng, Z. (2020). Clinical features of patients infected with 2019 novel coronavirus in Wuhan, China. *The Lancet, 395*(10223), 497–506. [CrossRef]

Husain, M. O., Gratzer, D., Husain, M. I., & Naeem, F. (2021). Mental Illness in the Post-pandemic World: Digital Psychiatry and the Future. *Frontiers in Psychology, 12*, 567426. [CrossRef]

Instituto Nacional de Estadística. (2020). *Defunciones por suicidio. Año 2019* [dataset]. Spanish Statistical Office Database. Available online: https://www.ine.es/jaxi/Datos.htm?tpx=48293 (accessed on 27 January 2025).

Instituto Nacional de Estadística. (2021). *Defunciones por suicidio. Año 2020* [dataset]. Spanish Statistical Office Database. Available online: https://www.ine.es/jaxi/Datos.htm?tpx=49948 (accessed on 27 January 2025).

Instituto Nacional de Estadística. (2023). *Estadísticas de suicidio en España*. Spanish Statistical Office Database. Available online: https://n9.cl/kml7b (accessed on 14 February 2025).

Instituto Nacional de Estadística. (2024). *Estadística de defunciones según causa de muerte* [dataset]. Spanish Statistical Office Database. Available online: https://www.ine.es/dyngs/INEbase/es/operacion.htm?c=Estadistica_C&cid=1254736176780&menu=ultiDatos&idp=1254735573175 (accessed on 14 February 2025).

Ji, X., Zhan, T., & Zhu, T. (2024). Impact of COVID-19 on negative body image: Evidence based on social media data. *Social Science & Medicine, 340*, 116461. [CrossRef]

Johns Hopkins University. (2023). *COVID-19 dashboard*. Available online: https://n9.cl/gj7w (accessed on 27 January 2025).

Kasal, A., Táborská, R., Juríková, L., Grabenhofer-Eggerth, A., Pichler, M., Gruber, B., Tomášková, H., & Niederkrotenthaler, T. (2023). Facilitators and barriers to implementation of suicide prevention interventions: Scoping review. *Global Mental Health, 10*, e15. [CrossRef] [PubMed]

Kawohl, W., & Nordt, C. (2020). COVID-19, unemployment, and suicide. *The Lancet Psychiatry, 7*(5), 389–390. [CrossRef] [PubMed]

Keohane, A., & Richardson, N. (2018). Negotiating Gender Norms to Support Men in Psychological Distress. *American Journal of Men's Health, 12*(1), 160–171. [CrossRef]

Kim, A. M. (2022). The impact of the COVID-19 pandemic on suicides: A population study. *Psychiatry Research, 314*, 114663. [CrossRef]

Krishnamoorthy, S., Mathieu, S., Armstrong, G., Ross, V., Francis, J., Reifels, L., & Kõlves, K. (2024). Implementation of complex suicide prevention interventions: Insights into barriers, facilitators and lessons learned. *Archives of Suicide Research: Official Journal of the International Academy for Suicide Research, 9*, 1–24. [CrossRef]

Kwon, J. W., Chun, H., & Cho, S. I. (2009). A closer look at the increase in suicide rates in South Korea from 1986–2005. *BMC Public Health, 9*, 1–9. [CrossRef]

Kwong, A. S. F., Pearson, R. M., Adams, M. J., Northstone, K., Tilling, K., Smith, D., Fawns-Ritchie, C., Bould, H., Warne, N., Zammit, S., Gunnell, D., Moran, P., Micali, N., & Timpson, N. J. (2021). Mental health before and during the COVID-19 pandemic in two longitudinal UK population cohorts. *The British Journal of Psychiatry, 218*(6), 334–343. [CrossRef]

Lee, H., & Singh, G. K. (2021). Monthly trends in self-reported health status and depression by race/ethnicity and socioeconomic status during the COVID-19 Pandemic, United States, April 2020–May 2021. *Annals of Epidemiology, 63*, 52–62. [CrossRef]

Lopes, J., Damasceno, A. B. P., da Costa, G. S., Silva, V. D. O., Filho, V. A. D. B., & De Lima, J. C. M. G. (2022). A Influência da Pandemia da COVID-19 na Pronunciação de Sinais Neurológicos e Cognitivos de Crianças e Adolescentes com TDAH: Uma Revisão Integrativa. *Brazilian Medical Students, 7*(10), 1–11. [CrossRef]

Manchia, M., Gathier, A. W., Yapici-Eser, H., Schmidt, M. V., de Quervain, D., van Amelsvoort, T., Bisson, J. I., Cryan, J. F., Howes, O. D., Pinto, L., van der Wee, N. J., Domschke, K., Branchi, I., & Vinkers, C. H. (2022). The impact of the prolonged COVID-19 pandemic on stress resilience and mental health: A critical review across waves. *European Neuropsychopharmacology: The Journal of the European College of Neuropsychopharmacology, 55*, 22–83. [CrossRef] [PubMed]

Martini, M., da Fonseca, R. C., de Sousa, M. H., de Azambuja Farias, C., Cardoso, T. A., Kunz, M., Longaray, V. K., & Magalhães, P. V. D. S. (2019). Age and sex trends for suicide in Brazil between 2000 and 2016. *Social Psychiatry and Psychiatric Epidemiology, 54*(7), 857–860. [CrossRef] [PubMed]

Mauss, M. (1990). *The gift: Forms and functions of exchange in archaic societies*. Routledge. (originally in French 1925).

Mayo Clinic. (2023). *Mental illness. Symptoms and causes*. Available online: https://www.mayoclinic.org/diseases-conditions/mental-illness/in-depth/mental-health/art-20046477 (accessed on 20 February 2025).

Meltzer, H., Bebbington, P., Brugha, T., Jenkins, R., McManus, S., & Dennis, M. S. (2011). Personal debt and suicidal ideation. *Psychological Medicine, 41*(4), 771–778. [CrossRef] [PubMed]

Mental Health and Substance Use. (2013). *Mental health action plan 2013–2020*. World Health Organization.

Mental Health and Substance Use. (2021). *Suicide worldwide in 2019. Global Health Estimates*. World Health Organization.

Merayo-Cano, J. M., Porras-Segovia, A. A., & Baca-García, E. (2023). COVID-19 impact vs. suicide impact in Spain. *Spanish Journal of Psychiatry and Mental Health, 16*(2), 129–130. [CrossRef]

Minian, N., Gayapersad, A., Coroiu, A., Dragonetti, R., Zawertailo, L., Zaheer, J., O'Neill, B., Lange, S., Thomson, N., Crawford, A., Kennedy, S. H., & Selby, P. (2024). Prototyping the implementation of a suicide prevention protocol in primary care settings using PDSA cycles: A mixed method study. *Frontiers in Psychiatry, 15*, 1286078. [CrossRef]

Ministerio de Sanidad. (2024). *Defunciones por suicidio en España, 2022–2024*. Available online: https://www.sanidad.gob.es/estadEstudios/estadisticas/estadisticas/estMinisterio/mortalidad/docs/DefunSuicidio2022-2024_NOTA__TEC.pdf (accessed on 20 February 2025).

Mościcki, E. K. (1994). Gender differences in completed and attempted suicides. *Annals of Epidemiology, 4*(2), 152–158. [CrossRef]

Motillon-Toudic, C., Walter, M., Séguin, M., Carrier, J. D., Berrouiguet, S., & Lemey, C. (2022). Social isolation and suicide risk: Literature review and perspectives. *European psychiatry: The journal of the Association of European Psychiatrists, 65*(1), e65. [CrossRef]

Möller-Leimkühler, A. M. (2003). The gender gap in suicide and premature death or: Why are men so vulnerable? *European Archives of Psychiatry and Clinical Neuroscience, 253*(1), 1–8. [CrossRef]

Mueller, A. S., Abrutyn, S., Pescosolido, B., & Diefendorf, S. (2021). The social roots of suicide: Theorizing how the external social world matters to suicide and suicide prevention. *Frontiers in Psychology, 12*, 621569. [CrossRef]

National Institutes of Health. (2023). *Suicide prevention*. Available online: https://www.nimh.nih.gov/health/topics/suicide-prevention (accessed on 20 February 2025).

Nettleton, S. (2021). *The sociology of health and illness*. Polity.

Nicolini, H. (2020). Depression and anxiety during COVID-19 pandemic. *Cirugía y Cirujanos, 88*(5), 542–547. [CrossRef]

Niedzwiedz, C. L., Green, M. J., Benzeval, M., Campbell, D., Craig, P., Demou, E., Leyland, A. H., Pearce, A., Thomson, R., & Whitley, E. (2021). Mental health and health behaviours before and during the initial phase of the COVID-19 lockdown: Longitudinal analyses of the UK Household Longitudinal Study. *Journal of Epidemiology & Community Health, 75*(3), 224–231. [CrossRef]

O'Connor, R. C., Wetherall, K., Cleare, S., McClelland, H., Melson, A. J., Niedzwiedz, C. L., O'Carroll, R. E., O'Connor, D. B., Platt, S., Scowcroft, E., Watson, B., Zortea, T., Ferguson, E., & Robb, K. A. (2021). Mental health and well-being during the COVID-19 pandemic: Longitudinal analyses of adults in the UK COVID-19 Mental Health & Wellbeing study. *The British Journal of Psychiatry: The Journal of Mental Science, 218*(6), 326–333. [CrossRef] [PubMed]

Pappa, S., Ntella, V., Giannakas, T., Giannakoulis, V. G., Papoutsi, E., & Katsaounou, P. (2020). Prevalence of depression, anxiety, and insomnia among healthcare workers during the COVID-19 pandemic: A systematic review and meta-analysis. *Brain, Behavior, and Immunity, 88*, 901–907. [CrossRef] [PubMed]

Paricio del Castillo, R., del Sol-Calderón, P., García-Murillo, L., Mallol-Castaño, L., Pascual-Aranda, A., & Palanca-Maresca, I. (2024). Suicidio infanto-juvenil tras la pandemia de COVID-19: Análisis de un fenómeno trágico. *Revista de la Asociación Española de Neuropsiquiatría, 44*(145), 19–45.

Pathirathna, M. L., Nandasena, H. M. R. K. G., Atapattu, A. M. M. P., & Weerasekara, I. (2022). Impact of the COVID-19 pandemic on suicidal attempts and death rates: A systematic review. *BMC Psychiatry, 22*(1), 506. [CrossRef]

Patwa, P., Sharma, S., Pykl, S., Guptha, V., Kumari, G., Akhtar, M. S., Ekbal, A., Das, A., & Chakraborty, T. (2021). Fighting an infodemic: COVID-19 fake news dataset. In *combating online hostile posts in regional languages during emergency situation: First international workshop, constraint 2021, collocated with AAAI 2021, virtual event, 8 February 2021, revised selected papers 1* (pp. 21–29). Springer International Publishing.

Pearman, A., Hughes, M. L., Smith, E. L., & Neupert, S. D. (2020). Mental health challenges of United States healthcare professionals during COVID-19. *Frontiers in Psychology, 11*, 2065. [CrossRef]

Pierce, M., Hope, H., Ford, T., Hatch, S., Hotopf, M., John, A., Kontopantelis, E., Webb, R., Wessely, S., McManus, S., & Abel, K. M. (2020). Mental health before and during the COVID-19 pandemic: A longitudinal probability sample survey of the UK population. *The Lancet Psychiatry, 7*(10), 883–892. [CrossRef]

Radhakrishnan, R., & Andrade, C. (2012). Suicide: An Indian perspective. *Indian Journal of Psychiatry, 54*(4), 304–319. [CrossRef]

Reger, M. A., Stanley, I. H., & Joiner, T. E. (2020). Suicide Mortality and Coronavirus Disease 2019-A Perfect Storm? *JAMA Psychiatry, 77*(11), 1093–1094. [CrossRef]

Schnitzer, P. G., Dykstra, H., & Collier, A. (2023). The COVID-19 Pandemic and Youth Suicide: 2020–2021. *Pediatrics, 151*(3), e2022058716. [CrossRef]

Schrijvers, D. L., Bollen, J., & Sabbe, B. G. (2012). The gender paradox in suicidal behavior and its impact on the suicidal process. *Journal of Affective Disorders, 138*(1–2), 19–26. [CrossRef] [PubMed]

Sher, L. (2020). The impact of the COVID-19 pandemic on suicide rates. *QJM: Monthly Journal of the Association of Physicians, 113*(10), 707–712. [CrossRef] [PubMed]

Shi, P., Yang, A., Zhao, Q., Chen, Z., Ren, X., & Dai, Q. (2021). A Hypothesis of Gender Differences in Self-Reporting Symptom of Depression: Implications to Solve Under-Diagnosis and Under-Treatment of Depression in Males. *Frontiers in Psychiatry, 12*, 589687. [CrossRef] [PubMed]

Shidhaye, R. (2023). Global priorities for improving access to mental health services for adolescents in the post-pandemic world. *Current Opinion in Psychology, 53*, 101661. [CrossRef]

Shinn, A. K., & Viron, M. (2020). Perspectives on the COVID-19 pandemic and individuals with serious mental illness. *The Journal of Clinical Psychiatry, 81*(3), 20com13412. [CrossRef]

Sohn, M., Koo, H., Choi, H., Cho, H., & Han, E. (2022). Collateral impact of the COVID−19 pandemic on the use of healthcare resources among people with disabilities. *Frontiers Public Health, 10*, 922043. [CrossRef]

Solomonov, N., Green, J., Quintana, A., Lin, J., Ognyanova, K., Santillana, M., Druckman, J. N., Baum, M. A., Lazer, D., Gunning, F. M., & Perlis, R. H. (2023). A 50-state survey study of thoughts of suicide and social isolation among older adults in the United States. *Journal of Affective Disorders, 334*, 43–49. [CrossRef]

Soria, K. M., & Horgos, B. (2020). *Social class differences in students' experiences during the COVID-19 pandemic*. University of California-Berkeley and University of Minnesota.

Substance Abuse and Mental Health Services Administration. (2023). *Key substance use and mental health indicators in the United States: Results from the 2022 national survey on drug use and health*. Available online: https://www.samhsa.gov/data/report/2022-nsduh-annual-national-report (accessed on 15 February 2025).

Tanaka, T., & Okamoto, S. (2021). Increase in suicide following an initial decline during the COVID-19 pandemic in Japan. *Nature Human Behaviour, 5*(2), 229–238. [CrossRef]

Toribio-Caballero, S., Cardenal, V., Ávila, A., & Ovejero, M. (2022). Gender roles and women's mental health: Their influence on the demand for psychological care. *Anales de Psicología, 38*(1), 7–16. [CrossRef]

Vadivel, R., Shoib, S., El Halabi, S., El Hayek, S., Essam, L., Gashi Bytyçi, D., Karaliuniene, R., Schuh Teixeira, A. L., Nagendrappa, S., Ramalho, R., Ransing, R., Pereira-Sanchez, V., Jatchavala, C., Adiukwu, F. N., & Kudva Kundadak, G. (2021). Mental health in the post-COVID-19 era: Challenges and the way forward. *General Psychiatry, 34*(1), e100424. [CrossRef]

van Bavel, J. J., Baicker, K., Boggio, P. S., Capraro, V., Cichocka, A., Cikara, M., Crockett, M. J., Crum, A. J., Douglas, K. M., Druckman, J. N., Drury, J., Dube, O., Ellemers, N., Finkel, E. J., Fowler, J. H., Gelfand, M., Han, S., Haslam, S. A., Jetten, J., . . . Willer, R. (2020). Using social and behavioural science to support COVID-19 pandemic response. *Nature Human Behaviour, 4*(5), 460–471. [CrossRef] [PubMed]

Werdin, S., & Wyss, K. (2024). Challenges in the evaluation of suicide prevention measures and quality of suicide data in Germany, Austria, and Switzerland: Findings from qualitative expert interviews. *BMC Public Health, 24*(1), 2209. [CrossRef] [PubMed]

Wetherall, K., & O'Connor, R. (2023). Suicide prevention targeting middle-aged males: The role of primary care. *The British Journal of General Practice: The Journal of the Royal College of General Practitioners, 73*(732), 292–294. [CrossRef]

Winkler, P., Formanek, T., Mlada, K., Kagstrom, A., Mohrova, Z., Mohr, P., & Csemy, L. (2020). Prevalence of depressive symptoms during the COVID-19 pandemic in the Czech Republic: A cross-sectional survey. *Journal of Affective Disorders, 277*, 251–257. [CrossRef]

World Health Organization. (2021). *Live life: An implementation guide for suicide prevention in countries*. Available online: https://n9.cl/9ygqy (accessed on 14 February 2025).

World Health Organization. (2023a). *Digital health*. Available online: https://www.who.int/health-topics/digital-health#tab=tab_1 (accessed on 20 February 2025).

World Health Organization. (2023b). *Fact sheets: Suicide*. Available online: https://www.who.int/news-room/fact-sheets/detail/suicide (accessed on 14 February 2025).

World Health Organization. (2023c). *With the international public health emergency ending, WHO/Europe launches its transition plan for COVID-19*. Available online: https://n9.cl/sb0t1 (accessed on 20 February 2025).

Wu, C., & Qian, Y. (2022). The gender peak effect: Women are most vulnerable to infections during COVID-19 peaks. *Frontiers Public Health, 10*, 937179. [CrossRef]

Yan, Y., Hou, J., Li, Q., & Yu, N. X. (2023). Suicide before and during the COVID-19 pandemic: A systematic review with meta-analysis. *International Journal of Environmental Research and Public Health, 20*(4), 3346. [CrossRef]

behavioral sciences

MDPI

Review

The Prevention of Suicide in Older Military Veterans

Joshua Levine [1,2] and Leo Sher [3,4,*]

1 Veterans' Administration New York Harbor Healthcare System, Brooklyn, NY 11209, USA; jpl2158@columbia.edu
2 School of Social Work, Columbia University, New York, NY 10027, USA
3 James J. Peters Veterans' Administration Medical Center, Bronx, NY 10468, USA
4 Department of Psychiatry, Icahn School of Medicine at Mount Sinai, New York, NY 10029, USA
* Correspondence: leo.sher@mssm.edu; Tel.: +1-718-584-9000

Abstract: Suicidal behavior among older military veterans is an important medical and social problem. The goal of this literature review is to discuss this underappreciated issue and identify suicide preventive interventions that can be utilized with the older military veteran population. Older veterans experience psychiatric, medical, and social problems associated with their age and/or military experience that can contribute to suicide risk. These problems include relationship losses through death or estrangement, depression, cognitive decline, loneliness, isolation, frailty, mobility issues, and chronic pain. Therefore, older veterans face a unique set of challenges. Suicide prevention in older veterans should take a multipronged approach which includes screening for suicidality, management of psychiatric and medical disorders, social assistance, safety planning, lethal means restriction, and involving family members in the veteran's healthcare. Family members should be included in the safety planning process when possible. Gatekeeper training programs can be utilized to train individuals who are working with older veterans to reduce suicides amongst this age group.

Keywords: suicide; public health; depression; stress; military veterans; older

1. Introduction: Geriatric Suicide—A Major Public Health Problem

The World Health Organization (WHO) reported that nearly one in six people will be 60 years or older by the year 2030 (World Health Organization, 2023). Suicide among the older adult population is a multinational problem. In 2019, 256,953 (36.53%) of the 703,220 people who were estimated to die by suicide globally were aged 60 and older (World Health Organization, 2020). It is possible that suicide rates are underestimated. Many suicide deaths may be incorrectly documented as "unnatural" or "undetermined" deaths (Sher & Oquendo, 2023; Tøllefson et al., 2015). Actual suicide rates may be 10–50% higher than reported. This makes suicide prevention efforts among the older population a crucial undertaking. Older adults experience problems associated with their age that can contribute to suicide risk. These problems consist of relationship losses through death or estrangement, mental health disorders (i.e., anxiety or depression), medical problems, cognitive decline, loneliness, isolation, frailty, mobility issues, and chronic pain (Conwell et al., 2011; O'Malley et al., 2020). Older persons are also at risk for neglect and elder abuse (i.e., physical, psychological, sexual, or financial) (Cooper et al., 2008; Yunus et al., 2019). For example, one review found that 6% of older people reported abuse in the last month, and nearly 25% of vulnerable older persons were at risk for abuse (Cooper et al., 2008).

Oftentimes, a considerable amount of attention is given in cases of adolescent suicide (Carballo et al., 2020; S. Kim et al., 2024; Zartaloudi, 2024). This may be because of the thought of years of potential life lost. From a humanitarian standpoint, geriatric suicide is an important problem, and should be a focus of suicide prevention efforts.

Suicide among older people, including older veterans, does not receive enough attention. The goal of this paper is to discuss this underappreciated issue and identify suicide preventive interventions that can be utilized with the older military veteran population.

2. Definitions

As noted above, this review is dedicated to the issue of suicidal behavior among older veterans. Suicidal behavior suggests suicide death but also includes different kinds of suicide attempts that range from highly lethal attempts to low-lethality attempts that may occur during a psychosocial crisis (Naguy et al., 2020; Sher & Oquendo, 2023; Turecki et al., 2019). A suicide attempt is commonly defined as a self-destructive act carried out with some degree of intent to end one's life. Suicidal ideation is a term used to describe suicidal thoughts (Harmer et al., 2024). Some suicide ideation definitions incorporate suicide planning thoughts, while others regard planning to be a separate phase. Suicidal ideation is associated with both suicide attempts and deaths and is a significant risk factor for future suicide attempts (Baca-Garcia et al., 2011; Sher & Oquendo, 2023). Suicidal ideation and suicidal behaviors can be conceptualized as taking place over a continuum from suicidal ideation, development of a suicide plan, nonfatal suicide attempt(s), or death from suicide, although the evolution from one to the other is not necessarily linear (Baca-Garcia et al., 2011). Multiple risk factors such as recent onset of suicidal ideation, the presence and recent onset of suicide plan, extreme risk taking, and failure to answer questions about the characteristics of one's suicidal thoughts predict transition from suicidal ideation to suicide attempt (Nock et al., 2018).

In the United States (U.S.), a military veteran is an individual who has served in the Armed Forces, including the Reserve (United States Census Bureau, 2021). Combat veterans are individuals who served in a conflict/war zone while in the military. In many countries, individuals are classified as military veterans if they served during wartime and/or participated in combat operations; i.e., only combat veterans are regarded as veterans (EUROMIL, 2022).

The U.S. National Institute on Aging defines older adults as people aged 65 or older (National Institutes of Health, 2024). However, definitions of older adulthood differ. For example, an older person is defined by the United Nations as an individual who is over 60 years of age (The UN Refugee Agency, 2024). It has also been suggested that "While age 60 was considered "old" in many peoples' grandparents' time, 80 is the median age considered "old" today" (Stagwell Global, 2024). For the purposes of this article, we assume that older adulthood is the stage of life usually beginning around age 65 and is characterized by different physical, cognitive, and social changes associated with aging.

3. Suicide Among the Military Veteran Population

As per the recent reports released by the U.S. Census Bureau, there are around 18 million military veterans and 2.1 million active-duty and Reserve service members in the U.S. (United States Census Bureau, 2020). More than 6% of the US population has served or is currently serving in the Armed Forces.

Suicide amongst the military veteran population is a significant public health problem (Department of Veterans Affairs, 2023; Levine & Sher, 2021c; Shen et al., 2016). Before 2000, the suicide rates among military servicemembers and veterans were lower than those among civilians. However, these rates have increased over the last 20 years and exceed the current rate among civilians (Moore et al., 2023). The National Veteran Suicide Prevention Annual Report revealed that 6278 U.S. military veterans died by suicide in 2020, and this number raised to 6392 in 2021 (Department of Veterans Affairs, 2023). This accounts for an increase of 17.2 to 17.5 average veteran suicides per day from 2020 to 2021 (Department of Veterans Affairs, 2023). Unfortunately, the COVID-19 pandemic may account for an increase in veteran suicide rates (Levine & Sher, 2021b).

Military veterans are at greater risk for medical problems, psychiatric disorders, and psychosocial stressors as compared to the general population (Bruce, 2010; Levine & Sher, 2021c; Pew Research Center, 2019; Rice & Sher, 2012). Research indicates that the presence of these conditions can increase suicidality in military veterans (Bruce, 2010).

4. What Makes Older Veterans Suicidal?

Older veterans may face a unique set of challenges as compared to their younger counterparts. They have more severe medical disorders, psychiatric problems, and psychosocial difficulties than younger veterans. The presentation of psychiatric and physical disorders may be different in the elderly population in comparison to the younger individuals. Considerable evidence suggests that older veterans are at elevated risk for suicide (Kaplan et al., 2012; Mills et al., 2013; Sullivan et al., 2023; Zivin et al., 2007).

4.1. Psychiatric Disorders

Many military veterans have unique experiences that the general population will not encounter. These circumstances might consist of combat exposure, being exposed to a chemical or toxin (i.e., Agent Orange or radiation), or deployment to a harsh terrain (i.e., desert or jungle). Combat exposure could lead to posttraumatic stress disorder (PTSD), physical injury, or being captured as a prisoner of war. Research shows that approximately 14–16% of U.S. military personnel who were deployed have a PTSD diagnosis (Gates et al., 2012). Comparatively, PTSD only affects about 7–8% of the U.S. general population (Gates et al., 2012). Among veterans older than 60, the prevalence of PTSD in combat veterans is 16.9%, and it is 5.5% among non-combat veterans (Goldberg et al., 2016). Combat exposure is not the only factor that contributes to PTSD in military veterans. Unfortunately, military veterans can also be victims of Military Sexual Trauma (MST). MST refers to sexual harassment or sexual assault that was experienced during military service (Kimerling et al., 2007). Additionally, military veterans who have never had a combat deployment might experience an incident on base that can result in PTSD, such as accidental death of a counterpart. PTSD has been shown to increase suicide risk in veteran populations (Bruce, 2010; Pompili et al., 2013; Sher, 2024b). Most studies, but not all studies, indicate that combat veterans are at higher risk for suicide than non-combat veterans or the general population (Bullman & Schneiderman, 2021; Schoenbaum et al., 2014; Shen et al., 2016; Sher, 2024b). For example, one study found that Operation Enduring Freedom and Operation Iraqi Freedom (OEF/OIF) war veterans had elevated suicide rates for the first 4 years after their deployment, in comparison with veterans who had not been deployed (Shen et al., 2016). It is a debatable issue that veterans who have had combat deployments are at the highest risk of suicide. One study reviewed data of 3.9 million U.S. military personnel who served in OEF/OIF (Reger et al., 2015). The study found that military personnel who were deployed were not at higher risk for suicide, as compared to those who were not deployed (Reger et al., 2015).

A meta-analysis and systematic review that reviewed eleven studies of veterans aged >65 years found that older veterans had a higher prevalence of alcohol and substance use disorders as compared to community estimates (Williamson et al., 2018). Veterans who experienced traumatic events earlier in their life might experience re-emerging PTSD symptoms during their geriatric years (Davison et al., 2016).

PTSD is not the only psychiatric disorder that is prevalent amongst military veterans. Seal et al. (2007) reviewed healthcare data of 103,788 U.S. military veterans who served in OEF/OIF (Seal et al., 2007). The researchers concluded that 25% (25,658) of these veterans had at least one mental health diagnosis consisting of either PTSD (13%), adjustment disorder (6%), anxiety disorder (6%), depression (5%), substance use disorder (5%), or other mental health disorder (12%) (Seal et al., 2007). Another study reviewed data of 821 United Kingdom (UK) OEF/OIF military veterans and identified the presence of the following mental health disorders: PTSD (4.8%), neurotic disorders (13.5%), depression disorders (11%), anxiety disorders (4.5%), somatization disorders (1.8%), and alcohol abuse (18%) (Iversen et al., 2009). All these psychiatric conditions are associated with suicidal ideation and behavior (Sher & Oquendo, 2023) and may increase suicide risk in older military veterans.

4.2. Medical Illnesses

Aging is associated with the development of multiple medical disorders including cardiovascular disease, metabolic conditions, chronic obstructive pulmonary disease, hearing loss, eye diseases, and pain syndromes including back and neck pain and osteoarthritis (Callahan et al., 2002; Fillit et al., 2016; Straus, 2001). All these conditions are associated with elevated suicide risk (Choi et al., 2023; Sher, 2024a). Medical issues that lead to functional limitations are associated with significantly increased suicide risk among the general population and are more prevalent among veterans ages 65 and older than in the general population (Bongar et al., 2017; Kaplan et al., 2007; Kaplan et al., 2012). All medical and neurological conditions, especially pain syndromes and traumatic brain injury (TBI), increase suicide risk in older veterans (Elman et al., 2013; Kirtley et al., 2020; Kuffel et al., 2023; Pakniyat-Jahromi et al., 2022; Rice & Sher, 2012). Higher lethality of suicide attempts among older adults is related to declines in physical condition (D. W. Kim et al., 2021).

Additionally, older veterans may have physical limitations, such as frailty, that make it difficult for them to ambulate to their healthcare appointments. One study found that frailty is associated with increased risk of suicide attempts and higher rates of suicide deaths in U.S. military veterans (Kuffel et al., 2023).

Suicidality in older veterans may be affected by combat-related injuries, medical disorders or a combination of both (Bullman & Kang, 1996; Kaplan et al., 2012; Rice & Sher, 2012). A 19-year post-War World II study of American veterans with spinal cord injury showed that suicide was the third most common cause of death, ranking behind only renal failure and secondary amyloidosis (Nyquist & Bors, 1967). In American Vietnam veterans, sustaining wounds that required hospitalization or sustaining two or more wounds was observed to increase the risk of suicide by 1.2- and 1.6-fold, respectively (Bullman & Kang, 1996). Combat or non-combat TBIs may increase suicide risk among military veterans (Brenner et al., 2011; Campbell-Sills et al., 2020; Silver et al., 2001).

4.3. Psychosocial Stressors

Older veterans have a lot of strengths and significant life experience to cope with challenges that are frequent in later life. However, psychosocial difficulties may negatively affect the mental and/or physical health of some older veterans and result in suicidal behavior (Beydoun et al., 2024; Fletcher et al., 2023; Wilson et al., 2018; Wirtz & von Känel, 2017). The VA Behavioral Health Autopsy Program (BHAP) reviewed 2545 U.S. military veteran suicides between 2019 and 2021 and found that 24.7% of veterans who died by suicide experienced financial loss, 12.6% had legal problems or arrest, and 11.5% were at risk for homelessness (Department of Veterans Affairs, 2023).

In older veterans, psychosocial stressors can be related to multiple life problems, including loneliness, loss of loved ones, financial difficulties, poor living conditions/homelessness, traumatic life events, low neighbor cohesion, and lower subjective and objective social status (Wilson et al., 2018; Wirtz & von Känel, 2017). A review of loneliness and social isolation of military veterans has demonstrated that older veterans present unique experiences of loneliness and social isolation (Fletcher et al., 2023; Wilson et al., 2018). The authors have also noted that there are differences between military cultures of the Armed Forces of different nations which may affect veterans' perception of social isolation and loneliness.

Population-based studies indicate that the risk for suicide grows with an increase in the number of risk factors present. In other words, when more risk factors are present at any one time, the more likely it is that they indicate an increased risk for suicidal behaviors at that time.

5. Prevention of Suicidal Behavior in Older Veterans

Suicide prevention efforts should take a multipronged approach when addressing the needs of older veterans. This approach should incorporate community education through gatekeeper training programs, involving family members in the veteran's healthcare, the use of technology, lethal means restriction, safety planning, treatment and management of medical and psychiatric disorders, the use of screening instruments and interviews, and the interdisciplinary team framework.

6. Diagnosis/Recognition

A psychiatric interview performed by a competent medical professional is the foundation of suicide risk evaluations (Lake et al., 1984; Sher, 2011). Healthcare professionals need to be able to estimate suicide risk based on all available information including patient answers to direct and indirect questions, known risk factors, information on how the patient behaved under similar circumstances in the past, and collateral information. It is vital to educate medical professionals that not all suicidal patients including older veterans report suicidal ideation, intent, or plan to clinicians. Screening questionnaires may help identify veterans at risk for suicidal behavior (National Institutes of Health, 2015). It has been suggested that a brief screening tool can identify individuals at risk for suicide, more reliably than leaving the identification up to a clinician's judgment (The Joint Commission, 2016). The Patient Health Questionnaire (PHQ-9) is a screening instrument that can assess suicide risk. One study that used the PHQ-9 found that individuals who expressed thoughts of self-harm or death were 10× more likely to attempt suicide than those who did not report those thoughts (Kroenke et al., 2001). Another screening tool that can be utilized to assess suicide risk is the Columbia Suicide Severity Rating Scale (C-SSRS). Researchers evaluated the C-SSRS over three multi-site studies and found it to be effective in assessing for suicidal ideation and behavior in clinical and research settings (Posner et al., 2011).

Once a veteran screens positive on a brief screening tool, a comprehensive suicide risk assessment should be completed. The suicide risk assessment should incorporate suicidal ideation, suicide plan, means available, preparatory acts, level of intent, reasons for living/lying/dying, previous suicide attempts, warning signs, risk/protective factors, and collateral information (Fowler, 2012). When assessing suicidal ideation, it is important to obtain as much detail as possible about the frequency, duration and intensity of the ideation.

7. Interventions

7.1. The Treatment of Psychiatric Conditions and Management of Medical Disorders

Effective management of psychiatric disorders is the foundation of suicide prevention in any patient population including older veterans (Mann et al., 2005; Rihmer & Gonda, 2013; Sher & Oquendo, 2023). Different pharmacological and psychological treatment modalities can be used. Pharmacological interventions need to take into account the age and medical conditions of the veterans; i.e., doses of psychotropic medications need to be adjusted (Bednarczyk et al., 2022; Varma et al., 2010). Older adults may have greater medication effects compared to younger people given the same doses of drugs. Aging is usually associated with an increase in the proportion of body fat in the body, causing an increase in the elimination half-life of many psychotropic and non-psychotropic medications. It should be noted that older adults are at significantly higher risk of having pharmacodynamic drug–drug interactions due to polypharmacy than younger people (Varma et al., 2010). Pharmacodynamic interactions occur when two or more drugs influence each other's effects at the cellular or molecular level (Varma et al., 2010).

Psychological treatment modalities should be carefully chosen specifically for the disorder that is being treated. For example, one pilot study found that prolonged exposure therapy was effective in treating PTSD in older veterans (Thorp et al., 2012). However, some researchers caution against the use of intensive exposure therapies with older adults (Owens et al., 2005). These interventions may trigger an autonomic arousal, which, combined with other medical comorbidities such as cardiovascular disease, could pose life-threatening consequences (Owens et al., 2005).

Treatment of medical disorders, especially conditions associated with pain, can also decrease suicide risk (Huang et al., 2022; Rice & Sher, 2012). Older veterans with chronic pain may have decreased mobility, which limits their ability to work or participate in daily activities, and successful treatment of these veterans may improve their mobility and consequently reduce suicidality.

7.2. Safety Planning

The suicide prevention safety plan is an effective tool that could be utilized in a crisis situation involving an older veteran (Matthieu et al., 2023; Stanley & Brown, 2012). It is a prioritized list of coping strategies that is tailored to an individual's specific mental health needs. Mental health professionals should complete the suicide prevention safety plan synchronously and in collaboration with the veteran. The safety plan should not be completed if the individual is actively experiencing a crisis situation, and it should be completed more so as a preventative measure. Each step of the safety plan should be reviewed in detail, and the veteran should be encouraged to utilize their safety plan in a crisis situation. The safety plan should be periodically reviewed through the course of treatment and updated with any relevant changes.

A review of the literature found that safety plans were effective in preventing suicidal behavior (Nuij et al., 2021). The researchers mentioned that there was no evidence that suicide prevention safety plans reduced suicidal ideation (Nuij et al., 2021). They recommended the use of other interventions, such as cognitive behavioral therapy or dialectical behavior therapy, to treat suicidal ideation (Nuij et al., 2021).

7.3. Social Help

Older veterans who are experiencing psychosocial stressors should be provided with social help. As noted above, research shows that psychosocial stressors may increase suicidality (Pompili et al., 2013). Levine and Sher propose increasing the role of social workers in global suicide prevention efforts (Levine & Sher, 2020). Social workers can assist older veterans with obtaining government benefits, case management, care coordination, referrals to community resources (i.e., home healthcare), housing placement (i.e., assisted living or nursing home), and legal assistance (Levine & Sher, 2021a). In cases of elder abuse, financial exploitation, or neglect, social workers can help older veterans navigate the appropriate legal channels or get connected to government resources.

7.4. Family Education

Family members should be included in an older veteran's healthcare, when applicable (Jazieh et al., 2018; Sandi et al., 2020; Shimange et al., 2024). Healthcare professionals can educate family members on lethal means restriction and include them in the safety planning process. Family members can assist with or provide confirmation of the disposal of lethal means, such as the disposal of expired or unused medications. They can also safely administer medications to older veterans with the use of daily pill organizers or medication lockboxes. In cases where older veterans are no longer able to live independently, social workers can work with family members to assist with placement in an assisted living or nursing home setting.

7.5. Public Education and Role of Gatekeepers

Public education can be effective in suicide prevention efforts with older military veterans (Levine & Sher, 2020; Mann et al., 2005). Healthcare professionals can educate the public on suicide risk factors and warning signs with the use of gatekeeper training programs or lectures (Levine & Sher, 2020). If community members have a general understanding of the scope of suicide amongst veterans, they can better screen the veteran and connect them to the appropriate resources. Employing the use of social workers to educate the public has been proposed as a means to decrease the overall suicides in a given area (Levine & Sher, 2020).

Gatekeeper training is an effective suicide prevention intervention (Mann et al., 2005). Gatekeepers are people who are trained to identify suicide risk factors and connect suicidal persons to appropriate services (Mann et al., 2005). Question, Persuade, and Referral (QPR) is one example of a gatekeeper training program (Quinnett, 1995). Researchers evaluated the QPR program amongst clinical and non-clinical U.S. Department of Veterans Affairs staff (Matthieu et al., 2008). The study found a significant increase in self-efficacy and knowledge amongst both clinical and non-clinical staff, with non-clinical staff having larger effect sizes in both areas (Matthieu et al., 2008). Gatekeeper training programs can be utilized to train individuals who are working with older veterans as a way to reduce suicides amongst this age group.

7.6. Lethal Means Restriction

Research shows that lethal means restriction is one of the most effective societal interventions for preventing suicides (Yip et al., 2012). In September 1998, the United Kingdom introduced new legislation to limit the size of over-the-counter analgesic packs (salicylates, paracetamol, and their compounds) in an effort to reduce suicides (Hawton et al., 2004). This resulted in a 22% decrease in suicide deaths from paracetamol and salicylate overdoses in the succeeding year, with the trend continuing for three years after the legislation

(Hawton et al., 2004). In 2006, Israel created the Israeli Defense Force (IDF) Suicide Prevention Program, which was designed to reduce firearm-related suicides amongst military personnel (Shelef et al., 2015). One of the aspects of this program was that IDF soldiers were required to lock their firearms in storage when on leave (Shelef et al., 2015). Suicide rates among IDF soldiers dropped by nearly 50% from 2006 to 2014 (Shelef et al., 2015).

Military veterans often have access to firearms and knowledge on how to use them from their military experience (Levine & Sher, 2021c). Firearm ownership in the U.S. is more prevalent amongst the veteran population (45% ownership) compared to the non-veteran population (19% ownership) (Department of Veterans Affairs, 2023). In 2021, the U.S. Department of Veterans Affairs reported that 73.4% of suicides among male veterans and 51.7% of suicides among female veterans involved the use of a firearm (Department of Veterans Affairs, 2023). Lethal means restriction can be utilized in cases of firearm ownership. Veterans can be encouraged to relinquish their firearms through a law enforcement agency. If the veteran is unwilling to give up their firearm, they can be encouraged to utilize a gunlock and/or gun locker. Ammunition can be stored separately from the firearm, ideally in an inconvenient location, or disposed of altogether. Firearms can be disassembled, so they cannot be easily used in a suicide attempt.

Older people often have access to a lot of medications due to medical issues related to old age. Lethal means restriction can also be utilized with medications. Medications can be portioned in weekly pill organizers, and excess medications can be stored in a medication lockbox. A family member or friend can administer the medications to the veteran as prescribed. Additionally, prescribers can limit the amount or refills or quantity of pills. Veterans can also be given information on where to dispose of unused or expired medications, such as at the local pharmacy or with the use of Deterra pouches. In cases when veterans are prescribed opioid medications, they should be provided with Narcan kits and information on how to use these kits.

7.7. Technology

Technology can play an important role in suicide preventive efforts with older military veterans. Following the COVID-19 outbreak, telehealth interventions have been increasingly used to increase access to healthcare (Bracken et al., 2024; Haderlein et al., 2024; Woon et al., 2024). Although it is preferred for healthcare services to be delivered in-person, especially for individuals who are at high risk for suicide, the use of technology can provide support to older veterans with mobility issues or who reside in rural areas. One study reviewed the efficacy of telehealth interventions in suicide prevention and found that telehealth was effective in reducing suicidal ideation, suicide reattempts, and suicide rates (Shoib et al., 2024). The researchers recommended that mental health professionals provide monthly telehealth outreaches for at least 12 months following an index suicide attempt (Shoib et al., 2024). A recent study in the Bronx, New York, showed that telehealth-delivered horticultural therapy significantly reduces risk factors for suicidality among veterans including stress, depression, and loneliness (Meore et al., 2024). Horticultural therapy utilizes gardening as a way to promote physical, emotional, mental and social well-being, which is especially important in older veterans (Meore et al., 2024).

It has been recommended to use social media in suicide preventive efforts (Levine & Sher, 2020; Robinson et al., 2016). Social media can provide support through online forums or support groups, identify older veterans who make suicidal statements over the internet, or reach individuals who are otherwise difficult to engage (Robinson et al., 2016). On the contrary, some researchers suggest that social media could increase suicide risk by posing a risk for contagion, increasing isolation, or normalizing suicidal behaviors (Robinson et al., 2016). Mental health providers should provide education on the positive and negative impacts of social media when working with older veterans (Levine & Sher, 2020).

Mobile apps that are designed for mental health can be utilized to reduce suicide risk, as they are publicly available and highly scalable (Melia et al., 2020). The Department of Veterans Affairs has created several mobile apps to support the overall well-being of U.S. military veterans. These apps consist of self-care activities, mindfulness or meditation exercises, physical exercises (i.e., Tai Chi, yoga), smoking cessation, suicide prevention safety plans, and resources related to various medical or mental health disorders (Department of Veterans Affairs, 2023).

Technology can also be incorporated through wearable alert systems and smart home technology that can actively and passively monitor physiological, emotional, behavioral and cognitive changes that may lead to suicidal behavior (Stanley & Mann, 2020). Older veterans need to be educated regarding the use of modern technology.

7.8. Interdisciplinary Approach

An interdisciplinary approach should be utilized when working with older military veterans at risk for suicide (Levine & Sher, 2021a). This approach should incorporate the collaboration of mental health professionals, medical professionals, caseworkers, lawyers, and other community professionals involved in the veteran's care (Holmes et al., 2020). One study evaluated an interdisciplinary care management intervention for individuals aged 60 years or older with minor or major depression (Alexopoulos et al., 2009). Study participants received case management and treatment services from social workers, nurses, psychologists and physicians over a two-year span (Alexopoulos et al., 2009). The researchers found that participants who received the interdisciplinary care management intervention had a 2.2-fold decrease in suicidal ideation, as compared to those who did not receive the intervention (Alexopoulos et al., 2009).

8. Conclusions

Suicide among the geriatric population is an underappreciated topic, particularly among military veterans. Older veterans may be hesitant to address their mental health issues due to generational influences, such as stigma associated with having a mental illness. Challenges that older male and female veterans may experience may include low mobility, frailty, isolation, loneliness, loss of loved ones, and cognitive decline. Researchers suggest that there is a paucity of data on suicide prevention research for military veterans aged 65 and older (Sullivan et al., 2023). Older veterans with suicidal behavior should not be neglected. It has been argued that it is a moral obligation for society to ensure that older persons are provided with comfort, health and security (Upadhyaya & Sher, 2019).

Author Contributions: Conceptualization, L.S.; methodology, J.L. and L.S.; validation, J.L. and L.S.; investigation, J.L. and L.S.; writing—original draft preparation, J.L.; writing—review and editing, J.L. and L.S.; visualization, J.L. and L.S.; supervision, L.S.; project administration, J.L. and L.S. All authors have read and agreed to the published version of the manuscript.

Funding: This research received no external funding.

Institutional Review Board Statement: Not applicable.

Informed Consent Statement: Not applicable.

Data Availability Statement: Not applicable.

Conflicts of Interest: The authors declare no conflicts of interest.

References

Alexopoulos, G. S., Reynolds, C. F., Bruce, M. L., Katz, I. R., Raue, P. J., Mulsant, B. H., Oslin, D. W., & Have, T. T. (2009). Reducing suicidal ideation and depression in older primary care patients: 24-month outcomes of the PROSPECT study. *American Journal of Psychiatry*, *166*(8), 882–890. [CrossRef]

Baca-Garcia, E., Perez-Rodriguez, M. M., Oquendo, M. A., Keyes, K. M., Hasin, D. S., Grant, B. F., & Blanco, C. (2011). Estimating risk for suicide attempt: Are we asking the right questions? Passive suicidal ideation as a marker for suicidal behavior. *Journal of Affective Disorders*, *134*(1–3), 327–332. [CrossRef] [PubMed]

Bednarczyk, E., Cook, S., Brauer, R., & Garfield, S. (2022). Stakeholders' views on the use of psychotropic medication in older people: A systematic review. *Age Ageing*, *51*(3), afac060. [CrossRef] [PubMed]

Beydoun, H. A., Szymkowiak, D., Pietrzak, R. H., Beydoun, M. A., Treadwell, R. M., & Tsai, J. (2024). Role of homelessness and psychiatric disorders in suicide deaths among veterans: A four-way decomposition analysis. *Psychiatry Research*, *340*, 116120. [CrossRef] [PubMed]

Bongar, B., Sullivan, G., & James, L. (2017). *Handbook of military and veteran suicide: Assessment, treatment, and prevention*. Oxford University Press.

Bracken, K., Salerno, J., & Yang, L. (2024). Physician-led synchronous telemedicine compared to face-to-face care in primary care: A systematic review. *Evaluation & the Health Professions*. [CrossRef]

Brenner, L. A., Ignacio, R. V., & Blow, F. C. (2011). Suicide and traumatic brain injury among individuals seeking Veterans Health Administration services. *The Journal of Head Trauma Rehabilitation*, *26*(4), 257–264. [CrossRef]

Bruce, M. L. (2010). Suicide risk and prevention in veteran populations. *Annals of the New York Academy of Sciences*, *1208*(1), 98–103. [CrossRef]

Bullman, T. A., & Kang, H. K. (1996). The risk of suicide among wounded Vietnam veterans. *American Journal of Public Health*, *86*(5), 662–667. [CrossRef]

Bullman, T. A., & Schneiderman, A. (2021). Risk of suicide among U.S. veterans who deployed as part of Operation Enduring Freedom, Operation Iraqi Freedom, and Operation New Dawn. *Injury Epidemiology*, *8*(1), 40. [CrossRef]

Callahan, E. H., Thomas, D. C., Goldhirsch, S. L., & Leipzig, R. M. (2002). Geriatric hospital medicine. *Medical Clinics North American*, *86*(4), 707–729. [CrossRef]

Campbell-Sills, L., Stein, M. B., Liu, H., Agtarap, S., Heeringa, S. G., Nock, M. K., Ursano, R. J., & Kessler, R. C. (2020). Associations of lifetime traumatic brain injury characteristics with prospective suicide attempt among deployed US Army soldiers. *The Journal of Head Trauma Rehabilitation*, *35*(1), 14–26. [CrossRef] [PubMed]

Carballo, J. J., Llorente, C., Kehrmann, L., Flamarique, I., Zuddas, A., Purper-Ouakil, D., Hoekstra, P. J., Coghill, D., Schulze, U. M. E., Dittmann, R. W., Buitelaar, J. K., Castro-Fornieles, J., Lievesley, K., Santosh, P., Arango, C., & STOP Consortium. (2020). Psychosocial risk factors for suicidality in children and adolescents. *European Child & Adolescent Psychiatry*, *29*(6), 759–776. [CrossRef]

Choi, N. G., Choi, B. Y., & Marti, C. N. (2023). Physical health problems as a suicide precipitant: Associations with other risk factors and suicide methods in three age groups of older decedents. *Innovation in Aging*, *7*(6), igad073. [CrossRef] [PubMed]

Conwell, Y., Van Orden, K., & Caine, E. D. (2011). Suicide in older adults. *Psychiatric Clinics North American*, *34*(2), 451–468. [CrossRef] [PubMed]

Cooper, C., Selwood, A., & Livingston, G. (2008). The prevalence of elder abuse and neglect: A systematic review. *Age Ageing*, *37*(2), 151–160. [CrossRef]

Davison, E. H., Kaiser, A. P., Spiro, A., Moye, J., King, L. A., & King, D. W. (2016). From late-onset stress symptomatology to later-adulthood trauma reengagement in aging combat veterans: Taking a broader view. *Gerontologist*, *56*(1), 14–21. [CrossRef]

Department of Veterans Affairs. (2023). *2023 national veteran suicide prevention annual report*. Available online: https://www.mentalhealth.va.gov/docs/data-sheets/2023/2023-National-Veteran-Suicide-Prevention-Annual-Report-FINAL-508.pdf (accessed on 9 December 2024).

Elman, I., Borsook, D., & Volkow, N. D. (2013). Pain and suicidality: Insights from reward and addiction neuroscience. *Progress in Neurobiology*, *109*, 1–27. [CrossRef]

EUROMIL. (2022). *Veterans*. Available online: https://euromil.org/wp-content/uploads/2022/06/2205_Southern_members_Veterans_Vero.pdf (accessed on 9 December 2024).

Fillit, H. M., Rockwood, K., & Young, J. B. (2016). *Brocklehurst's textbook of geriatric medicine and gerontology* (8th ed.). Elsevier.

Fletcher, K. L., Martin, J. A., Black, E. R., Dekel, R., Rooney, M., & Albright, D. L. (2023). Older veterans. In J. T. McDaniel, E. R. Seamone, & S. N. Xenakis (Eds.), *Preventing and treating the invisible wounds of war* (pp. 85–105). Oxford University Press.

Fowler, J. C. (2012). Suicide risk assessment in clinical practice: Pragmatic guidelines for imperfect assessments. *Psychother*, *49*(1), 81–90. [CrossRef]

Gates, M. A., Holowka, D. W., Vasterling, J. J., Keane, T. M., Marx, B. P., & Rosen, R. C. (2012). Posttraumatic stress disorder in veterans and military personnel: Epidemiology, screening, and case recognition. *Psychological Services, 9*(4), 361–382. [CrossRef]

Goldberg, J., Magruder, K. M., Forsberg, C. W., Friedman, M. J., Litz, B. T., Vaccarino, V., Heagerty, P. J., Gleason, T. C., Huang, G. D., & Smith, N. L. (2016). Prevalence of Post-Traumatic Stress Disorder in aging Vietnam-era veterans: Veterans Administration cooperative study 569: Course and consequences of Post-Traumatic Stress Disorder in Vietnam-era veteran twins. *The American Journal of Geriatric Psychiatry, 24*(3), 181–191. [CrossRef]

Haderlein, T. P., Guzman-Clark, J., Dardashti, N. S., McMahon, N., Duran, E. L., Huan, J. N., Robinson, S. A., Blok, A. C., Cutrona, S. L., Lindsay, J. A., Armstrong, C. M., Nazi, K. M., Shimada, S. L., Wilck, N. R., Reilly, E., Kuhn, E., & Hogan, T. P. (2024). Improving veteran engagement with virtual care technologies: A Veterans Health Administration state of the art conference research agenda. *Journal of General Internal Medicine, 39*(Suppl. S1), 21–28. [CrossRef] [PubMed]

Harmer, B., Lee, S., Rizvi, A., & Saadabadi, A. (2024). Suicidal ideation. In *StatPearls*. StatPearls Publishing.

Hawton, K., Simkin, S., Deeks, J., Cooper, J., Johnston, A. M., Waters, K., Arundel, M., Bernal, W., Gunson, B., Hudson, M., Suri, D., & Simpson, K. (2004). UK legislation on analgesic packs: Before and after study of long term effect on poisonings. *BMJ, 329*(7474), 1076. [CrossRef] [PubMed]

Holmes, E. A., O'Connor, R. C., Perry, V. H., Tracey, I., Wessely, S., Arseneault, L., Ballard, C., Christensen, H., Silver, R. C., Everall, I., Ford, T., John, A., Kabir, T., King, K., Madan, I., Michie, S., Przybylski, A. K., Shafran, R., Sweeney, A., … Bullmore, E. (2020). Multidisciplinary research priorities for the COVID-19 pandemic: A call for action for mental health science. *The Lancet Psychiatry, 7*(6), 547–560. [CrossRef]

Huang, S., Lewis, M. O., Bao, Y., Adekkanattu, P., Adkins, L. E., Banerjee, S., Bian, J., Gellad, W. F., Goodin, A. J., Luo, Y., Fairless, J. A., Walunas, T. L., Wilson, D. L., Wu, Y., Yin, P., Oslin, D. W., Pathak, J., & Lo-Ciganic, W. H. (2022). Predictive modeling for suicide-related outcomes and risk factors among patients with pain conditions: A systematic review. *Journal of Clinical Medicine, 11*(16), 4813. [CrossRef]

Iversen, A. C., van Staden, L., Hughes, J. H., Browne, T., Hull, L., Hall, J., Greenberg, N., Rona, R. J., Hotopf, M., Wessely, S., & Fear, N. T. (2009). The prevalence of common mental disorders and PTSD in the UK military: Using data from a clinical interview-based study. *BMC Psychiatry, 9*, 1–12. [CrossRef]

Jazieh, A. R., Volker, S., & Taher, S. (2018). Involving the family in patient care: A culturally tailored communication model. *Global Journal on Quality and Safety in Healthcare, 1*(2), 33–37. [CrossRef]

Kaplan, M. S., McFarland, B. H., Huguet, N., & Newsom, J. T. (2007). Physical illness, functional limitations, and suicide risk: A population-based study. *American Journal of Orthopsychiatry, 77*(1), 56–60. [CrossRef]

Kaplan, M. S., McFarland, B. H., Huguet, N., & Valenstein, M. (2012). Suicide risk and precipitating circumstances among young, middle-aged, and older male veterans. *American Journal of Public Health, 102*(S1), S131–S137. [CrossRef]

Kim, D. W., Cho, S. E., Kang, J. M., Woo, S. K., Kang, S. G., Yeon, B. K., & Cho, S. J. (2021). Risk factors for serious suicide attempts: Difference between older and younger attempters in the emergency department. *Frontiers in Psychiatry, 11*, 607811. [CrossRef]

Kim, S., Park, J., Lee, H., Lee, H., Woo, S., Kwon, R., Kim, S., Koyanagi, A., Smith, L., Rahmati, M., Fond, G., Boyer, L., Kang, J., Lee, J. H., Oh, J., & Yon, D. K. (2024). Global public concern of childhood and adolescence suicide: A new perspective and new strategies for suicide prevention in the post-pandemic era. *World Journal of Pediatrics, 20*(9), 872–900. [CrossRef]

Kimerling, R., Gima, K., Smith, M. W., Street, A., & Frayne, S. (2007). The Veterans Health Administration and military sexual trauma. *American Journal of Public Health, 97*(12), 2160–2166. [CrossRef]

Kirtley, O. J., Rodham, K., & Crane, C. (2020). Understanding suicidal ideation and behaviour in individuals with chronic pain: A review of the role of novel transdiagnostic psychological factors. *The Lancet Psychiatry, 7*(3), 282–290. [CrossRef]

Kroenke, K., Spitzer, R. L., & Williams, J. B. W. (2001). Patient Health Questionnaire-9 (PHQ-9). The PHQ-9: Validity of a brief depression severity measure. *Journal of general internal medicine, 16*(9), 606–613. [CrossRef] [PubMed]

Kuffel, R. L., Morin, R. T., Covinsky, K. E., Boscardin, W. J., Lohman, M. C., Li, Y., & Byers, A. L. (2023). Association of frailty with risk of suicide attempt in a national cohort of US veterans aged 65 years or older. *JAMA Psychiatry, 80*(4), 287–295. [CrossRef] [PubMed]

Lake, C. R., Moriarty, K. M., & Alagna, S. W. (1984). The acute psychiatric diagnostic interview. *Psychiatric Clinics North American, 7*(4), 657–670. [CrossRef]

Levine, J., & Sher, L. (2020). How to increase the role of social workers in suicide preventive interventions. *Acta Neuropsychiatrica, 32*(4), 186–195. [CrossRef]

Levine, J., & Sher, L. (2021a). Interdisciplinary approach and suicide prevention amongst U.S. military veterans. *Psychiatria Danubina, 33*(2), 200.

Levine, J., & Sher, L. (2021b). The prevention of suicide among military veterans during the COVID-19 pandemic. *European Archives of Psychiatry and Clinical Neuroscience, 271*(2), 405–406. [CrossRef]

Levine, J., & Sher, L. (2021c). The role of social workers in suicide prevention among military veterans. In M. Pompili (Ed.), *Suicide risk assessment and prevention* (pp. 1–21). Springer International Publishing.

Mann, J. J., Apter, A., Bertolote, J., Beautrais, A., Currier, D., Haas, A., Hegerl, U., Lonnqvist, J., Malone, K., Marusic, A., Mehlum, L., Patton, G., Phillips, M., Rutz, W., Rihmer, Z., Schmidtke, A., Shaffer, D., Silverman, M., Takahashi, Y., . . . Hendin, H. (2005). Suicide prevention strategies: A systematic review. *JAMA, 294*(16), 2064–2074. [CrossRef]

Matthieu, M. M., Cross, W., Batres, A. R., Flora, C. M., & Knox, K. L. (2008). Evaluation of gatekeeper training for suicide prevention in veterans. *Archives of Suicide Research, 12*(2), 148–154. [CrossRef]

Matthieu, M. M., Morissette, S. B., Clafferty, S., Degutis, L., Oliver, C. M., Adkins, D. A., & DeBeer, B. B. (2023). Veteran experiences with suicide ideation, suicide attempt, and social support in safety planning within the Department of Veterans Affairs. *Military Medicine, 188*(11–12), e3289–e3294. [CrossRef] [PubMed]

Melia, R., Francis, K., Hickey, E., Bogue, J., Duggan, J., O'Sullivan, M., & Young, K. (2020). Mobile health technology interventions for suicide prevention: Systematic review. *JMIR mHealth and uHealth, 8*(1), e12516. [CrossRef] [PubMed]

Meore, A., Ganesh, N., Sun, S., Singer, A., Byma, L., Lorenzetti, B., Feder, A., Adams, T., Galfalvy, H., Boyer, J., & Haghighi, F. (2024). Pilot study of telehealth delivery of horticultural therapy (TeleHT) as an acceptable intervention and in reducing suicide risk factors in veterans. *Complementary Therapies in Medicine, 85*, 103075. [CrossRef] [PubMed]

Mills, P. D., Watts, B. V., Huh, T. J., Boar, S., & Kemp, J. (2013). Helping elderly patients to avoid suicide: A review of case reports from a National Veterans Affairs database. *The Journal of Nervous and Mental Disease, 201*(1), 12–16. [CrossRef]

Moore, M. J., Shawler, E., Jordan, C. H., & Jackson, C. A. (2023). Veteran and military mental health issues. In *StatPearls*. StatPearls Publishing.

Naguy, A., Elbadry, H., & Salem, H. (2020). Suicide: A précis! *Journal of Family Medicine and Primary Care, 9*(8), 4009–4015. [CrossRef]

National Institutes of Health. (2015). *Swedish council on health technology assessment. Instruments for suicide risk assessment*. Available online: https://www.ncbi.nlm.nih.gov/books/NBK350492/ (accessed on 9 December 2024).

National Institutes of Health. (2024). *Age*. Available online: https://www.nih.gov/nih-style-guide/age (accessed on 9 December 2024).

Nock, M. K., Millner, A. J., Joiner, T. E., Gutierrez, P. M., Han, G., Hwang, I., King, A., Naifeh, J. A., Sampson, N. A., Zaslavsky, A. M., Stein, M. B., Ursano, R. J., & Kessler, R. C. (2018). Risk factors for the transition from suicide ideation to suicide attempt: Results from the Army Study to Assess Risk and Resilience in Servicemembers (Army STARRS). *Journal of Abnormal Psychology, 127*(2), 139–149. [CrossRef]

Nuij, C., van Ballegooijen, W., De Beurs, D., Juniar, D., Erlangsen, A., Portzky, G., O'Connor, R. C., Smit, J. H., Kerkhof, A., & Riper, H. (2021). Safety planning-type interventions for suicide prevention: Meta-analysis. *British Journal of Psychiatry, 219*(2), 419–426. [CrossRef]

Nyquist, R., & Bors, E. (1967). Mortality and survival in traumatic myelopathy during nineteen years from 1946–1965. *Paraplegia, 5*, 22–48. [CrossRef]

O'Malley, K. A., Vinson, L., Pless Kaiser, A., Sager, Z., & Hinrichs, K. (2020). Mental health and aging veterans: How the veterans health administration meets the needs of aging veterans. *Public Policy & Aging Report, 30*(1), 19–23. [CrossRef]

Owens, G. P., Baker, D. G., Kasckow, J., Ciesla, J. A., & Mohamed, S. (2005). Review of assessment and treatment of PTSD among elderly American armed forces veterans. *International Journal of Geriatric Psychiatry, 20*(12), 1118–1130. [CrossRef]

Pakniyat-Jahromi, S., Korenis, P., & Sher, L. (2022). Pain and suicide: What should we tell our trainees? *Acta Neuropsychiatrica, 34*(3), 127–131. [CrossRef]

Pew Research Center. (2019). *The American veteran experience and the Post-9/11 generation*. Available online: https://www.pewresearch.org/wp-content/uploads/sites/20/2019/09/09.10.19_veteransexperiences_full_report_updated.pdf (accessed on 9 December 2024).

Pompili, M., Sher, L., Serafini, G., Forte, A., Innamorati, M., Dominici, G., Lester, D., Amore, M., & Girardi, P. (2013). Posttraumatic stress disorder and suicide risk among veterans: A literature review. *The Journal of Nervous and Mental Disease, 201*(9), 802–812. [CrossRef] [PubMed]

Posner, K., Brown, G. K., Stanley, B., Brent, D. A., Yershova, K. V., Oquendo, M. A., Currier, G. W., Melvin, G. A., Greenhill, L., Shen, S., & Mann, J. J. (2011). The Columbia-Suicide Severity Rating Scale: Initial validity and internal consistency findings from three multisite studies with adolescents and adults. *American Journal of Psychiatry, 168*(12), 1266–1277. [CrossRef]

Quinnett, P. (1995). *QPR: Ask a question, save a life*. The QPR Institute.

Reger, M. A., Smolenski, D. J., Skopp, N. A., Metzger-Abamukang, M. J., Kang, H. K., Bullman, T. A., Perdue, S., & Gahm, G. A. (2015). Risk of suicide among US military service members following Operation Enduring Freedom or Operation Iraqi Freedom deployment and separation from the US military. *JAMA Psychiatry, 72*(6), 561–569. [CrossRef] [PubMed]

Rice, T. R., & Sher, L. (2012). Suicidal behavior in war veterans. *Expert Review of Neurotherapeutics, 12*(5), 611–624. [CrossRef] [PubMed]

Rihmer, Z., & Gonda, X. (2013). Pharmacological prevention of suicide in patients with major mood disorders. *Neuroscience & Biobehavioral Reviews, 37*(10 Pt 1), 2398–2403. [CrossRef]

Robinson, J., Cox, G., & Bailey, E. (2016). Social media and suicide prevention: A systematic review. *Early Intervention in Psychiatry, 10*(2), 103–121. [CrossRef]

Sandi, R., Nasir, S., Moedjiono, A. I., & Ibrahim, E. (2020). Knowledge and understanding of mental disorders in families of people with mental disorders. *Open Access Macedonian Journal of Medical Sciences, 8*(T2), 136–140. [CrossRef]

Schoenbaum, M., Kessler, R. C., Gilman, S. E., Colpe, L. J., Heeringa, S. G., Stein, M. B., Ursano, R. J., Cox, K. L., & Army STARRS Collaborators. (2014). Predictors of suicide and accident death in the army study to assess risk and resilience in servicemembers (Army STARRS): Results from the army study to assess risk and resilience in servicemembers (ArmySTARRS). *JAMA Psychiatry, 71*(5), 493–503. [CrossRef]

Seal, K. H., Bertenthal, D., Miner, C. R., Sen, S., & Marmar, C. (2007). Bringing the war back home: Mental health disorders among 103,788 US veterans returning from Iraq and Afghanistan seen at Department of Veterans Affairs facilities. *Archives of Internal Medicine, 167*(5), 476–482. [CrossRef]

Shelef, L., Laur, L., Raviv, G., & Fruchter, E. (2015). A military suicide prevention program in the Israeli Defense Force: A review of an important military medical procedure. *Disaster and Military Medicine, 1*, 16. [CrossRef]

Shen, Y. C., Cunha, J. M., & Williams, T. V. (2016). Time-varying associations of suicide with deployments, mental health conditions, and stressful life events among current and former US military personnel: A retrospective multivariate analysis. *The Lancet Psychiatry, 3*(11), 1039–1048. [CrossRef]

Sher, L. (2011). Teaching medical professionals about suicide prevention: What's missing? *QJM, 104*(11), 1005–1008. [CrossRef] [PubMed]

Sher, L. (2024a). Suicide in individuals with no psychiatric disorders: What makes you vulnerable? *QJM: An International Journal of Medicine, 117*(5), 313–316. [CrossRef]

Sher, L. (2024b). The uncounted casualties of war: Suicide in combat veterans. *QJM, 117*(3), 163–167. [CrossRef]

Sher, L., & Oquendo, M. A. (2023). Suicide: An overview for clinicians. *Medical Clinics North American, 107*(1), 119–130. [CrossRef] [PubMed]

Shimange, M. E., Shilubane, H. N., Ndou, N. D., & Mulondo, A. S. (2024). Mental healthcare consumers' experiences of mental health care: Variation in knowledge by the family members and support. *SAGE Open Nursing, 10*, 23779608241272489. [CrossRef] [PubMed]

Shoib, S., Shaheen, N., Anwar, A., Saad, A. M., Akr, L. M., Saud, A. I., Kundu, M., Nahidi, M., Chandradasa, M., Swed, S., & Saeed, F. (2024). The effectiveness of telehealth interventions in suicide prevention: A systematic review and meta-analysis. *International Journal of Social Psychiatry, 70*(3), 415–423. [CrossRef]

Silver, J. M., Kramer, R., Greenwald, S., & Weissman, M. (2001). The association between head injuries and psychiatric disorders: Findings from the New Haven NIMH Epidemiologic Catchment Area Study. *Brain Injury, 15*(11), 935–945. [CrossRef]

Stagwell Global. (2024). *What the data say: Age 80 replaces 60 as today's definition of 'old'*. Available online: https://www.stagwellglobal.com/what-the-data-say-age-80-replaces-60-as-todays-definition-of-old/ (accessed on 9 December 2024).

Stanley, B., & Brown, G. K. (2012). Safety planning intervention: A brief intervention to mitigate suicide risk. *Cognitive and Behavioral Practice, 19*(2), 256–264. [CrossRef]

Stanley, B., & Mann, J. J. (2020). The need for innovation in health care systems to improve suicide prevention. *JAMA Psychiatry, 77*(1), 96–98. [CrossRef]

Straus, S. E. (2001). Geriatric medicine. *BMJ, 322*(7278), 86–89. [CrossRef] [PubMed]

Sullivan, J. L., Simons, K. V., Mills, W. L., Hilgeman, M. M., Freytes, I. M., Morin, R. T., Bower, E. S., Clark, R., & Byers, A. L. (2023). A paucity of data on veterans 65 and older and risk of suicide: A systematic review. *The American Journal of Geriatric Psychiatry, 31*(7), 525–539. [CrossRef] [PubMed]

The Joint Commission. (2016). *Sentinel event alert 56: Detecting and treating suicidal ideation in all settings*. Available online: https://jointcommission.org/sea_issue_56/ (accessed on 9 December 2024).

The UN Refugee Agency. (2024, June 13). *Older persons*. Available online: https://emergency.unhcr.org/protection/persons-risk/older-persons (accessed on 9 December 2024).

Thorp, S. R., Stein, M. B., Jeste, D. V., Patterson, T. L., & Wetherell, J. L. (2012). Prolonged exposure therapy for older veterans with posttraumatic stress disorder: A pilot study. *The American Journal of Geriatric Psychiatry, 20*(3), 276–280. [CrossRef] [PubMed]

Tøllefson, I. M., Helweg-Larsen, K., Thiblin, I., Hem, E., Kastrup, M. C., Nyberg, U., Rogde, S., Zahl, P.-H., Østevold, G., & Ekeberg, Ø. (2015). Are suicide deaths under-reported? Nationwide re-evaluations of 1800 deaths in Scandinavia. *BMJ Open, 5*(11), e009120. [CrossRef]

Turecki, G., Brent, D. A., Gunnell, D., O'Connor, R. C., Oquendo, M. A., Pirkis, J., & Stanley, B. H. (2019). Suicide and suicide risk. *Nature Reviews Disease Primers*, *5*(1), 74. [CrossRef]

United States Census Bureau. (2020). *Census bureau releases new report on veterans*. Available online: https://www.census.gov/newsroom/press-releases/2020/veterans-report.html (accessed on 9 December 2024).

United States Census Bureau. (2021). *Veterans glossary*. Available online: https://www.census.gov/topics/population/veterans/about/glossary.html (accessed on 9 December 2024).

Upadhyaya, M., & Sher, L. (2019). Prevention of suicide in older adults. *Brazilian Journal of Psychiatry*, *41*(4), 365–366. [CrossRef]

Varma, S., Sareen, H., & Trivedi, J. K. (2010). The geriatric population and psychiatric medication. *Mens Sana Monographs*, *8*(1), 30–51. [CrossRef]

Williamson, V., Stevelink, S. A. M., Greenberg, K., & Greenberg, N. (2018). Prevalence of mental health disorders in elderly U.S. military veterans: A meta-analysis and systematic review. *The American Journal of Geriatric Psychiatry*, *26*(5), 534–545. [CrossRef]

Wilson, G., Hill, M., & Kiernan, M. D. (2018). Loneliness and social isolation of military veterans: Systematic narrative review. *Occupational Medicine*, *68*(9), 600–609. [CrossRef]

Wirtz, P. H., & von Känel, R. (2017). Psychological stress, inflammation, and coronary heart disease. *Current Cardiology Reports*, *19*(11), 111. [CrossRef] [PubMed]

Woon, L. S., Maguire, P. A., Reay, R. E., & Looi, J. C. L. (2024). Telepsychiatry in Australia: A scoping review. *Inquiry*, *61*, 469580241237116. [CrossRef]

World Health Organization. (2020). *Global health estimates 2020: Deaths by cause, age, sex, by country and by region, 2000–2019*. Available online: https://www.who.int/data/gho/data/themes/mortality-and-global-health-estimates (accessed on 9 December 2024).

World Health Organization. (2023). *Mental health of older adults*. Available online: https://www.who.int/news-room/fact-sheets/detail/mental-health-of-older-adults#:~:text=The%20most%20common%20mental%20health,people%20aged%2060%20or%20over (accessed on 9 December 2024).

Yip, P. S., Caine, E., Yousuf, S., Chang, S. S., Wu, K. C. C., & Chen, Y. Y. (2012). Means restriction for suicide prevention. *The Lancet*, *379*(9834), 2393–2399. [CrossRef] [PubMed]

Yunus, R. M., Hairi, N. N., & Choo, W. Y. (2019). Consequences of elder abuse and neglect: A systematic review of observational studies. *Trauma, Violence, & Abuse*, *20*(2), 197–213. [CrossRef]

Zartaloudi, A. E. (2024). Adolescent suicide: A major mental health issue in pediatric care. *Minerva Pediatrics*, *76*(5), 660–678. [CrossRef]

Zivin, K., Kim, M., McCarthy, J. F., Austin, K. L., Hoggatt, K. J., Walters, H., & Valenstein, M. (2007). Suicide mortality among individuals receiving treatment for depression in the veteran affairs health system: Associations with patients and treatment setting characteristics. *American Journal of Public Health*, *97*(12), 2193–2198. [CrossRef]

behavioral sciences

MDPI

Review

The Impact of Relationships Within Combat Units on Post-Deployment Suicide Risk

Leo Sher [1,2,3]

[1] Inpatient Psychiatry, James J. Peters VA Medical Center, New York, NY 10468, USA; leo.sher@mssm.edu
[2] Department of Psychiatry, Icahn School of Medicine at Mount Sinai, New York, NY 10029, USA
[3] Department of Psychiatry, Columbia University Vagelos College of Physicians and Surgeons, New York, NY 10032, USA

Abstract: Multiple deployment factors may affect suicidality in combat veterans. The relationships between combat deployments and suicidality are complex and not completely understood. Studies of stress in the military and psychological effects of military actions are mostly focused on stressors relating to combat operations. However, many studies suggest that interactions within combat units affect post-deployment psychiatric conditions, suicidal ideation, and behavior. The goal of this article is to review and discuss how relationships within combat units may influence post-deployment suicide risk. Studies of the relationships within combat units are generally focused on two aspects: unit cohesion and harassment/abuse. Considerable evidence suggests that service members who report strong unit cohesion have a lower risk of post-deployment psychiatric disorders and suicidal behavior. Studies examining deployment sexual and non-sexual harassment and abuse have found that combat veterans who experience harassment and abuse during deployment are at heightened post-deployment suicide risk. Sound post-deployment social support and the efficient treatment of psychiatric disorders may mitigate the suicide risk associated with adverse relationships within combat units. Improvements in units' cohesion and the prevention of harassment/abuse during a military deployment are necessary to reduce post-deployment psychiatric pathology, including suicidal behavior.

Keywords: combat veteran; deployment; unit cohesion; harassment; suicide

1. Introduction

Wars have been a part of the history of humankind. Regretfully, there is no evidence that a time free of war will become a reality in the foreseeable future. According to a recently published report, "Global Peace Index 2024: Measuring Peace in a Complex World" there are 56 military conflicts around world at the present time [1]. This is the largest number of military conflicts since the Second World War. According to this report, 92 countries are engaged in military actions beyond their borders. The number of minor military conflicts is increasing. This raises the possibility that there will be more major wars in the future.

There are millions of combat veterans around the globe. For example, after the terrorist attacks of 11 September 2001, between 1.9 and 3 million members of the U.S. Armed Forces served in military operations in Iraq and Afghanistan and over half of them were deployed more than once [2]. It should be noted that in the U.S., a military veteran is a person who served in the Armed Forces [3]. In the U.S., combat veterans are those who served in an area of conflict/war while in the Armed Forces. In many countries, individuals are regarded as military veterans if they served during wartime and/or participated in combat operations; i.e., only combat veterans are classified as veterans [4].

Combat conditions are characterized by violence, brutality, physical and emotional strain, separation from families and friends, and other adversities. Major physical combat injuries are associated with psychiatric disorders including post-traumatic stress disorder

(PTSD), depression, anxiety, and suicidality [5–7]. For example, a study of the UK military servicemembers who were deployed to Afghanistan showed that servicemembers who had physical combat injuries were 46–67% more likely to report PTSD, depression, and anxiety in comparison with uninjured servicemembers [7].

Multiple deployment factors may affect suicidality in combat veterans [8]. The relationships between combat deployments and suicidality are complex and not completely understood. Studies of stress in the military and the psychological effects of military actions are mostly focused on stressors relating to combat operations, such as traumatic exposure to death and injuries, exhaustion, and being exposed to extreme climates [9]. However, many studies performed over the last several decades suggest that interactions within combat units affect post-deployment psychiatric conditions and suicidal ideation and behavior [10–21]. These studies are generally focused on two aspects: unit cohesion and harassment/abuse (See Table 1) The goal of this article is to review and to discuss how relationships within combat units may influence post-deployment suicide risk.

Table 1. Studies on the relations between suicidality and combat unit cohesion and between suicidality and deployment harassment/abuse.

Authors	Purpose	Study Design	Sample	Main Findings
Anderson et al. [19]	To evaluate prospective associations of perceived unit cohesion with mental health outcomes following combat deployment	A survey before and after deployment to Afghanistan	4645 soldiers	Soldiers who reported strong unit cohesion before deployment had a lower risk of post-deployment mental disorders and suicidal ideation
Bryan and Heron [15]	To study factors that protect against depression in military servicemembers	Self-report measures of depression, posttraumatic stress, and sense of "belonging" before and after deploying to Iraq	168 Air Force convoy operators	A sense of belonging may protect service members from depression at all stages of the deployment cycle
Du Preez et al. [12]	To examine the association between unit cohesion and probability of PTSD or other mental disorders	Information was collected on socio-demographic and military characteristics and deployment experiences	4901 male UK armed forces personnel deployed to Iraq	Unit cohesion had a linear association with less probable PTSD and common mental disorder
Ejdesgaard et al. [16]	To identify risk and protective factors for suicidal ideation and suicide attempts among deployed Danish soldiers	A questionnaire survey	1264 Danish soldiers deployed from 1990 to 2009	A heavy workload was associated with suicidal ideation. Pointless tasks were a predictor for suicide attempts
Gradus et al. [14]	To examine the role of post-deployment mental health in associations between deployment stressors and post-deployment suicidal ideation	A questionnaire survey	A national sample of 2321 female and male OEF/OIF veterans	Among female veterans, sexual harassment was the only deployment stressor to have an independent association with suicidal ideation

Table 1. *Cont.*

Authors	Purpose	Study Design	Sample	Main Findings
Griffith [17]	To examine relationships among combat exposure, post-deployment stressors, social support, and unit cohesion	A questionnaire survey	4567 combat soldiers who were members of 50 company-sized units	At the group level, a diminished risk for suicidal ideation was associated with units having better than typical cohesion
Kimerling et al. [18]	To assess associations between military sexual trauma screen results and subsequent suicide mortality	Screening for military sexual trauma	Veterans who received Veterans Health Administration services in the fiscal years 2007–2011: 5,991,080 men and 360,774 women	A total of 9017 veterans died by suicide during the follow-up period. The hazard ratios for military sexual trauma were 1.69 (95% CI = 1.45, 1.97) among men and 2.27 (95% CI = 1.76, 2.94) among women
Kovacic et al. [22]	To examine platelet serotonin concentration in male combat veterans and non-veterans	A survey and determination of platelet serotonin concentration	73 suicidal and 47 non-suicidal veterans with current and chronic combat-related PTSD, 45 suicidal and 30 non-suicidal comparative non-PTSD subjects, and 147 healthy men	A reduced platelet serotonin concentration is related to suicidal behavior in PTSD
Lemaire and Graham [11]	To examine factors associated with suicidal ideation in returning Iraq and Afghanistan war veterans	A cross-sectional review of veterans' initial mental health screening evaluations	1740 OEF/OIF veterans	General (non-sexual) harassment was associated with post-deployment suicidal ideation
Mitchell et al. [13]	To test the associations between combat exposure, unit cohesion, and their interaction in predicting suicide-related ideation	A survey using rating scales	1663 recently redeployed soldiers	Soldiers who experienced greater combat exposure but also had higher levels of unit cohesion had relatively lower levels of suicide-related ideation. Soldiers who had higher levels of combat exposure and lower unit cohesion were most at risk for suicide-related ideation
Monteith et al. [20]	To evaluate whether military sexual trauma is associated with post-military suicidal ideation and suicide attempt history	A secondary analysis of quantitative data collected from a survey	2250 post-9/11 female veterans	An elevated prevalence of suicidal ideation after military service was associated with both military sexual harassment and assault

Table 1. *Cont.*

Authors	Purpose	Study Design	Sample	Main Findings
Pietrzak et al. [10]	To examine variables associated with suicidality in OEF/OIF veterans	A questionnaire survey	272 OEF/OIF veterans	Veterans who reported post-deployment suicidal ideation had lower scores on measures of unit support
Sher et al. [21]	To test the hypothesis that harassment during a combat deployment is associated with post-deployment suicidality and testosterone function	An interview using rating scales	32 male combat veterans with or without a history of suicide attempts	Harassment scores were higher and free testosterone levels were lower among suicide attempters in comparison with non-attempters

2. Suicidality in Combat Veterans

Suicide among combat and non-combat veterans is a critical public health issue that causes incalculable pain among individuals, families, and communities [8,23,24]. According to the 2022 VA National Veteran Suicide Prevention Annual Report published by the Office of Mental Health and Suicide Prevention of the U.S. Department of Veterans Affairs, there were 6146 veteran suicide deaths in the U.S. in 2020 [24]. Military veterans have higher rates of suicide than individuals in the general population. According to the above-mentioned report, the suicide rate for veterans was 57.3% higher than non-veteran U.S. adults in 2020, after adjusting for age and sex differences [24]. An epidemiological study performed by psychiatric researchers in Michigan found that among veterans from different periods of military service treated in the U.S. Veterans Health Administration (VHA) medical facilities, male veterans were 1.66 times more likely to die by suicide than males in the general population, and female veterans were 1.87 times more likely to die by suicide than females in the general population [23].

Studies of the U.S. veterans of Operation Enduring Freedom (OEF), Operation Iraqi Freedom (OIF), and Operation New Dawn (OND), and other U.S. and international veterans, suggest that many combat veterans exhibit suicidal ideation and behavior [8,10,25,26]. A survey of 272 OEF/OIF veterans in Connecticut found that 12.5 percent of study participants had contemplated suicide in the 2 weeks preceding the study [10]. The Army Study to Assess Risk and Resilience in Servicemembers performed by a large group of U.S. researchers found a higher suicide rate in service members who were currently deployed or had been previously deployed compared with those who had never been deployed [27].

A more recent study of the risk of suicide among U.S. combat veterans found that there was an increased risk of suicide when all OEF/OIF/OND veterans were compared with the U.S. general population [28]. Researchers from the U.S. Department of Veterans Affairs used records from the U.S. Department of Defense to identify the study cohort. They found that both male and female veterans had an increased risk of suicide when compared to their gender-specific non-veteran counterparts. About 70 percent of veterans who died by suicide killed themselves using a firearm. After 15 years of follow-up, OEF/OIF/OND veterans continued to have a suicide rate that exceeded a suicide rate in the U.S. general population. A retrospective multivariate analysis of all U.S. military personnel between 2001 and 2011 that included about 3.8 million service members found that OEF and OIF veterans had elevated suicide rates for the first 4 years after their deployment in comparison with military personnel who had not been deployed [29]. This indicates that the risk of suicide is the highest during the first years after a war-zone deployment. Although some studies did not find relationships between suicide and deployments to OEF or OIF, some subgroups of combat veterans appeared to be more vulnerable to suicide than other combat veterans [30,31].

In 2002, U.K. veterans of the Falklands War (April-June 1982) claimed that more Falklands veterans had died by suicide (N = 264) since the conflict ended than died during the conflict itself (N = 256) [32]. Suicide rates among U.K. veterans of the 1991 Gulf War were also significant [32].

3. Unit Cohesion

Unit cohesion refers to the ties that preserve service members' dedication to each other, the unit, and the mission [33]. The concept of unit cohesion includes trust, reliance, and comradeship among peers (horizontal cohesion), as well as support, help and encouragement from, and respect for, unit leadership (vertical cohesion) [33,34]. Vertical cohesion can be described as leader-led support. Unit cohesion in the Armed Forces is critically integral to individual and group well-being, functioning, and security. Military unit cohesion strongly affects psychological and physical outcomes [12,35–37].

One of the important experiences of the Second World War was the identification of the critical significance of team cohesion in preventing psychiatric issues among the soldiers [35,36]. It has been suggested that "WWII clearly showed that interpersonal relationships and other social and situational circumstances were at least as important as personality configuration or individual assets and liabilities in the effectiveness of coping behavior" [35].

Considerable evidence suggests that servicemembers who report strong unit cohesion have a lower risk of psychiatric disorders and suicidal ideation [10,12,15,17,19]. A study showed that among U.S. Army soldiers, a higher perceived unit cohesion approximately 1–2 months before deployment to Afghanistan was associated with a lower risk of PTSD, major depression, generalized anxiety disorder, substance use disorder, and suicidal ideation 3 and 9 months after return from deployment [19]. In one study mentioned above [10], the authors used the Unit Support Scale (USS), a 12-item self-report instrument from the Deployment Risk and Resilience Inventory (DRRI) [34,38] that assesses the amount of assistance and encouragement in the war-zone from unit leaders and members and the military in general. The authors found that veterans who reported post-deployment suicidal ideation had lower scores on measures of unit support [10].

Griffith [17] from the U.S. National Center for Veterans Studies examined relationships among combat exposure, post-deployment problems, social help, and unit cohesion. In all, 4567 formerly deployed U.S. servicemembers who were soldiers of 50 company-sized units were surveyed. The study showed that at the group level, a diminished risk for suicidal ideation was associated with units having better than typical cohesion [17]. A study of 1663 U.S. servicemembers performed by a research group from the U.S. Army Institute of Public Health showed that combat exposure was a significant risk factor for suicidal ideation, while unit cohesion was a significant protective factor [13]. The significant interaction between the two factors indicated that soldiers who experienced greater combat exposure but also had higher levels of unit cohesion had relatively lower levels of suicide-related ideation. In addition, those who had higher levels of combat exposure and lower unit cohesion were most at risk for suicide-related ideation.

A study of risk and protective factors for suicidal ideation and suicide attempts among deployed Danish soldiers found that a heavy workload was associated with suicidal ideation and pointless tasks were a predictor for suicide attempts [16]. Pointless tasks can include repetitive chores when no military duties are available or military operations that are illogical from the soldiers' point of view. The perception or presence of heavy workloads and/or pointless tasks may be related to weak vertical cohesion.

4. Sexual and Non-Sexual Harassment and Abuse

Studies examining deployment sexual and non-sexual harassment and abuse have found that combat veterans who experience harassment and abuse are at heightened suicide risk [11,14,18,20,21]. This is consistent with observations among civilians indicating that different types of harassment and abuse lead to mental health issues and suicidality [39–42].

This underlines the importance of the prevention of harassment and abuse in different groups of the population.

A cross-sectional retrospective analysis of psychological evaluations of 1740 OEF/OIF veterans performed by researchers in Texas showed that general (non-sexual) harassment was associated with post-deployment suicidal ideation [11]. We performed a study on the relation of harassment during a combat deployment with post-deployment suicidality and testosterone function in male veterans [21]. We found that harassment scores were higher, and free testosterone levels were lower, among veterans who made post-deployment suicide attempts in comparison with veteran non-attempters. In the whole sample, harassment scores positively correlated with suicidal ideation scores ($r = 0.40$, $p = 0.02$) and negatively correlated with free testosterone levels ($r = -0.36$, $p = 0.04$). Free testosterone levels negatively correlated with suicidal ideation scores ($r = -0.57$, $p < 0.001$). Our observations may indicate that there is a link between deployment harassment, testosterone function, and suicidality. Our study is consistent with previous observations indicating that suicidal behavior in combat veterans has a neurobiological basis [8,22,43].

Kimerling et al. [18] examined data on veterans who received VHA services in the fiscal years 2007–2011 and were screened for military sexual trauma (MST; 5,991,080 men; 360,774 women). In the VHA, the term MST is used to refer to sexual assault or repeated, threatening sexual harassment during military service [44]. MST was reported by 1.1% of men and 21.2% of women. A total of 9017 veterans died by suicide during the follow-up period. Hazard ratios for military sexual trauma were 1.69 (95% CI = 1.45, 1.97) among men and 2.27 (95% CI = 1.76, 2.94) among women. Another study found that among female veterans, sexual harassment was the only deployment stressor to have an independent association with suicidal ideation, even when accounting for depression and alcohol-use symptoms [14]. Sexual harassment occurring during deployment may have an especially harmful effect on female veterans above and beyond its impact on psychiatric symptoms. A more recent study of women veterans who use VHA reproductive health care services performed by researchers in Colorado showed that the elevated prevalence of suicidal ideation after military service was associated with both military sexual harassment and assault [20]. Post-military suicide attempts were associated with military sexual assault. Studies by Kimerling et al. [18] and Monteith et al. [20] included both combat and non-combat veterans.

5. Post-Deployment Interventions to Decrease Suicidality

Sound post-deployment social support and the efficient treatment of psychiatric disorders may mitigate the suicide risk associated with adverse relationships within combat units [10,45–47]. A study on a longitudinal cohort derived from the Survey of Experiences of Returning Veterans that included 824 (480 men, 344 women) previously deployed OEF/OIF/OND veterans showed that among men, the association between deployment sexual trauma and suicidal ideation was moderated by post-deployment social support [47]. The authors also found that deployment sexual trauma predicted suicidal ideation only for men reporting that their post-deployment social support was low. Among women, post-deployment support mediated the association between deployment sexual trauma and suicidal ideation. The inclusion of post-deployment support in the model decreased the magnitude of the association between deployment sexual trauma and suicidal ideation. Another study showed that increased post-deployment social support and feelings of purpose and control were associated with fewer suicidal thoughts [10].

A study of 145 OEF/OIF veterans revealed that symptoms of PTSD and depression had almost no effect on suicidal ideation when post-deployment social support was high; however, when post-deployment social support was low, symptoms of PTSD and depression were positively associated with suicidal ideation [46]. Therefore, it is crucial to help veterans who have suffered deployment harassment and/or abuse to obtain social support after returning from deployment. A sense of purpose is frequently essential to recovery for these veterans. Also, for veterans reporting poor perceived post-deployment support, evaluating suicidality may be especially important. It is also very important to provide psychoeducation for the families and friends of returning veterans to emphasize the significance of post-deployment support and to educate them on how to recognize the warning signs of suicide [48,49]. Families are vital to recovery and are often the first to recognize suicidality in veterans.

The effective psychological and pharmacological treatment of psychiatric symptoms is a useful point of intervention for veterans experiencing suicidality after deployment. Psychotherapeutic interventions including cognitive–behavioral therapy and supportive therapy may reduce symptoms of depression, PTSD, and other psychiatric disorders and, consequently, reduce suicidality [50,51].

Antidepressants and other medications may reduce symptoms of depression, anxiety, PTSD, and other psychiatric disorders and, therefore, reduce the suicide risk in veterans [45,50,51]. It is important to note that even mild symptoms of depression and PTSD may increase the risk of suicide. The continuity of care is critical when dealing with veterans who have suicidal ideation or a history of attempted suicide. Such veterans need an effective outpatient follow-up upon discharge from the emergency department or inpatient care.

6. Organizational Changes

As described above, considerable evidence suggests that relations within combat units influence the development of post-deployment psychiatric illnesses, including suicidal ideation and behavior. More specifically, it has been shown that poor unit cohesion and the presence of harassment and/or abuse may have a deleterious effect on the mental health of combat veterans. Therefore, improvement in units' cohesion and the prevention of harassment/abuse during a military deployment are necessary to reduce post-deployment psychiatric pathology, including suicidal behavior [8,9,11,12,35–37]. This should be a priority in the military.

Commanding officers can prevent harassing behavior, because they monitor and manage military servicemembers [17,52]. In 2018, the U.S. Department of Defense established a policy on harassment, "Harassment Prevention and Response in the Armed Forces" [52]. This policy comprises all types of harassment, including general harassment, "discriminatory" harassment (based on race, color, religion, sex, etc.), sexual harassment, bullying, hazing, retaliation, and reprisals. According to this policy, military leadership is expected to take appropriate disciplinary or administrative actions against the harasser if harassment complaints are confirmed.

Effective leaders that recognize psychiatric problems among service members and address mental health stigma, collaborate with mental health professionals, and support ethical and spiritual practices may reduce suicidal ideation and behavior among military personnel [53,54]. Some service members may have had an undiagnosed psychiatric disorder upon entry into the Armed Forces, and the distress related to that disorder only became evident during their time in military service. Some service members may have also had a predisposition to a psychiatric condition that developed during military service because of the stress. For example, the military environment can serve as a facilitator for the development and progression of depression [54]. The actions of military leaders toward servicemembers with mental health problems and communication strategies surrounding suicidal behavior may significantly influence the psychological condition of affected soldiers. It is important to support public health interventions, with a view to fostering screening, enhanced access, and greater coordination with unit leaders. Also, it is essential that military personnel are educated about the importance of a non-judgmental and supportive attitude toward their peers with mental health issues.

Sexual minority service members encounter distinct stressors and issues which may affect the mental health of this demographic group. For example, a cross-sectional survey by McDonald et al. [55] showed that a higher proportion of lesbian, gay, or bisexual soldiers than heterosexual soldiers screened positive for anxiety, PTSD, and suicidality.

The mental health of sexual-minority individuals in the military represents a crucial area of investigation.

Military commanders influence service members and activities that make up the Armed Forces. The diligent selection and effective training of military leaders are of utmost importance. Effective military leaders are expected to value their subordinates, protect them from harassment, and efficiently work to improve vertical and horizontal cohesion [9,17,52,56]. Trustworthiness, credibility, skills, knowledge, concern for morale, instilling a sense of purpose, and providing regular feedback are vital to successful military leadership.

The studies referenced in this review cover a wide chronological span. It is important to note that conditions in the military may change over time, especially considering that weapons of war are becoming more powerful, sophisticated, accurate, and destructive.

7. Conclusions

Weak unit cohesion and the existence of harassment and/or abuse have a harmful impact on the psychological health of servicemembers and veterans. Moreover, such adverse circumstances may negatively affect the ability of combat units to perform military tasks. Therefore, efforts should be made to reduce harmful relations within combat teams. Mental and non-mental health medical practitioners need to be educated in the importance of identifying servicemembers and veterans who are victims of adverse relations within military units and proving them with appropriate psychiatric and medical treatment. Military leaders and policy makers should try to improve team cohesion and to reduce harassment/abuse in combat units. The prevention of mental health issues including suicidal behavior in military personnel and veterans is of utmost importance.

Funding: This research received no external funding.

Institutional Review Board Statement: Not applicable.

Informed Consent Statement: Not applicable.

Data Availability Statement: Not applicable.

Conflicts of Interest: The author declares no conflicts of interest.

References

1. Institute for Economics & Peace. Global Peace Index 2024: Measuring Peace in a Complex World. Sydney, June 2024. Available online: http://visionofhumanity.org/resources (accessed on 17 August 2024).
2. Brown University Watson Institute for International and Public Affairs. Costs of War. August 2024. Available online: https://watson.brown.edu/costsofwar/costs/human/veterans (accessed on 14 August 2024).
3. U.S. Census Bureau. Veterans Glossary. December 2021. Available online: https://www.census.gov/topics/population/veterans/about/glossary.html (accessed on 14 August 2024).
4. EUROMIL. EUROMIL Position Paper on Veterans. June 2020. Available online: https://euromil.org/wp-content/uploads/2020/05/2010_Position_Paper_Veterans.pdf (accessed on 4 November 2024).
5. Rice, T.R.; Sher, L. Suicidal behavior in war veterans. *Expert Rev. Neurother.* **2012**, *12*, 611–624. [CrossRef] [PubMed]
6. Macgregor, A.J.; Tang, J.J.; Dougherty, A.L.; Galarneau, M.R. Deployment-related injury and posttraumatic stress disorder in US military personnel. *Injury* **2013**, *44*, 1458–1464. [CrossRef] [PubMed]
7. Dyball, D.; Bennett, A.N.; Schofield, S.; Cullinan, P.; Boos, C.J.; Bull, A.M.J.; Wessely, S.; Stevelink, S.A.M.; Fear, N.T.; ADVANCE study. Mental health outcomes of male UK military personnel deployed to Afghanistan and the role of combat injury: Analysis of baseline data from the ADVANCE cohort study. *Lancet Psychiatry* **2022**, *9*, 547–554. [CrossRef] [PubMed]
8. Sher, L. The uncounted casualties of war: Suicide in combat veterans. *QJM* **2024**, *117*, 163–167. [CrossRef]
9. Brooks, S.K.; Greenberg, N. Non-deployment factors affecting psychological wellbeing in military personnel: Literature review. *J. Ment. Health.* **2018**, *27*, 80–90. [CrossRef]
10. Pietrzak, R.H.; Goldstein, M.B.; Malley, J.C.; Rivers, A.J.; Johnson, D.C.; Southwick, S.M. Risk and protective factors associated with suicidal ideation in veterans of Operations Enduring Freedom and Iraqi Freedom. *J. Affect. Disord.* **2010**, *123*, 102–107. [CrossRef]
11. Lemaire, C.M.; Graham, D.P. Factors associated with suicidal ideation in OEF/OIF veterans. *J. Affect. Disord.* **2011**, *130*, 231–238. [CrossRef]

12. Du Preez, J.; Sundin, J.; Wessely, S.; Fear, N.T. Unit cohesion and mental health in the UK armed forces. *Occup. Med.* **2012**, *62*, 47–53. [CrossRef]
13. Mitchell, M.M.; Gallaway, M.S.; Millikan, A.M.; Bell, M. Interaction of combat exposure and unit cohesion in predicting suicide-related ideation among post-deployment soldiers. *Suicide Life Threat. Behav.* **2012**, *42*, 486–494. [CrossRef]
14. Gradus, J.L.; Street, A.E.; Suvak, M.K.; Resick, P.A. Predictors of suicidal ideation in a gender-stratified sample of OEF/OIF veterans. *Suicide Life Threat. Behav.* **2013**, *45*, 574–588. [CrossRef]
15. Bryan, C.J.; Heron, E.A. Belonging protects against postdeployment depression in military personnel. *Depress. Anxiety* **2015**, *32*, 349–355. [CrossRef] [PubMed]
16. Ejdesgaard, B.A.; Zøllner, L.; Jensen, B.F.; Jørgensen, H.O.; Kähler, H. Risk and protective factors for suicidal ideation and suicide attempts among deployed Danish soldiers from 1990 to 2009. *Mil. Med.* **2015**, *180*, 61–67. [CrossRef] [PubMed]
17. Griffith, J. Cross (Unit)-Level Effects of Cohesion on Relationships of Suicide Thoughts to Combat Exposure, Postdeployment Stressors, and Postdeployment Social Support. *Behav. Med.* **2015**, *41*, 98–106. [CrossRef]
18. Kimerling, R.; Makin-Byrd, K.; Louzon, S.; Ignacio, R.V.; McCarthy, J.F. Military Sexual Trauma and Suicide Mortality. *Am. J. Prev. Med.* **2016**, *50*, 684–691. [CrossRef] [PubMed]
19. Anderson, L.; Campbell-Sills, L.; Ursano, R.J.; Kessler, R.C.; Sun, X.; Heeringa, S.G.; Nock, M.K.; Bliese, P.D.; Gonzalez, O.I.; Wynn, G.H.; et al. Prospective associations of perceived unit cohesion with postdeployment mental health outcomes. *Depress. Anxiety* **2019**, *36*, 511–521. [CrossRef] [PubMed]
20. Monteith, L.L.; Kittel, J.A.; Schneider, A.L.; Miller, C.N.; Holliday, R.; Katon, J.G.; Brenner, L.A.; Hoffmire, C.A. Military sexual trauma among women Veterans using Veterans Health Administration Reproductive Health Care: Screening challenges and associations with post-Military suicidal ideation and suicide attempts. *J. Interpers. Violence* **2023**, *38*, 7578–7601. [CrossRef]
21. Sher, L.; Bierer, L.M.; Flory, J.; Makotkine, I.; Yehuda, R. Interplay of combat deployment harassment, testosterone concentrations and post-deployment suicide risk in male veterans. *Acta Neuropsychiatr.* **2024**, *36*, 167–171. [CrossRef]
22. Kovacic, Z.; Henigsberg, N.; Pivac, N.; Nedic, G.; Borovecki, A. Platelet serotonin concentration and suicidal behavior in combat related posttraumatic stress disorder. *Prog. Neuropsychopharmacol. Biol. Psychiatry* **2008**, *32*, 544–551. [CrossRef]
23. McCarthy, J.F.; Valenstein, M.; Kim, H.M.; Ilgen, M.; Zivin, K.; Blow, F.C. Suicide mortality among patients receiving care in the veterans health administration health system. *Am. J. Epidemiol.* **2009**, *169*, 1033–1038. [CrossRef]
24. Department of Veterans Affairs, Office of Mental Health and Suicide Prevention. 2022 National Veteran Suicide Prevention Annual Report. September 2022. Available online: https://www.mentalhealth.va.gov/suicide_prevention/data.asp (accessed on 31 July 2024).
25. Sher, L.; Yehuda, R. Preventing suicide among returning combat veterans: A moral imperative. *Mil. Med.* **2011**, *176*, 601–602. [CrossRef]
26. Orak, U.; Yildiz, M.; Aydogdu, R.; Koenig, H.G.; Pietrzak, R.H. The relationship between combat exposure and suicide risk in U.S. military veterans: Exploring the role of posttraumatic stress symptoms and religious coping. *J. Affect Disord.* **2023**, *341*, 77–87. [CrossRef] [PubMed]
27. Schoenbaum, M.; Kessler, R.C.; Gilman, S.E.; Colpe, L.J.; Heeringa, S.G.; Stein, M.B.; Ursano, R.J.; Cox, K.L.; Army STARRS Collaborators. Predictors of suicide and accident death in the Army Study to Assess Risk and Resilience in Servicemembers (Army STARRS): Results from the Army Study to Assess Risk and Resilience in Servicemembers (Army STARRS). *JAMA Psychiatry* **2014**, *71*, 493–503. [CrossRef] [PubMed]
28. Bullman, T.; Schneiderman, A. Risk of suicide among U.S. veterans who deployed as part of Operation Enduring Freedom, Operation Iraqi Freedom, and Operation New Dawn. *Inj. Epidemiol.* **2021**, *8*, 40. [CrossRef] [PubMed]
29. Shen, Y.C.; Cunha, J.M.; Williams, T.V. Time-varying associations of suicide with deployments, mental health conditions, and stressful life events among current and former US military personnel: A retrospective multivariate analysis. *Lancet Psychiatry* **2016**, *3*, 1039–1048. [CrossRef] [PubMed]
30. Kang, H.K.; Bullman, T.A. Risk of suicide among US veterans after returning from the Iraq or Afghanistan war zones. *JAMA* **2008**, *300*, 652–653. [CrossRef]
31. Reger, M.A.; Tucker, R.P.; Carter, S.P.; Ammerman, B.A. Military deployments and suicide: A critical examination. *Perspect. Psychol. Sci.* **2018**, *13*, 688–699. [CrossRef]
32. Spooner, M.H. Suicide claiming more British Falkland veterans than fighting did. *CMAJ* **2002**, *166*, 1453.
33. Van Epps, G. Relooking Unit Cohesion: A Sensemaking Approach. *Mil. Rev.* **2008**, *88*, 102–110.
34. King, L.A.; King, D.W.; Vogt, D.S.; Knight, J.; Samper, R.E. Deployment Risk and Resilience Inventory: A collection of measures for studying deployment related experiences of military personnel and veterans. *Mil. Psychol.* **2006**, *18*, 89–120. [CrossRef]
35. Glass, A.J. Lessons learned. In *Neuropsychiatry in World War II, Overseas Theaters*; Glass, A.J., Ed.; Office of the Surgeon General, U.S. Army: Washington, DC, USA, 1973; Volume 2, pp. 989–1027.
36. Institute of Medicine (US) Medical Follow-Up Agency; Joellenbeck, L.M.; Russell, P.K.; Guze, S.B. (Eds.) Strategies to Protect the Health of Deployed U.S. Forces: Medical Surveillance, Record Keeping, and Risk Reduction. In *Risks to Deployed Forces*; National Academies Press (US): Washington, DC, USA, 1999; Volume 2. Available online: https://www.ncbi.nlm.nih.gov/books/NBK225082/ (accessed on 9 August 2024).
37. Williams, J.; Brown, J.M.; Bray, R.M.; Anderson Goodell, E.M.; Rae Olmsted, K.; Adler, A.B. Unit cohesion, resilience, and mental health of soldiers in basic combat training. *Mil. Psychol.* **2016**, *28*, 241–250. [CrossRef]

38. Vogt, D.S.; Proctor, S.P.; King, D.W.; King, L.A.; Vasterling, J.J. Validation of scales from the Deployment Risk and Resilience Inventory in a sample of Operation Iraqi Freedom veterans. *Assessment* **2008**, *15*, 391–403. [CrossRef] [PubMed]
39. Makhija, N.; Sher, L. Childhood abuse, adult alcohol use disorders and suicidal behaviour. *QJM* **2007**, *100*, 305–309. [CrossRef] [PubMed]
40. Wolford-Clevenger, C.; Vann, N.C.; Smith, P.N. The Association of Partner Abuse Types and Suicidal Ideation Among Men and Women College Students. *Violence Vict.* **2016**, *31*, 471–485. [CrossRef] [PubMed]
41. Gårdvik, K.S.; Torgersen, T.; Rygg, M.; Lydersen, S.; Indredavik, M.S. Suicidality, function and associated negative life events in an adolescent psychiatric population at 3-year follow-up. *BMC Psychiatry* **2021**, *21*, 109. [CrossRef]
42. Magnusson Hanson, L.L.; Pentti, J.; Nordentoft, M.; Xu, T.; Rugulies, R.; Madsen, I.E.H.; Conway, P.M.; Westerlund, H.; Vahtera, J.; Ervasti, J.; et al. Association of workplace violence and bullying with later suicide risk: A multicohort study and meta-analysis of published data. *Lancet Public Health* **2023**, *8*, e494–e503. [CrossRef]
43. Sher, L. Neurobiology of suicidal behavior in combat veterans. *Braz. J. Psychiatry* **2020**, *42*, 465–466. [CrossRef]
44. U.S. Department of Veteran Affairs. Veterans Health Administration. Military Sexual Trauma. May 2021. Available online: https://www.mentalhealth.va.gov/docs/mst_general_factsheet.pdf (accessed on 10 September 2024).
45. Kudler, H.; Straits-Tröster, K. Identifying and treating post deployment mental health problems among new combat veterans. *N. C. Med. J.* **2008**, *69*, 39–42. [CrossRef]
46. DeBeer, B.B.; Kimbrel, N.A.; Meyer, E.C.; Gulliver, S.B.; Morissette, S.B. Combined PTSD and depressive symptoms interact with post-deployment social support to predict suicidal ideation in Operation Enduring Freedom and Operation Iraqi Freedom veterans. *Psychiatry Res.* **2014**, *216*, 357–362. [CrossRef]
47. Monteith, L.L.; Hoffmire, C.A.; Holliday, R.; Park, C.L.; Mazure, C.M.; Hoff, R.A. Do unit and post-deployment social support influence the association between deployment sexual trauma and suicidal ideation? *Psychiatry Res.* **2018**, *270*, 673–681. [CrossRef]
48. Debeer, B.B.; Matthieu, M.M.; Kittel, J.A.; Degutis, L.C.; Clafferty, S.; Qualls, N.; Morissette, S.B. Quality improvement evaluation of the feasibility and acceptability of adding a concerned significant other to safety planning for suicide prevention with veterans. *J. Ment. Health Couns.* **2019**, *4*, 4–20. [CrossRef]
49. DuBois, D.; Richmond, R.; Stephanie Roberts, L.; Mahar, A.; Fear, N.; Gill, K.; Samantha Leroux, J.; Cramm, H. A scoping review of military and Veteran families within international suicidality and suicide prevention research. *Prev. Med. Rep.* **2023**, *33*, 102206. [CrossRef] [PubMed]
50. Lazar, S.G. The mental health needs of military service members and veterans. *Psychodyn. Psychiatry* **2014**, *42*, 459–478. [CrossRef] [PubMed]
51. Sher, L.; Oquendo, M.A. Suicide: An Overview for Clinicians. *Med. Clin. N. Am.* **2023**, *107*, 119–130. [CrossRef] [PubMed]
52. Gilberg, K. New Military Policy on Harassment. Military Law Task Force. 17 March 2018. Available online: https://nlgmltf.org/military-law/2018/new-military-policy-on-harassment/ (accessed on 14 August 2024).
53. Umbrasas, K. Rediscovering Leadership as an Antidote to Adjustment Problems in the Army. *Mil. Rev.* **2022**, 97–105. Available online: https://www.armyupress.army.mil/Journals/Military-Review/English-Edition-Archives/July-August-2022/Umbrasas/ (accessed on 9 September 2024).
54. Moore, M.J.; Shawler, E.; Jordan, C.H.; Jackson, C.A. Veteran and Military Mental Health Issues. In *StatPearls [Internet]*; StatPearls Publishing: Treasure Island, FL, USA, 2024; [Updated 17 August 2023]. Available online: https://www.ncbi.nlm.nih.gov/books/NBK572092/ (accessed on 31 July 2024).
55. McDonald, J.L.; Ganulin, M.L.; Dretsch, M.N.; Taylor, M.R.; Cabrera, O.A. Assessing the Well-being of Sexual Minority Soldiers at a Military Academic Institution. *Mil. Med.* **2020**, *185* (Suppl. S1), 342–347. [CrossRef]
56. Pflanz, S.E.; Ogle, A.D. Job stress, depression, work performance, and perceptions of supervisors in military personnel. *Mil. Med.* **2006**, *171*, 861–865. [CrossRef]

behavioral sciences

MDPI

Review

Grief Intervention in Suicide Loss Survivors through Cognitive-Behavioral Therapy: A Systematic Review

José Carlos Romero-Moreno [1], María Cantero-García [2,*], Ana Huertes-del Arco [2,3], Eva Izquierdo-Sotorrío [2], María Rueda-Extremera [2] and Jesús González-Moreno [1]

1 Psicología, Facultad de Ciencias de la Salud, Universidad Internacional de Valencia (VIU), 46003 Valencia, Spain; josecarlosromeromoreno@gmail.com (J.C.R.-M.); jesus.gonzalezm@professor.universidadviu.com (J.G.-M.)
2 Psicología, Facultad de Ciencias de la Salud y Educación, Universidad a Distancia de Madrid (UDIMA), 28400 Madrid, Spain; ana.huertes@udima.es (A.H.-d.A.); eva.izquierdo@udima.es (E.I.-S.); maria.rueda@udima.es (M.R.-E.)
3 Facultad de Psicología, Universidad Nacional de Educación a Distancia (UNED), 28040 Madrid, Spain
* Correspondence: mariafrancisca.cantero.g@udima.es or maria.canterogar@gmail.com

Abstract: Suicide is one of the leading causes of death worldwide, affecting numerous individuals close to the person who died by suicide, including family members, friends, and colleagues. Those affected by the suicide of someone are referred to as "suicide survivors", and the psychological consequences they face are particularly severe. One of these consequences is grief, which is more complicated in survivors of suicide compared with those grieving deaths from other causes, mainly because of the stigma that continues to surround them. Therefore, psychotherapeutic intervention for suicide loss survivors is crucial. This study examines the efficacy of cognitive-behavioral programs for addressing grief and other related variables in suicide loss survivors. The search was conducted in databases including Psycinfo, Academic Search Premier, Medline, APA PsycArticles, E-Journals, Scopus, and PubMed. Five randomized controlled trials were selected, one of which focused exclusively on minors. The results reveal that cognitive-behavioral therapy is effective, although the methodological quality of these studies is not adequate, and the representativeness of the samples is very low. More RCTs are needed on the application of cognitive-behavioral programs to treat grief in suicide loss survivors.

Keywords: survivor of suicide; grief; depression; cognitive-behavioral therapy; systematic review

1. Introduction

Every 40 s, a suicide occurs globally, totaling over 700,000 completed suicides annually [1–3]. In the United States alone, suicide rates increased by approximately 36% between 2000 and 2022, with 49,476 deaths in 2022—equating to about one death every 11 min [4]. Each suicide affects an estimated 60 individuals, including family, friends, and colleagues, known as "suicide survivors" [5]. The grief experienced by suicide loss survivors is often more complex because of the stigma surrounding suicide, impacting not only those directly affected by the attempts but also their loved ones, ultimately leading to complicated grief [6–8].

Previous reviews have highlighted the cognitive-behavioral model by Boelen et al. [9] as a key theoretical framework for addressing complicated grief. Although these reviews noted a scarcity of studies examining the effectiveness of cognitive-behavioral interventions (CBT) through randomized controlled trials, these reviews are outdated. Therefore, new reviews are necessary to identify recent randomized controlled trials employing cognitive-behavioral therapies in suicide loss survivors to alleviate grief and assess the effectiveness of such therapies in reducing grief in this population.

Suicide can be defined as any self-inflicted behavior performed with the intention of causing oneself intentional death [10,11]. The World Health Organization [3] defines it as an "act with a fatal outcome, deliberately initiated and performed by the deceased in the knowledge or expectation of a fatal outcome through which changes he or she desired to achieve". According to global data, suicide claims the lives of more than 700,000 people annually [1–3], with one suicide attempt every three seconds [3], making it one of the top ten leading causes of non-natural deaths in Europe, America, and much of Asia [2]. These figures have increased because of the situation caused by the COVID-19 pandemic [12].

The etiology of suicide is multifactorial, resulting from the combination of biological, psychological, and social factors that interact differentially according to the individual and culture [13–15]. However, studies that seek to establish a "general risk profile" for suicide often focus on middle-aged Caucasian populations, making this profile not globally representative [13]. Additionally, many suicides are not classified as such when "passive" methods are used, such as overdoses or traffic collisions, which are often mistaken for accidental events [8].

The Impact of Suicide: Addressing Complicated Grief in Survivors

It has been noted that a single suicide typically affects at least six closely related individuals [8,16]; however, these figures could be higher [7], potentially reaching up to 40, including family members and other acquaintances [17]. Based on this, the term "suicide survivor" has become popular, referring to someone close to a person who has died by suicide, attempting to "understand the reasons for the death and learn to continue with their life" [5]. This definition emphasizes the change that the suicide of a loved one brings to the survivor's life [6]. Despite being a term frequently used by researchers, it also has certain limitations, including confusion about who the term refers to (whether it refers to those who survive the suicide or an individual who attempts suicide and survives) and the difficulty in delimiting the social network to which this term may refer (family members, friends, someone who indirectly collaborates in the suicidal act such as a train conductor when someone jumps onto the tracks to death by suicide, etc.) [6,7]. Based on the conception of this definition, Shneidman [16] used the term "postvention" to refer to all activities and/or interventions carried out to address the psychological consequences arising from the suicide of a loved one.

The death of a loved one is a universally stressful event, which favors the appearance of a set of unpleasant emotional, cognitive, behavioral, and physiological symptoms that can contribute to the development of subsequent psychological problems [18]. It has been estimated that between 6 and 15% of people who experience grief over the loss of a loved one may develop greater complications such as complicated grief [19]. However, in the case of suicide, this probability increases considerably [6–8]. For example, a higher risk of suicidal behaviors and a high prevalence of complicated grief have been observed in suicide loss survivors, with feelings of guilt, rumination on the reason for the loved one's suicide, post-traumatic symptoms, and anger being prominent in this type of grief [7,8]. Complicated grief is defined as a prolongation over time of the normal grief reaction, where feelings of concern, sadness, and emotional pain persist, and positive memories of the deceased are blocked, hindering the recovery of normal life [8]. Although the presence of complicated grief is quite common in suicide loss survivors, in some cases, such as when the deceased was diagnosed with a psychiatric disorder, the process is more manageable, and understanding of the suicidal act by their loved ones is facilitated [6]. Additionally, as noted by Ali [6] and Jordan [7], grief after suicide is experienced in solitude; suicide is still highly stigmatized, so survivors are often blamed for not having done enough to save the individual, leading to grief that is experienced in isolation and shame, even hiding what happened to avoid feeling more responsible than the survivor already feels. Complicated grief in suicide loss survivors is greater the closer the relationship with the deceased; Mitchell et al. [8] observed that the prevalence of complicated grief in suicide loss survivors was twice as high in those who were closely related to the suicide victim compared with those who had a less intimate relationship with them.

In addition to grief, post-traumatic symptoms, guilt, stigma, and depressive and anxious symptoms are also frequent [6]. Hopelessness and yearning, characteristics present in depressive episodes, are very common in complicated grief, which may be related to suicidal ideation and behaviors with the intention of avoiding suffering and reuniting with the deceased [8], explaining the elevated risk of suicide in suicide loss survivors.

Boelen et al. [9] describe the development and maintenance of complicated grief from a cognitive-behavioral perspective, highlighting the following three key phases in this process: (a) Poor elaboration and integration of the death into the subject's autobiographical information: Individuals with complicated grief, despite being exposed to numerous stimuli reminding them of the deceased, are unable to assimilate the loss, continuing to perceive it as "unreal". (b) Global and negative beliefs about oneself, life, and the future and erroneous interpretations of grief: The loss of a loved one and the role they played in the mourner's life can disrupt the stable and global beliefs the mourner had about life and the future. As Boelen et al. [9] point out, the death of a child can affect beliefs about the meaning of life, while the death of a romantic partner can alter expectations for the future. This disruption of "future-directed stability" can affect daily functioning. Furthermore, the loss may not only affect future expectations but also reactivate negative beliefs about oneself that the presence of the deceased had previously mitigated. The authors provide an example of how the death of a romantic partner can trigger latent negative beliefs that were suppressed while the partner was alive. These beliefs, combined with the interpretation that the loved one's death is an unbearable pain and intrusive memories of the deceased (erroneous interpretations of grief), lead to avoidance, which in turn sustains complicated grief. Guilt and anger are also central to this process, especially in cases of suicide grief, where the mourner may feel responsible for the death or struggle to understand why it happened. (c) Avoidance of grief-related reactions: These strategies include anxious and depressive behaviors, such as avoiding thoughts, memories, and feelings related to the deceased in order to prevent "going crazy".

Examples of these are avoiding exposure to places the mourner visited with the deceased, to people who may talk about the deceased, or to objects that remind them of the deceased (although, sometimes the opposite effect occurs, where avoidance occurs towards "no contact" with those objects, people, or situations, with the intention of avoiding contact with a reality without the deceased), and rumination on the reason for the loss. Among the latter, depressive strategies stand out, including those in which the mourner enters a state of hypoactivity, ceasing to participate in social events and pleasurable activities; in this case, the goal is not to avoid stimuli, but rather the cause is the lack of reinforcement or guilt for "enjoying without the deceased".

The authors include in this model other variables such as individual vulnerability factors, event characteristics, and the consequences of loss, along with another set of variables and processes that make up the Boelen et al. [9] model. Based on the cognitive-behavioral model of complicated grief developed by Boelen et al. [9], cognitive-behavioral therapy has frequently been applied to treat complicated grief, finding positive effects of this intervention [20]. However, fewer studies have analyzed, with adequate methodological quality, the efficacy of cognitive-behavioral therapy and other types of interventions in cases of complicated grief due to suicide [21].

In 2008, Jordan [7] noted the lack of empirical support with controlled designs on interventions for grief in suicide loss survivors while highlighting that individual therapy, joint family therapy, and support groups appear to be useful for these survivors. Similarly, considering the high prevalence of post-traumatic symptoms in these individuals, some behavioral interventions such as exposure therapy, techniques like empty chair or narrative therapy, and interventions such as eye movement desensitization and reprocessing (EMDR) could be useful [7]. Linde et al. [1] conducted a systematic review of interventions used in grief among suicide loss survivors, finding that cognitive-behavioral interventions were effective in suicide loss survivors with high suicidal ideation, although only two cognitive-behavioral programs were identified in their review. In a systematic review conducted by Andriessen et al. [22], promising results were also found for cognitive-behavioral programs, although the review was conducted only a year after Linde et al.'s study [1], so they did not find many more publications regarding this type of program because of the short time lapse between one review and the other.

Taking into consideration that the most recent review available was conducted by Andriessen et al. [22] and was performed in 2018, it is important to conduct new systematic reviews to determine if there are more recent studies applying cognitive-behavioral programs in grief among suicide loss survivors, as well as the efficacy of such programs. Based on the PICO questions, the general objective of this work is to determine the efficacy of cognitive-behavioral programs (intervention) compared to control groups (comparison) in reducing grief (outcome) in suicide loss survivors (patients). The specific objectives of this systematic review are as follows: 1. Determine how many RCTs have been conducted to analyze the efficacy of cognitive behavioral interventions in reducing complicated grief in suicide loss survivors. 2. Identify the types of relatives to whom these cognitive-behavioral programs have been applied. 3. Determine the types of cognitive behavioral programs used in the reviewed RCTs (format, duration, and components). 4. Identify the types of controls used in the reviewed RCTs. 5. Determine if cognitive-behavioral programs are effective in reducing grief related to suicide.

2. Materials and Methods

This systematic review was conducted according to PRISMA criteria [23]. The search process began on 1 April and ended on 20 April 2024, using Psycinfo, Academic Search Premier, Medline, APA PSycArticles, E-Journals, Scopus, and Pubmed databases. The following search equation was used in all databases: (cognitive-behavioral therapy OR cognitive-behaviour therapy) AND (grief OR mourning OR bereavement OR depression) AND suicide AND intervention AND controlled. No temporal restrictions were established regarding publications. RCTs were accepted only if they included suicide loss survivors in grief as participants and if their primary measure was related to grief (depression, suicidal ideation, post-traumatic symptoms, rumination, and/or guilt). Samples of both adult and child participants were accepted, and survivors with both familial and non-familial close relationships with the deceased were admitted. Studies using intervention programs that, while not exclusively cognitive behavioral, were largely based on this theoretical framework were also accepted. Qualitative studies, systematic reviews, meta-analyses (although consulted for new records), single case studies, books, book chapters, studies not focusing on survivors, and the gray literature were excluded from this review. Studies published in languages other than English and Spanish were also excluded. After performing all the aforementioned searches, the obtained records were identified, and duplicate records were removed. Subsequently, the first screening was conducted based on the title and abstract of each identified record. Studies that did not meet the criteria were eliminated after this screening and, in the second screening, each record was read in its entirety to eliminate records that did not meet the criteria or were inaccessible. The selection of relevant studies involved a three-phase process carried out by two reviewers (R.M.J.C. and M.C.G.). First, the titles and abstracts of all identified papers were assessed according to the pre-established inclusion and exclusion criteria. In the second phase, the full texts of papers deemed potentially relevant were examined. This phase concluded with a cross-reference check.

Data analysis was performed using qualitative synthesis, and the risk of bias of each accepted study in the review was analyzed based on Cochrane criteria [24] aimed at evaluating the risk of selection, performance, detection, attrition, and reporting bias.

The authors registered this manuscript in Open Science Framework (OSF) at 24 July 2024.

3. Results

During the search process, a total of 405 records were identified, with 109 identified in the Scopus database, 99 in Psycinfo, 93 in Medline, 65 in Academic Search Premier, 29 in E-Journals, 7 in Pubmed, and 3 in APA Psycarticles. Additionally, an additional record was identified from the previous reviews. Of these 406 records, 166 were duplicates, resulting in 240 unique records after removing duplicates. In the first screening, titles and abstracts of each record were analyzed, leading to the elimination of 235 studies that did not meet the criteria (219 of them either addressed grief but not suicide or addressed suicide but not survivor grief, 7 were responses to other authors, editorials, or conference posters, 6 were not in English or Spanish, 2 were systematic reviews, and 1 was a protocol for intervention for survivor grief but had not yet been implemented). Thus, five records passed the first screening and were read in their entirety in the second screening, and they were accepted for meeting all selection criteria, with four of them coming from database searches and one being an additional record. In Figure 1, the flowchart is shown.

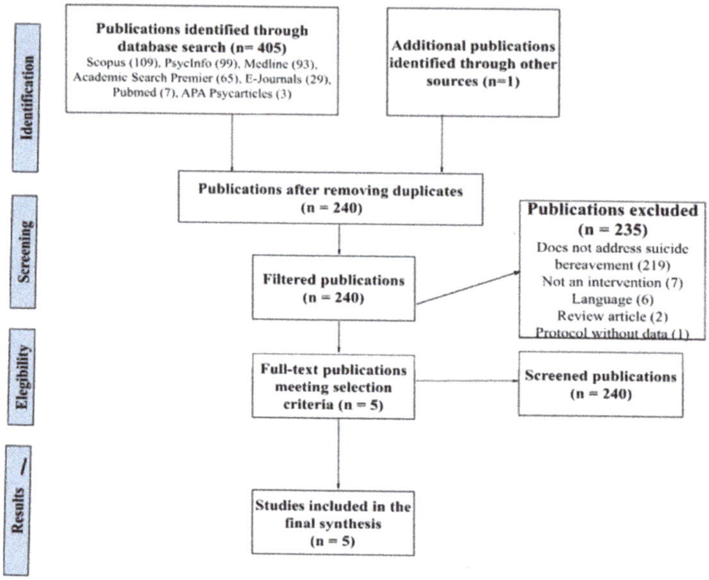

Figure 1. PRISMA-based systematic review process flowchart.

A qualitative analysis of the accepted studies was conducted, and the data obtained were synthesized based on the following four themes: study design, description of interventions, assessment instruments used, and results obtained. Table 1 presents the synthesis of these data.

Table 1. Summary of results.

Author and Year	Design	Intervention	Measurements	Results
Pfeffer et al. [25]	A total of 75 children ($N_{experimental}$ = 39; $N_{control}$ = 36). Mean age = 10.5 years old, SD = 3.2; 28 men. Pre- and post-intervention measures	Experimental group: BGI × 10 weekly group sessions, 1.5 h per session. Two components: psychoeducation and support. Groups of two–five children, organized by age (6–9 years old; 10–12 years old; 13–15 years old). Control group: Waiting list.	CPTSRI for post-traumatic symptomatology, CDI for depressive symptomatology, RCMAS for anxious symptomatology, SAICA to assess social adjustment.	Between-group comparisons: Significantly greater reductions in anxiety symptoms ($p < 0.009$; d = 0.80) and depressive symptoms ($p < 0.01$; d = 0.70) were observed in the experimental group compared with the control group, with larger reductions observed in middle-aged children (11 years old) compared with younger (6 years old) and older (14 years old) children. No significant differences were found in post-traumatic symptomatology or social adjustment. Within-group comparisons: Significant reductions were observed in post-measure anxiety symptoms ($p < 0.04$) and depressive symptoms ($p < 0.003$) in the experimental group, with a non-significant reduction in post-traumatic symptomatology ($p < 0.06$).
De Groot et al. [26]	A total of 134 participants > 15 years old ($N_{experimental}$ = 74; $N_{control}$ = 60). Mean age = 43 years old, SD= 13.6; 40 men. Preintervention measures (2.5 months after the suicide) and post-intervention measures (13 months after the suicide).	Experimental group: CBT counseling × four sessions of 2 h each, one session every 2–3 weeks. Intervention for the entire family system. Components: Psychoeducation, emotional processing, effective interaction, and problem-solving. Based on the theory of Boelen et al. [9]. Control group: Waiting list.	ITG complicated grief, CESD depressive symptomatology, PSI suicidal ideation, responsibility for suicide feelings with ad hoc questionnaire, TRGR2L maladaptive grief reactions.	Between-group comparisons: No effect on complicated grief ($p = 0.82$), depression levels ($p = 0.28$), or the presence of suicidal ideation, but there was an effect on maladaptive grief reactions with a notable but not significant reduction ($p = 0.056$) and on guilt perception with a significant reduction ($p = 0.01$). No within-group comparisons either each group.
De Groot et al. [27]	A total of 134 participants > 15 years old ($N_{experimental}$ = 74; $N_{control}$ = 60). Mean age= 43 years old, SD= 13.6; 40 men. Preintervention measures (2.5 months after the suicide) and post-intervention measures (13 months after the suicide).	Experimental group: CBT counseling × four sessions of 2 h each, one session every 2–3 weeks. Intervention for the entire family system. Components: Psychoeducation, emotional processing, effective interaction, and problem-solving. Based on the theory of Boelen et al. [9]. Control group: Waiting list.	EPQ-RSS, neuroticism; perceived sense of control over one's life; self-esteem with RSES; family history of suicide; subjective expectation of suicide index; responsibility for suicide feelings with ad hoc scales; complicated grief with ITG; depressive symptoms with CESD; suicidal ideation with PSI; maladaptive grief reactions with TRGR2L; anxiety and depression with SCAN 2.1	Survivors with suicidal ideation had a higher history of anxiety ($p < 0.05$), depression ($p < 0.01$), suicidal behavior ($p < 0.001$), and neuroticism ($p < 0.001$) and lower self-esteem ($p < 0.001$) compared with survivors without suicidal ideation. No significant differences were found in the interaction between suicidal ideation and intervention factors on the variables of complicated grief ($p = 0.33$), depressive symptoms ($p = 0.57$), or guilt perception ($p = 0.60$). There was a significantly greater reduction in maladaptive grief reactions ($p = 0.03$) and suicidal behavior ($p = 0.03$) among relatives with suicidal ideation
Wittouck et al. [28]	A total of 83 adult participants ($N_{experimental}$ = 47; $N_{control}$ = 36). Mean age = 48.6 years old, SD = 13.3; 20 men. Measures pre- and post-intervention. Four additional visits during the intervention in the experimental group.	Experimental group: CBT × home sessions lasting 2 h each session. Components: Psychoeducation about suicide, grief, specific aspects of grief due to suicide, and coping with grief. Based on the theory of Boelen et al. [9]. Control group: Waiting list.	Maladaptive grief symptomatology with ITG, depressive symptomatology with BDI-II, hopelessness with BHS, negative cognitions related to grief distress with CGQ, maladaptive coping with UCL.	Reducción significativa en el grupo experimental en sintomatología desadaptativa de duelo ($p = 0.021$) y en sintomatología depresiva ($p = 0.006$), pero no en desesperanza ($p = 0.231$). Sin reducción en grupo control ni en sintomatología de duelo ($p = 0.503$), ni en sintomatología depresiva ($p = 0.250$) ni en desesperanza ($p = 0.688$). Sin reducción en ninguna de las dimensiones del GCQ ni en grupo experimental ni en control. Reducción significativa en grupo experimental en las dimensiones del UCL "apoyo social" (p = 0.002), "reacción pasiva" (p = 0.013) y "expresión emocional" (p = 0.004).

Table 1. *Cont.*

Author and Year	Design	Intervention	Measurements	Results
Treml et al. [29]	A total of 58 adults ($N_{experimental}$ = 30; $N_{control}$ = 29). Mean age = 44.57 years old, SD= 14.25; 8 men. Measures pre- and post-intervention and follow-up at 3, 6, and 12 months after completing the intervention.	Experimental group: Online CBT × psychoeducation about suicide and suicide grief + 10 writing tasks (narrative therapy). Three phases: Coping, cognitive restructuring, and social exchange. Control group: Waiting list.	Severity of grief symptomatology with ICG, grief reaction after loss by suicide with GEQ, depressive symptomatology with BDI-II, general psychopathology with BSI.	Significant reductions in the follow-up measure at 12 months with respect to the post-measure in the experimental group versus the control in the GEQ subscales "guilt" (p = 0.043) and "shame" (p = 0.015), without differences among follow-up measures. No differences in follow-up in depressive symptoms or psychopathology in general.

Abbreviation Index: Depression Inventory-II; BHS: Beck Hopelessness Scale; BSI: Brief Symptom Inventory; CESD: Center for Epidemiologic Studies depression scale; CGQ: Grief Cognitions Questionnaire; EPQ-RSS: Eysenck Personality Questionnaire; GEQ: Grief Experience Questionnaire; ICG: Inventory of Complicated Grief; ITG: Inventory of Traumatic Grief; PSI: Paykel's Suicidality Items; RSES: Rosenberg Self Esteem Scale; SCAN 2.1: Schedules for Clinical Assessment in Neuropsychiatry; TRGR2L: Traumatic Grief Evaluation of Response to Loss; UCL: Utrecht Coping List.

3.1. Methodological Quality Assessment

A study was conducted to assess the methodological quality of the reviewed studies. Reporting bias was high in all studies, as significance data were frequently not provided for non-significant differences or effect sizes were not reported. Only the study by Treml et al. [29] provided information on the method of handling dropouts during the intervention. All studies, except for Pfeffer et al. [25], reported the method of randomization used. However, there were no guarantees regarding the blinding of participants and personnel in most studies. Pfeffer et al. [25] had the lowest methodological quality as it did not provide data on any of the analyzed criteria. In Figures 2 and 3, the risk of bias graph and the summary risk of bias graph, respectively, of the reviewed RCTs are shown.

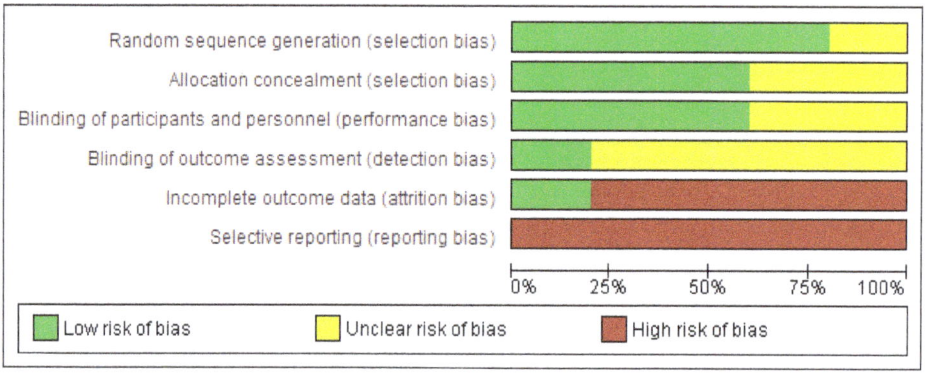

Figure 2. Risk of bias graph.

3.2. Participant Description

The mean age of the total sample obtained in the review was 36.67 years (SD = 11.08), with a total of 350 suicide loss survivors, of which 27.43% were male. All studies except for Pfeffer et al. [25] included adult survivors, although DeGroot et al. [26] and De Groot et al. [27] allowed participation from individuals aged 15 and above. Participants in De Groot et al. [26,27] were mainly spouses (36 participants), parents (29 participants), children (27 participants), and siblings (21 participants). In Wittouck et al. [28], most participants were children of the deceased (33 participants), spouses (20 participants), siblings (15 participants), and parents (8 participants). In Treml et al. [29], participants were primarily parents (19 participants), children (11 participants), siblings (11 participants), and spouses (10 participants). All studies accepted other participants with a close relationship with the deceased (friends, etc.). Finally, in Pfeffer et al. [25], participants were children (46 participants) and siblings of the deceased (25 participants).

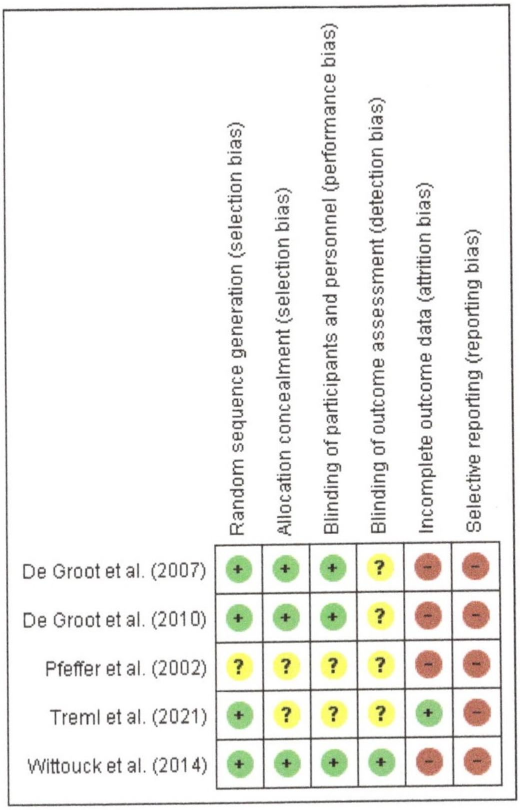

Figure 3. Risk of bias graph (see Figure 2 for explanation of symbols used) [25–29].

3.3. Description of Interventions

Only participants in the experimental conditions of each study received an intervention, while participants in the control conditions were placed on a waiting list. Notably, the study by De Groot et al. [27] is an extension of the study by De Groot et al. [26], analyzing differences in the effectiveness of the intervention between grieving survivors with and without suicidal ideation. Although all intervention programs were based on the cognitive-behavioral model, there was a great variety in the application format and structure of each program.

The interventions described in De Groot et al. [26,27] and Wittouck et al. [28] were conducted through home visits. Treml et al. [29] utilized an online format, while Pfeffer et al. [25] did not specify the location of the intervention. De Groot et al. [26,27] and Wittouck et al. [28] were based on the cognitive-behavioral model of Boelen et al. [9]. In De Groot et al.'s studies [26,27], the intervention involved psychotherapeutic counseling conducted by psychiatric nurses who had received prior training in this cognitive-behavioral intervention. Each family was assigned a specialized nurse who supervised each session conducted in the family's home. The intervention aimed to involve the entire family system, providing psychoeducation, emotional processing, effective interaction techniques, and problem-solving techniques. The program consisted of fixed modules (cognitive restructuring and support consolidation) and optional modules tailored to each family's needs. Wittouck et al. [28] mainly provided psychoeducation on suicide and discussions on various grief myths. Treml et al. [29] implemented an online narrative therapy program based on Lange et al. [30] and adapted by Wagner et al. [20] for individuals experiencing complicated grief.

Pfeffer et al. [25] used an eclectic program based on various theories and models, including Bowlby's attachment theory [31], Ness and Pfeffer's loss response theory [32], and Lazarus and Folkman's cognitive coping theory [33]. The program consisted of the following main components: psychoeducation and support, aimed at addressing the understanding of death and suicide, and the loss of psychosocial and personal resources.

3.4. Intervention Effectiveness

Most interventions were effective in reducing grief, both in direct grief measures and related symptoms (depressive, anxious, post-traumatic, or suicidal). While there was a non-significant reduction in maladaptive grief reactions, it was more pronounced in survivors with suicidal ideation. Significant reductions were observed in maladaptive grief symptoms post-intervention in Wittouck et al. [28] and in the severity of grief symptoms in Treml et al. [29], which persisted over time. Depressive symptom reduction was significant in all studies except for De Groot et al. [26,27]. Only Pfeffer et al. [25] included anxious symptomatology, showing a significant reduction after intervention. Post-traumatic symptomatology was included only in Pfeffer et al. [25], where no significant changes were found after intervention. Regarding suicidal symptomatology, no significant changes were found in the studies by De Groot et al. [26,27], although the intervention was more effective in those with suicidal ideation [27].

4. Discussion

This work aimed to systematically review randomized controlled trials using cognitive-behavioral therapy (CBT) interventions to alleviate grief and related symptoms in suicide loss survivors. It found a limited number of such trials, with generally low methodological quality. Despite the high risk of complications among suicide loss survivors, there is a lack of studies applying CBT, highlighting a gap in intervention research. While there is some evidence suggesting the effectiveness of CBT in alleviating grief-related symptoms, the mixed results across studies make it challenging to draw definitive conclusions.

It is crucial to recognize the importance of designing and implementing CBT interventions that are tailored to the specific characteristics of both younger and older adults. While most research tends to focus on younger populations, particularly because of concerns over rising suicide rates in this group, it is equally vital to consider older adults. This group often faces multiple risk factors, such as social isolation, the loss of loved ones, and the presence of chronic illnesses, and may benefit from interventions that specifically address their unique circumstances and challenges.

Adapting interventions to each age group would not only better meet their needs but could also enhance the effectiveness of the therapies applied. For example, younger individuals may require approaches that take into account emotional development and the influence of social networks, whereas older adults might benefit more from strategies that integrate social support and address loneliness and accumulated grief throughout life. Considering these differences in the design and implementation of future studies could provide more precise and applicable data for each demographic group.

These findings agree with Wilson and Marshall [34], who noted the insufficient availability and quality of psychological support services for grieving suicide loss survivors. The impact of cognitive-behavioral therapy on grief and related variables such as anxiety, depression, and post-traumatic symptoms shows mixed results in the literature. While some studies have reported significant reductions in grief symptoms, others have not, and the authors did not offer explanations for these discrepancies. Additionally, some studies only provided partial results without reporting effect sizes, and missing data were not addressed using specific analytical methods. Moreover, it was observed that suicidal ideation among suicide loss survivors influenced the interventions' effectiveness, with greater efficacy observed among individuals with suicidal ideation. However, this finding may be biased since individuals with higher suicidal ideation also tended to have higher levels of anxiety, depression, and neuroticism, suggesting a greater potential for improvement in these individuals.

In Pfeffer et al. [25], although no specific grief measure was included, significant reductions were found in depression and anxiety symptoms related to the suicide of parents or siblings, but not in post-traumatic symptoms. The authors suggested that the lack of an effect on post-traumatic symptoms could be due to low social adaptation, which might improve over time, leading to a reduction in post-traumatic symptoms. However, the authors noted potential biases due to the small sample size and high experimental mortality rate (i.e., loss of participants during the course of an experiment or study). They did not offer explanations for why the intervention seemed more effective in middle-aged children. In Wittouck et al. [28], although reductions in depressive symptoms and grief-related symptoms were observed post-intervention, there were no reductions in hopelessness or negative cognitions related to grief distress. The passive coping style (worrying, rumination, pessimism, etc.) decreased, which is crucial in the cognitive-behavioral model of complicated grief by Boelen et al. [9]. However, participants in the experimental group decreased their seeking of social support post-intervention, possibly because of the emotional support experienced during the intervention. The authors also noted a low sample size and potential selection bias among participants. In Treml et al. [29], positive results were found in grief symptoms, depression, guilt, and shame measures, common issues among suicide loss survivors because of the stigma associated with suicide, which interferes with normalization and adaptation. However, general psychopathology improved in both the experimental and control groups. The authors attributed these results to the online intervention's acceptance among users, suggesting that the protection of user data may reduce fear of judgment, encouraging more expression. However, the authors cautioned that this could increase the likelihood of misunderstandings. Despite the positive intervention results, caution is warranted because of the limited generalizability, as most of the sample were highly educated women living with a partner, which facilitates social support, a crucial variable in grief adaptation according to Boelen et al. [9]. Participants with various psychopathologies, including suicidal ideation, were excluded, potentially biasing the results.

This review has limitations, including the selection of only randomized controlled trials published in scientific journals, potentially reducing the number of studies obtained. Additionally, because of the variety of variables collected in each study, a meta-analysis was not performed, limiting specificity regarding intervention effectiveness. Therefore, while our findings suggest that CBT can be effective in certain contexts, more randomized controlled trials are needed to establish its full efficacy and to explore other potential strategies for supporting suicide loss survivors. The lack of a clinically significant cutoff point for complicated grief diagnosis and consideration of the time frame needed to classify grief as a mental disorder may have affected the observed reductions in grief symptoms. Future reviews should include more grief-related variables and focus on tertiary interventions targeting individuals clinically diagnosed with complicated grief. It is also essential to analyze intervention effectiveness by age, as studies specific to older adults were lacking.

While there is some evidence indicating that cognitive-behavioral therapy may be helpful in reducing grief symptoms in suicide loss survivors, along with other related symptoms, the methodological quality of the studies, small sample sizes, low representativeness, and high experimental mortality rate make it challenging to draw general conclusions about intervention effectiveness. More randomized controlled trials analyzing the efficacy of cognitive-behavioral therapy in suicide loss survivors, both in adults and children, with more representative samples, are needed.

Future research should focus on conducting higher-quality randomized controlled trials with larger and more diverse samples, including participants with various psychological profiles, such as those experiencing suicidal ideation, to improve the generalizability of the findings. It is also important to include diverse demographic groups, such as older adults, ethnic minorities, individuals from various socioeconomic backgrounds, and men, to better evaluate the generalizability of interventions for suicide loss survivors. Additionally, there is a critical need to develop and validate standardized measures for assessing grief, particularly in the context of suicide bereavement, which would enable more consistent comparisons of outcomes across studies. Investigating the long-term effectiveness of cognitive-behavioral therapy (CBT) interventions through follow-up assessments at multiple time points is recommended to determine whether the benefits are sustained or if additional interventions are required. Moreover, future research should compare the effectiveness of CBT with other psychological therapies, such as Acceptance and Commitment Therapy (ACT), Narrative Therapy, Dialectical Behavior Therapy (DBT), Client-Centered Therapy (CCT), or Brief Psychodynamic Psychotherapy (BPP). In addition to RCTs, non-RCT studies, such as large-scale cohort studies, real-world effectiveness trials, and case-control studies, should also be considered to explore the effectiveness of these interventions in practical, real-world settings. For example, cohort studies could track outcomes over time in naturalistic settings where randomization is not feasible, providing valuable insights into how these therapies perform outside controlled experimental conditions. Real-world effectiveness trials could assess the impact of these interventions across diverse healthcare settings, including community clinics and telehealth platforms, where conditions are less controlled than in traditional RCTs. Additionally, case-control studies could be used to investigate the effectiveness of interventions in specific subgroups, such as individuals with concurrent mental health disorders or those from underserved populations. This comparison would help identify the most effective strategies for different groups of suicide loss survivors. Furthermore, it is essential to delve deeper into the role of social support in grief adaptation, especially within online intervention contexts, and to establish clinically significant cutoff points for the diagnosis of complicated grief, taking into account the necessary time frame for classifying grief as a mental disorder. Future research should also explore the specific mechanisms through which these various therapies reduce grief and related symptoms to enhance the development of more targeted clinical interventions.

Author Contributions: Conceptualization, J.C.R.-M., M.C.-G., A.H.-d.A., E.I.-S., M.R.-E. and J.G.-M.; methodology, J.C.R.-M., M.C.-G., A.H.-d.A., E.I.-S., M.R.-E. and J.G.-M.; formal analysis, J.C.R.-M. and M.C.-G.; resources, J.C.R.-M., M.C.-G., A.H.-d.A., E.I.-S., M.R.-E. and J.G.-M.; data curation, J.C.R.-M., M.C.-G., A.H.-d.A., E.I.-S., M.R.-E. and J.G.-M.; writing—original draft preparation, J.C.R.-M., M.C.-G., A.H.-d.A., E.I.-S., M.R.-E. and J.G.-M.; writing—review and editing, J.C.R.-M., M.C.-G., A.H.-d.A., E.I.-S., M.R.-E. and J.G.-M. All authors have read and agreed to the published version of this manuscript.

Funding: This research received no external funding.

Institutional Review Board Statement: Not applicable.

Informed Consent Statement: Not applicable.

Data Availability Statement: The original data presented in the study are openly available in OSF at reference [35].

Conflicts of Interest: The authors declare no conflicts of interest.

References

1. Linde, K.; Treml, J.; Steinig, J.; Nagl, M.; Kersting, A. Grief interventions for people bereaved by suicide: A systematic review. *PLoS ONE* **2017**, *12*, e0179496. [CrossRef] [PubMed]
2. Naghavi, M. Global, regional, and national burden of suicide mortality 1990 to 2016: Systematic analysis for the Global Burden of Disease Study 2016. *BMJ* **2019**, *364*, l94. [CrossRef] [PubMed]
3. Organización Mundial de la Salud. Suicide Worldwide in 2019: Global Health Estimates. Organización Mundial de la Salud, 2021. Available online: https://iris.who.int/bitstream/handle/10665/341728/9789240026643-eng.pdf?sequence=1 (accessed on 16 April 2024).
4. Centers for Disease Control and Prevention (CDC). Facts About Suicide | Suicide Prevention. 25 April 2024. Available online: https://www.cdc.gov/suicide/facts (accessed on 30 August 2024).

5. Cerel, J.; Maple, M.; Aldrich, R.; van de Venne, J. Exposure to suicide and identification as survivor. *Crisis* **2013**, *34*, 413–419. Available online: https://www.researchgate.net/profile/Judy-Van-De-Venne/publication/250922980_Exposure_to_Suicide_and_Identification_as_Survivor/links/5697d08c08aea2d74375c733/Exposure-to-Suicide-and-Identification-as-Survivor.pdf (accessed on 18 April 2024). [CrossRef] [PubMed]
6. Ali, F. Exploring the complexities of suicide bereavement research. *Procedia Soc. Behav. Sci.* **2015**, *165*, 30–39. [CrossRef]
7. Jordan, J.R. Bereavement after suicide. *Psychiatr. Ann.* **2008**, *38*, 679–685. [CrossRef]
8. Shear, M.K.; Ghesquiere, A.; Katzke, M. Bereavement and complicated grief in older adults. *Late Life Mood Disord.* **2013**, *14*, 206–219. [CrossRef]
9. Boelen, P.A.; Van Den Hout, M.A.; Van Den Bout, J. A cognitive-behavioral conceptualization of complicated grief. *Clin. Psychol. Sci. Pract.* **2006**, *13*, 109–128. [CrossRef]
10. Crosby, A.; Gfroerer, J.; Han, B.; Ortega, L.; Parks, S.E. *Suicidal Thoughts and Behaviors among Adults Aged >18 Years—United States, 2008–2009*; US Department of Health and Human Services, Centers for Disease Control and Prevention: Atlanta, GA, USA, 2011.
11. Nizama, M. Suicidio. *Rev. Peru. Epidemiol.* **2011**, *15*, 1–5. Available online: https://pesquisa.bvsalud.org/portal/resource/pt/biblio-1111629 (accessed on 20 April 2024).
12. Castillo, A.E. Contención del suicidio en España: Evaluación del diseño de las políticas y Planes de Salud Mental de las Comunidades Autónomas. *Gest. Anál Polít Públicas* **2022**, *28*, 6–26. [CrossRef]
13. Knox, K.L.; Conwell, Y.; Caine, E.D. If suicide is a public health problem, what are we doing to prevent it? *Am. J. Public Health* **2004**, *94*, 37–45. [CrossRef]
14. Raschke, N.; Mohsenpour, A.; Aschentrup, L.; Fischer, F.; Wrona, K.J. Socioeconomic factors associated with suicidal behaviors in South Korea: Systematic review on the current state of evidence. *BMC Public Health* **2022**, *22*, 129. [CrossRef] [PubMed]
15. Zalsman, G. Suicide: Epidemiology, etiology, treatment and prevention. *Harefuah* **2019**, *158*, 468–472. Available online: https://europepmc.org/ (accessed on 20 April 2024). [PubMed]
16. Andriessen, K. Can Postvention Be Prevention? *Crisis* **2009**, *30*, 43–47. [CrossRef] [PubMed]
17. Berman, A.L. Estimating the population of survivors of suicide: Seeking an evidence base: Estimating the population of survivors of suicide. *Suicide Life Threat. Behav.* **2011**, *41*, 110–116. [CrossRef]
18. Enez, Ö. Complicated Grief: Epidemiology, Clinical Features, Assessment, and Diagnosis. *Psikiyatride Güncel Yaklaşımlar* **2018**, *10*, 269–279. [CrossRef]
19. Nam, I. Suicide Bereavement and Complicated Grief: Experiential Avoidance as a Mediating Mechanism. *J. Loss Trauma* **2016**, *21*, 325–334. [CrossRef]
20. Wagner, B.; Knaevelsrud, C.; Maercker, A. Internet-based cognitive-behavioral therapy for complicated grief: A randomized controlled trial. *Death Stud.* **2006**, *30*, 429–453. [CrossRef]
21. Jordan, J.R.; McMenamy, J. Interventions for suicide survivors: A review of the literature. *Suicide Life Threat. Behav.* **2004**, *34*, 337–349. [CrossRef]
22. Andriessen, K.; Krysinska, K.; Hill, N.T.M.; Reifels, L.; Robinson, J.; Reavley, N.; Pirkis, J. Effectiveness of interventions for people bereaved through suicide: A systematic review of controlled studies of grief, psychosocial and suicide-related outcomes. *BMC Psychiatry* **2019**, *19*, 49. [CrossRef]
23. Page, M.J.; McKenzie, J.E.; Bossuyt, P.M.; Boutron, I.; Hoffmann, T.C.; Mulrow, C.D.; Shamseer, L.; Tetzlaff, J.M.; Akl, E.A.; Brennan, S.E.; et al. Declaración PRISMA 2020: Una guía actualizada para la publicación de revisiones sistemáticas. *Rev. Esp. Cardiol.* **2021**, *74*, 790–799. [CrossRef]
24. Higgins, J.P.; Green, S. Cochrane Handbook for Systematic Reviews of Interventions (Version 5.1.0). The Cochrane Collaboration, 2011. Available online: www.handbook.cochrane.org (accessed on 20 April 2024).
25. Pfeffer, C.R.; Jiang, H.; Kakuma, T.; Hwang, J.; Metsch, M. Group intervention for children bereaved by the suicide of a relative. *J. Am. Acad. Child. Adolesc. Psychiatry* **2002**, *41*, 505–513. [CrossRef]
26. De Groot, M.; de Keijser, J.; Neeleman, J.; Kerkhof, A.; Nolen, W.; Burger, H. Cognitive behaviour therapy to prevent complicated grief among relatives and spouses bereaved by suicide: Cluster randomised controlled trial. *BMJ* **2007**, *334*, 994. [CrossRef]
27. De Groot, M.; Neeleman, J.; van der Meer, K.; Burger, H. The effectiveness of family-based cognitive-behavior grief therapy to prevent complicated grief in relatives of suicide victims: The mediating role of suicide ideation. *Suicide Life Threat. Behav.* **2010**, *40*, 425–437. [CrossRef] [PubMed]
28. Wittouck, C.; Van Autreve, S.; Portzky, G.; van Heeringen, K. A CBT-based psychoeducational intervention for suicide survivors. *Crisis* **2014**, *35*, 193–201. [CrossRef] [PubMed]
29. Treml, J.; Nagl, M.; Linde, K.; Kündiger, C.; Peterhänsel, C.; Kersting, A. Efficacy of an Internet-based cognitive-behavioural grief therapy for people bereaved by suicide: A randomized controlled trial. *Eur. J. Psychotraumatol.* **2021**, *12*, 1926650. [CrossRef] [PubMed]
30. Lange, T.M. Trans-affirmative narrative exposure therapy (TA-NET): A therapeutic approach for targeting minority stress, internalized stigma, and trauma reactions among gender diverse adults. *Pract. Innov.* **2020**, *5*, 230. [CrossRef]
31. Bowlby, J. The Bowlby-Ainsworth attachment theory. *Behav. Brain Sci.* **1979**, *2*, 637–638. [CrossRef]
32. Ness, D.; Pfeffer, C.R. Sequelae of bereavement resulting from suicide. *Am. J. Psychiatry* **1990**, *147*, 279–285.
33. Lazarus, R.S.; Folkman, S. Cognitive theories of stress and the issue of circularity. In *Dynamics of Stress: Physiological, Psychological, and Social Perspectives*; Appley, M.H., Trumbull, R., Eds.; Springer: Boston, MA, USA, 1986; pp. 63–80.

34. Wilson, A.; Marshall, A. The support needs and experiences of suicidally bereaved family and friends. *Death Stud.* **2010**, *34*, 625–640. [CrossRef]
35. Romero-Moreno, J.C.; Cantero-García, M.; Huertes-del Arco, A.; Izquierdo-Sotorrío, E.; Rueda-Extremera, M.; González-Moreno, J. Grief Intervention in Suicide Loss Survivors through Cognitive-Behavioral Therapy: A Systematic Review [Internet]. Available online: https://osf.io/ja3w4 (accessed on 24 July 2024).

behavioral sciences

MDPI

Systematic Review

Social Cognition in Suicidal Behavior in Psychosis: A Systematic Review

María Carcedo Herrero [1,2], Aina Sastre-Buades [1,3] and Maria Luisa Barrigón [4,5,6,7,*]

1 Department of Psychology, Universidad a Distancia de Madrid (UDIMA), 28400 Collado-Villalba, Spain; mariacarcedoherrero@gmail.com (M.C.H.); aina.sastre@hsll.es (A.S.-B.)
2 Private Practice, 48008 Bilbao, Spain
3 Department of Psychiatry, Son Llàtzer University Hospital, 07198 Palma, Spain
4 Centro de Investigación Biomédica en Red de Salud Mental (CIBERSAM), 28029 Madrid, Spain
5 Instituto de Psiquiatría y Salud Mental, Hospital General Universitario Gregorio Marañón, 28007 Madrid, Spain
6 Gregorio Marañón Health Research Institute, 28009 Madrid, Spain
7 School of Medicine, Universidad Complutense de Madrid, 28040 Madrid, Spain
* Correspondence: marialuisa.barrigon@salud.madrid.org

Abstract: Suicide is a major concern worldwide, especially in psychotic disorders that have an increased risk for suicidal behavior (SB). There are many well-established risk factors for SB in psychosis. Still, others, such as the domains of social cognition (SC)—the theory of mind, social perception, emotional processing, and attributional style—are unclarified. We aim to review evidence on SC and SB in psychosis and clarify their relationship, examining the differences between SC domains and the potential mediating variables in this relationship and proposing that worse performance in regard to SC is related to a higher risk of suicide. We searched databases for papers on SC and SB published between 2009 and 2024, resulting in the 18 articles included in this systematic review. Individuals with psychotic disorders and SB showed better emotional processing for basic emotional recognition—although they performed poorly on more complex tasks—and exhibited greater empathy within the affective theory of mind. Cognitive biases associated with attributional style and increased distrust as part of social perception were also found. Our findings cannot establish a relationship with the cognitive theory of mind. So, further studies are needed to integrate all domains of SC in longitudinal studies and examine the mediating variables of these relationships.

Keywords: psychosis; psychotic disorder; suicidal behavior; suicide; social cognition

1. Introduction

Suicide is one of the main public health problems worldwide, with over 700,000 people dying each year, making it a priority objective of the World Health Organization (WHO, 2021). In Spain, it is also treated as a major problem, since according to the latest data established by the National Institute of Statistics (INE), in 2023, it resulted in 4116 deaths by suicide, again placing it as the leading external cause of death in our country (INE, 2023). The WHO (2014) defines suicidal behavior as a continuum that extends from suicidal ideation to death by suicide, including suicidal planning and attempted suicide, and is the result of a complex interaction of biological, psychological, social, and environmental factors (Turecki et al., 2019). The inclusion of suicidal ideation in this continuum, as an aspect that involves cognitive changes or deficits (Keilp et al., 2013,

2014; Roca et al., 2019; Westheide et al., 2008), remains a complex issue. Although there are discrepancies among different authors, it has been concluded that suicidal ideation is associated with worse verbal learning in major depressive disorder (Lan et al., 2020) or impaired decision making (Westheide et al., 2008), and they could be considered a cognitive biomarker of suicide risk (Lan et al., 2020; Sastre-Buades et al., 2021). Among the diagnoses with higher rates of suicidal behavior, we find that severe mental disorders—among which psychotic disorders, major depressive disorder, and bipolar disorder stand out—have much higher rates than the general population, thereby increasing the risk by five to ten times (Fu et al., 2023). Despite the high risk of suicidal behavior in psychotic disorders, limited research has been conducted on this topic, partly because a diagnosis of psychotic disorder is often an exclusion criterion in studies on suicidal behavior (Villa et al., 2019).

Individuals with psychotic disorder have a life expectancy 15–20 years shorter than the general population, with suicide as the main cause, although they also have a higher mortality from natural causes due to comorbid factors. Taking into account mortality risk and associated risk factors, clinical practice is essential, as such risks must be addressed urgently from multiple levels (Correll et al., 2022). The lifetime risk of suicide in these individuals is 5% (Hor & Taylor, 2010); however, when suicide attempts are taken into account, this rate rises at the onset of the disorder to 45.9%, at 6 months to 38%, and over a lifetime, it would be around 26.8% (Lu et al., 2019). Over the years, research has identified different factors that are associated with an increased risk of suicidal tendencies in these individuals. These factors include depressive symptomatology, a higher number of both positive and negative psychotic symptoms, frequent hospitalizations, comorbid drug use, a psychiatric history, a family history of suicide attempts, being male and under 40 years of age, poor adherence to treatment, and previous suicide attempts (Cassidy et al., 2018; Yüksel et al., 2024). This elevated mortality is associated with risk factors for suicidal behavior. Many of these factors can be modified through clinical practice, particularly social cognition, which this paper focuses on (Correll et al., 2022).

Recent years have seen a growing interest in variables such as neurocognition or social cognition and their role in psychosis. Taking these factors into account allows us to propose new therapeutic approaches for individuals with psychotic disorders who are at risk of engaging in suicidal behavior. Social cognition refers to the mental operations through which we interpret, analyze, remember, and use information about the environment and relationships, and thanks to this, we deduce the emotions of others and put ourselves in their place to understand what they will think or how they will react to a given situation. There are discrepancies in the conceptualization of social cognition, and therefore the NIMH has sought to explain more operationally what social cognition encompasses by dividing it into different domains. The first domain is theory of mind, developed by Premack and Woodruff (1978), which refers to the ability to distinguish between one's mental states and those of others, including the understanding of false beliefs, intentions of others, deceptions, or metaphors. Within theory of mind, it is possible to differentiate between a more affective theory of mind related to the affective state, emotion, or feeling of others, and a more cognitive part about the beliefs, thoughts, or intentions of others (Jarvis et al., 2024). The second domain is social perception, defined as the identification and interpretation of different social situations based on the rules and roles in the social context, that is, the perceptual processes involved in directing attention to social signals. Third, attributional style refers to how the causes of social events and the intentions of others are usually understood, and involves the study of biases. Fourth, emotional processing encompasses the skills or strategies related to the perception and use of emotional information, including the identification, creation, understanding, and management of emotions and nonverbal language (Green et al., 2008; Pinkham, 2014).

Several studies have demonstrated deficits in social cognition in individuals with psychotic disorders, particularly in the categories of social perception, emotional processing, and theory of mind (Fortuny et al., 2023; Healey et al., 2016; Kohler et al., 2010; Savla et al., 2013). These deficits appear to be associated with negative symptoms, subsequent clinical depression (Pelizza et al., 2020), and poorer perceived quality of life in domains such as physical and psychological health, social relationships, and environment (Martín et al., 2017). Moreover, evidence suggests that social cognition impairment occurs both in early psychotic episodes and in chronic patients, showing stability throughout the disorder (Bora & Pantelis, 2013; Healey et al., 2016). Other studies have examined theory of mind in isolation and concluded that its impairment could predict a suicide attempt (Canal-Rivero et al., 2017). In line with this, without taking into account clinical diagnosis, differences have been found between deficits in social cognition and different levels of suicidal risk. That is, greater impairment is detected in individuals with a history of suicide attempts in comparison with individuals with suicidal ideation, who show worse performance than the general population, suggesting that social cognition may serve as a clinical marker associated with greater or lesser suicidal risk (Comparelli et al., 2022). Regarding social perception and attributional style, few studies are available in this population (Healey et al., 2016). However, other studies suggest that individuals with a history of suicide attempts may perform better on social cognition tasks, exhibiting a very low externalizing bias (attribution of positive events to external elements), similar to individuals with depressive disorder, and demonstrating better theory of mind performance (Sastre-Buades et al., 2023). Additionally, individuals with previous suicide attempts have been found to show better empathic performance (Ma et al., 2024). Similarly, another study by Dickhoff et al. (2021) reported that both individuals with previous suicide attempts and those with current suicidal ideation performed better on emotional face recognition and theory of mind tasks. This could suggest that the factor influencing suicidal behavior is not a deficit in social cognition, but rather an insufficient ability to regulate social stress as a result of increased sensitivity to social relationships, which is contrary to findings from other studies that have directly identified a deficit in this social perception (Fortuny et al., 2023; Healey et al., 2016; Kohler et al., 2010; Savla et al., 2013).

Current research on social cognition in this population has identified two contrasting perspectives. One perspective indicates a clear lack of social cognition that may directly or indirectly lead to a higher probability of suicide, while the other suggests that these individuals have better social cognition, which could trigger greater social stress leading to suicidal behavior.

The main objective of this study is to conduct a systematic review of the relationship between social cognition, and its distinct domains, and suicidal behavior in psychotic disorders. As secondary objectives, we examine whether differences exist between the specific domains that comprise social cognition and whether additional variables mediate this relationship. We hypothesize that social cognition performance is associated with increased suicidal behavior in individuals with psychotic disorders. Therefore, this review aims to clarify whether social cognition constitutes a risk factor for suicidal behavior, with the goal of optimizing and individualizing treatment approaches (Correll et al., 2022; WHO, 2021). In this review, different concepts along the suicidal behavior continuum are considered and clearly differentiated from one another (WHO, 2014).

2. Materials and Methods

The present review was conducted in accordance with the updated of Preferred Reporting Items for Systematic Reviews and Meta-Analyses (PRISMA) guidelines (Page et al., 2021).

2.1. Eligibility Criteria

The selection criteria for the articles were established based on the objective of this study; therefore, included studies were required to address social cognition in relation to suicidal behavior with in psychosis.

We adopted the WHO perspective, which defines suicidal behavior as a continuum ranging from suicidal ideation to death by suicide, taking into account and differentiating the various concepts along this continuum (WHO, 2014).

Social cognition refers to the mental operations by which individuals interpret, analyze, and use information from their environment. In this review, we included the following domains of social cognition: theory of mind, social perception, attributional style, and emotional processing (Green et al., 2008; Pinkham, 2014). Theory of mind, as developed by Premack and Woodruff (1978), is defined as the ability to distinguish between one's own mental states and those of others. Social perception is defined as the identification and interpretation of different social situations based on social rules and roles. Attributional style refers to the way in which individuals understand the causes of social events and the intentions of others. Emotional processing encompasses the skills and strategies related to the perception, understanding, and use of emotional information.

In addition, only scientific publications after 2009 were included. Meta-analyses or systematic reviews that did not specifically assess suicidal behavior in the psychotic population, did not measure social cognition, or focused solely on neuroimaging tests or other biological markers were excluded.

2.2. Information Sources

An exhaustive search was conducted in several databases, including ProQuest (which searches eight databases, such as PsycInfo), Web of Science (which also examines multiple databases), PubMed (which includes Medline and other resources), and Scopus. In addition to these four databases, a search was performed in Google Scholar, an academic search engine oriented towards scientific content. The search was conducted between 8 April 2024 and 22 April 2024.

2.3. Search Strategy

The search was limited to scientific articles published within the last 15 years (2009–2024) in English or Spanish, using keywords such as social cognition, theory of mind, social perception, attributional style, suicidal behavior, and psychosis. Articles not available in English or Spanish were excluded. A second-level search was performed by reviewing the bibliographic references of studies identified in the primary search that were relevant to the aim of this review. The same inclusion and exclusion criteria were applied as in the primary search.

The final search strategy was as follows: (psychosis OR schizophrenia) AND (suicide attempt OR suicidal behavior OR suicide risk) AND (social cognition OR theory of mind OR social perception OR social cognition OR attributional bias OR emotional processing). MeSH terms were not used, as the search was not limited to PubMed, and the strategy was replicated across multiple databases.

Initially, 730 articles were identified from the databases and four additional records from Google Scholar. All references were imported into Mendeley to remove duplicates, resulting in 566 unique publications. This process is illustrated in Figure 1, which presents the different phases followed during the two screening stages, culminating in a total of 18 articles included in the final qualitative synthesis.

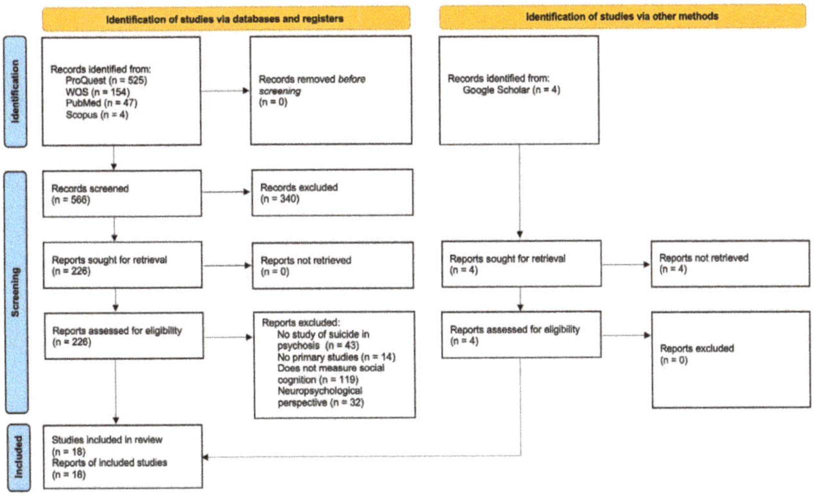

Figure 1. PRISMA 2020 flow diagram of studies on social cognition in psychosis and suicide behavior published between 2009 and 2024.

2.4. Selection Process

To determine study eligibility, one researcher (MCH) screened the abstracts of the selected papers. The full text of potentially eligible studies were then assessed by the same reviewer (MCH). A double eligibility check was not performed. The literature search yielded 566 papers, of which 18 met the inclusion criteria (Figure 1). Only original articles were included.

2.5. Data Collection Process

One researcher (MCH) independently collected data from all reports. No automation tools were used during this process.

2.6. Data Items

Once the studies had been selected, a standardized form was used to extract the following data: authors, publication date, study design (longitudinal or cross-sectional), sample size, age, sex, diagnostic condition, and the psychological instruments used to assess both suicidal behavior and social cognition. Quality assessment of the included studies was performed using a tool for longitudinal and cross-sectional observational studies developed by the NIH (2014). This tool evaluates key concepts relevant to assessing the internal validity of each selected studies. Higher methodological quality was observed in the longitudinal studies (Canal-Rivero et al., 2017; Cuesta et al., 2022; Depp et al., 2018; Dickhoff et al., 2021; Parrish et al., 2024; Wastler et al., 2022), while the studies by Rocca et al. (2016), and Abdo et al. (2021) were most likely to be biased. A double checking of the quality assessment was not performed. A summary of each study is provided in Table S1.

2.7. Study Risk of Bias Assessment

Risk of bias assessment was not conducted, as meta-analysis was not performed in this review. Conducting a meta-analysis was not an objective of this work due to the diversity of variables studied and the heterogeneity of the measurement instruments used across the included studies, which made it difficult to perform the corresponding statistical analyses.

2.8. Effect Measures

Due to the heterogeneity of the variables studied and the measurement instruments used across the included studies, no effect measures were selected or extracted in this review.

2.9. Synthesis Methods

The study characteristics, assessment measures, results and quality ratings were tabulated and are summarized in Table 1. Additionally, the measurement instruments used to assess social cognition, due to their variety, are presented in Table 2. No meta-analysis was performed in this review, as explained in Section 2.7.

Table 1. Summary of the studies included for the systematic review about the relationship between social cognition and suicidal behavior in psychosis.

Author and Year	Design and Sample	Measure of Suicidal Behavior	Social Cognition Assessment	Results	Quality Assessment by the NIH
Abdo et al. (2021)	Transversal n = 21; Mean age = 30.1; F = 100%; Schizophrenia = 100%	SPS	ToM: RMET	Suicidal ideation (hopelessness subdomain): lower affective theory of mind.	Fair
Canal-Rivero et al. (2017)	Longitudinal (12 months) n = 65; Mean age = 26.2; M = 67.7%; F = 32.3%; Schizophrenia = 70.8%	SCAN	ToM: FBT, Hinting task	History of suicide attempt: more errors in first- and second-order false belief tasks. Predictor: deficit in first-order tasks.	Good
Chalker et al. (2022)	Transversal n = 96; Mean age = 43.8; M = 44.8%; F = 55.2%; Schizophrenia = 38.5%	C-SSRS	AS: AIHQ	Suicidal ideation: tendency to blame others in individuals with history of emotional or physical abuse.	Fair
Comparelli et al. (2018)	Transversal n = 86; Mean age = 36.3; M = 74%; F = 26%	C-SSRS	EP: MSCEIT	Suicidal ideation: greater severity related to impairment in social cognition. Predictor: deficit in social cognition.	Fair
Cuesta et al. (2022)	Longitudinal (20 years) n = 172; Mean age = 48.1; M = 51.7%; F = 48.3%; Schizophrenia = 43.6%	Clinical interview	EP: MSCEIT	No statistically significant relationship.	Good
Depp et al. (2018)	Longitudinal (2 weeks) n = 179; Mean age = 42.1; M = 65.4%; F = 34.6%; Schizophrenia = 53.1%	BDI-2	EP: BLERT, ER-40 SP: Trustworthiness Task AS: AIHQ	Suicidal ideation: greater tendency to blame others, greater unreliability in unreliable faces, and greater accuracy in rating negative affect. Predictor: attribution of blame to others, especially in persistent ideation.	Good
Dickhoff et al. (2021)	Longitudinal (3 years) n = 715; Mean age = 27.2; M = 72.4%; F = 27.6%; Schizophrenia = 70.4%	Clinical interview, CANSAS	EP: DFAR, BFRT ToM: Hinting task	Suicide ideation/attempt: better performance in face detection, especially for fear emotion, and better performance in hinting task in participants with suicidal ideation and attempt.	Good
Duñó et al. (2009)	Transversal n = 57; Mean age = 31.2; M = 70.1%; F = 29.9%; Schizophrenia = 100%	Clinical interview	ToM: FBT	History of suicide attempt: worse performance in second-order false belief task. Predictor: second-order task.	Fair

Table 1. *Cont.*

Author and Year	Design and Sample	Measure of Suicidal Behavior	Social Cognition Assessment	Results	Quality Assessment by the NIH
Harenski et al. (2017)	Transversal *n* = 41; Mean age = 39.7; M = 100%; Schizophrenia = 46.3% Prison population	C-SSRS	EP: Empathic accuracy task	History of suicide attempt: lower empathic accuracy. Predictor: empathic accuracy.	Fair
Liu et al. (2023)	Transversal *n* = 301; Mean age = 33.9; M = 60.8%; F = 39.2%; Schizophrenia = 100%	BDI	ToM: IRI	Suicidal ideation: greater personal distress (affective empathy). Predictor: personal distress (affective empathy).	Fair
Parrish et al. (2024)	Longitudinal (10 days) *n* = 273; Mean age = 41.7; M = 62.6%; F = 37.4%; Schizophrenia = 26%	C-SSRS	EP: ER-40	No statistically significant relationship between ER-40 and suicide risk, but greater over attribution of threat related to interpersonal constructs related to suicidal behavior.	Good
Rocca et al. (2016)	Transversal *n* = 809; Mean age = 40.1; Schizophrenia = 100%	Clinical interview	EP: MSCEIT, FEIT ToM: TASIT	No statistically significant relationship.	Poor
Sastre-Buades et al. (2023)	Transversal *n* = 190; Mean age = 27.9; M = 67.2%; F = 32.8%; Schizophrenia = 38.4%	Clinical interview	EP: Baron Cohen's Face Test (CBC) ToM: Hinting task AS: IPSAQ	No statistically significant relationship. Small mean effect size for better performance in hinting tasks and very low externalizing bias in patients with suicide attemp history.	Fair
Villa et al. (2018)	Transversal *n* = 101; Mean age = 49.9; M = 45.5%; F = 54.5%; Schizophrenia + Schizoaffective = 74.3%	C-SSRS, MSSI	EP: ER-40	No statistically significant relationship. Tendency in patients with history of suicide to misattribute threat to neutral stimuli.	Fair
Wang et al. (2020)	Transversal *n* = 627; Mean age = 47.7; M = 63%; F = 37%; Schizophrenia = 100%	Clinical interview	ToM: IRI	Suicide attempt history: greater total empathy, fantasy (cognitive empathy) and personal distress (affective empathy). Predictor: personal distress (affective empathy).	Fair
Wastler et al. (2022)	Longitudinal (6 months) *n* = 65; Mean age = 23; M = 70.8%; F = 29.2%; Schizophrenia spectrum = 60%	CDSS	EP: MSCEIT	No statistically significant relationship	Good
Yin et al. (2020)	Transversal *n* = 159; Mean age = 27.1; M = 47.8%; F = 52.2%; Schizophrenia = 100%	Clinical interview	EP: MSCEIT	No statistically significant relationship	Fair
Zhu and Zhang (2024)	Transversal *n* = 554; Mean age = 46.4; M = 68.4%; F = 31.6%; Schizophrenia = 100%	Clinical interview; BDI	ToM: IRI	Suicidal ideation: greater personal anguish (affective empathy)	Fair

Note: F: female; M: male; ToM: theory of mind; AS: attributional style; SP: social perception; EP: emotional processing; NIH: National Institutes of Health.

Table 2. Summary of instruments for measuring different domains of social cognition.

	Description	Authors
Reading the Mind in the Eyes Test (RMET)	ToM. Recognition of emotions through photographs of the eyes; the participant must choose the word that most represents the emotion.	(Baron-Cohen et al., 2001; Fernández-Abascal et al., 2013)
The Awareness of Social Inference Test (TASIT)	ToM. Audiovisual tool integrating gestures, prosody, facial expression, and context to interpret meanings, emotions, beliefs and intentions.	(McDonald et al., 2006)

Table 2. *Cont.*

	Description	Authors
Hinting Task	ToM. Stories describing a social interaction with a hint that the participant must interpret.	(Corcoran et al., 1995; Gil et al., 2012)
False Belief Test (FBT)	ToM. First order task: predict the behavior of a character guided by a false belief. Second order task: predict the false belief that one character has about another character's belief.	(Frith & Corcoran, 1996)
Interpersonal Reactivity Index (IRI)	ToM. Divided into cognitive empathy (understanding another's perspective) and affective empathy (emotional response to another's affective state).	(Davis, 1983; Pérez-Albéniz et al., 2003)
Internal, Personal and Situational Attributions Questionnaire (IPSAQ)	AS. Ability to discriminate between external and internal attributions, both personal and situational, through hypothetical scenarios.	(Kinderman & Bentall, 1996)
Ambiguous Intentions and Hostility Questionnaire (AIHQ)	AS. Analyzes the tendency to overattribute negative intentions to others using vignettes of social situations, asking about the intentions of the characters and the participant's own likely response,	(Combs et al., 2007)
Trustworthiness Task (TT)	SP. Ability to make complex social judgments of trustworthiness from facial photographs.	(Adolphs et al., 1998)
Mayer-Salovey-Caruso Emotional Intelligence Test (MSCEIT)	EP. Tests assessing emotional perception, emotional facilitation, emotional understanding, and emotional management as skills for handling emotional problems.	(Mayer et al., 2002; Extremera et al., 2006)
The Bell Lysaker Emotion Recognition Task (BLERT)	EP. Identification of emotion through the intonation used by an actor interpreting emotions in videos.	(Bryson et al., 1997)
Penn Emotion Recognition task (ER-40)	EP. Recognition of basic emotions through facial photographs.	(Kohler et al., 2003)
Degraded Facial Affect Recognition Task (DFAR)	EP. Computer images of people displaying basic emotions, shown with increasing intensity to raise difficulty.	(Van't Wout et al., 2004)
Baron Cohen's Face Test (CBC)	EP. Photographs of an actress representing an emotion; the participant must choose the emotion that best fits.	(Baron-Cohen et al., 1997; Huerta-Ramos et al., 2021)
The Benton Facial Recognition Task (BFRT)	EP. Assesses face memory by showing a series of face cards, which the participant must identify among several photographs.	(Benton et al., 1983)
Facial Emotion Identification Test (FEIT)	EP. Identification of basic emotions through facial photographs.	(Kerr & Neale, 1993)

Note: ToM: Theory of mind; AS: attributional style; SP: social perception; EP: emotional processing.

2.10. Reporting Bias Assessment

As explained in Section 2.7, risk of bias assessment was not conducted because a meta-analysis was not performed in this review.

2.11. Certainty Assessment

The certainty in the body of evidence for outcomes in this review was assessed using the OCEBM Levels of Evidence Working Group (n.d.).

3. Results

Eighteen articles were included in this systematic review (Figure 1). The results and conclusions of the original studies and reviews are summarized in Table 1, highlighting the main findings of each work. Studies that identified important trends, such as effect sizes, were also included, as the limited number of studies and the controversial nature of the topic make these findings potentially valuable. Some studies performed regression analysis to predict suicidal behavior based on the variables examined or to analyze possible mediating variables; these variables are also described in the corresponding section.

3.1. Description of the Studies

Among the selected studies, 6 were longitudinal, involving repeated assessments over time, while 12 were cross-sectional, with a single measurement point. Cross-sectional studies, which account for 66.6% of the total number of studies, are less able to establish cause–effect relationships compared to longitudinal designs.

Regarding assessment instruments, numerous tools are available to assess suicidal behavior and social cognition; however, there is no consensus on the most appropriate tests for assessing these variables in schizophrenia (Gil-Sanz et al., 2019).

First, clinical interview is the most commonly used method to assess suicide, being employed on seven occasions to record the number of previous suicide attempts, quantitatively or dichotomously (Yes/No); the Schedule for Clinical Assessment in Neuropsychiatry (SCAN) is employed in similar circumstances (Vazquez-Barquero et al., 1994; Wing et al., 1990). The Columbia Suicide Severity Rating Scale (C-SSRS) (Al-Halabí et al., 2016; Posner et al., 2011) has also been widely used (on five occasions) to assess both suicide ideation and suicide attempt, as has The Suicide Probability Scale (SPS) (Cull & Gill, 1982). Other instruments, such as the Beck Depression Inventory (BDI-II) (Beck et al., 1961; Sanz et al., 2003), the Camberwell Questionnaire for Assessment of Needs (CANSAS) (Phelan et al., 1995; Rosales et al., 2002), the Modified Scale for Suicidal Ideation (MSSI) (Miller et al., 1986), and the Calgary Depression Scale (CDSS) (Addington et al., 1993; Sarró et al., 2004) are primarily used to assess suicidal ideation.

On the other hand, social cognition was assessed using 16 different instruments (Table 2). For theory of mind, the most widely used tools are the hinting task (Corcoran et al., 1995; Gil et al., 2012) and the Interpersonal Reactivity Index (IRI) (Davis, 1983; Pérez-Albéniz et al., 2003). For emotional processing, the Mayer–Salovey–Caruso Emotional Intelligence Test (MSCEIT) (Mayer et al., 2002; Extremera et al., 2006) and the Penn Emotion Recognition task (ER-40) (Kohler et al., 2003) are the most commonly used tools. For attributional style, the Ambiguous Intentions and Hostility Questionnaire (AIHQ) (Combs et al., 2007) and the Internal, Personal, and Situational Attributions Questionnaire (IPSAQ) (Kinderman & Bentall, 1996) are most common. Finally, the most commonly used tool for social perception is the Trustworthiness Task (Adolphs et al., 1998).

3.2. Sample

In all 18 original studies, there were 4511 participants. Sample sizes ranged from 21 to 809 participants, and seven studies included less than 100 participants. Sixteen of the eighteen studies involved an adult population aged 27–59 years, and two studies included a young adult population aged 23–26.2 years. Regarding sex distribution, one study included only males and another only females; in 12 studies, the majority of participants were male; in three studies, the majority were female; and one did not report on this information.

Regarding the diagnosis of the participants within the psychosis spectrum, only 50% of the studies considered this variable; the remaining studies did not apply consistent diagnostic classification, making it difficult to compare figures across variables. However, most samples consisted of individuals diagnosed with schizophrenia and schizoaffective disorder. Six studies included participants with bipolar disorder with psychotic symptoms, and four included individuals with major depressive disorder with psychotic symptoms.

According to the DSM-5, these diagnosis are not classified within the psychosis spectrum, despite the presence of psychotic symptoms. Therefore, for comparison purposes, only the percentages for schizophrenic are reported. Using this approach, we found that in 72.2% of the studies, more than 50% of the sample was diagnosed with schizophrenia.

Regarding suicidal behavior, 12 of the studies assessed this variable as previous suicide attempts, most often recorded retrospectively through clinical interviews. The percentage of participants with a history of suicide attempts varied widely, ranging from 11.3% to 64.6%, with an average of approximately 35.5%. Suicidal ideation was evaluated in ten studies, with an average prevalence of 31.9%. Chapman et al. (2015) conducted a meta-analysis that demonstrated a strong association between suicidal ideation and suicidal behavior in psychotic disorders.

3.3. Emotional Processing

Emotional processing was the most studied social cognition domain, examined in 61.1% (11) of the articles and assessed by eight different instruments. Depp et al. (2018), using the BLERT emotion identification task (Bryson et al., 1997), found that participants with current suicidal ideation were more accurate in rating negative affect (p = 0.042, d = 0.441). This finding agrees with Dickhoff et al. (2021), who also used the DFAR (Van't Wout et al., 2004) and obtained better performance in face detection, especially for fear expressions, in participants with a history of suicide attempts or current suicidal ideation (F (1,586) = 4.1, p = 0.04). Thus, we found a tendency toward better emotional processing for emotion recognition, particularly for negative emotions.

However, Harenski et al. (2017) found worse emotion identification using their ad hoc test of empathic accuracy in participants with a history of suicidal behavior, although this study only included a prison population (p = 0.032). Parrish et al. (2024) and Villa et al. (2018) found no significant relationship between emotion recognition and suicidal behavior but observed a misattribution of anger or fear to neutral faces ($p < 0.01$, d = 0.141). They also found an over-attribution bias for threat, which was related to perceived burden to others (t = 4.72, $p < 0.001$), reduced social motivation (t = 3.33, $p < 0.001$), and increased social avoidance (t = 3.70, $p < 0.001$). These constructs are related to suicide and may therefore indirectly contribute to suicidal behavior.

Comparelli et al. (2018) found that greater severity of suicidal ideation was associated with lower performance on the MSCEIT (r = 0.329, $p < 0.05$) (Mayer et al., 2002; Extremera et al., 2006), a test that assesses not only emotion recognition but also the ability to identify, understand and manage emotions. Furthermore, they indicated that this deficit may serve as a potential predictor of suicidal ideation (p = 0.015).

The evidence for emotional processing is supported by a relatively large number of studies (n = 11), with generally consistent findings regarding the association between emotional recognition—particularly of negative emotions—and suicidal behavior. However, the certainty of this evidence is limited by methodological heterogeneity, variability in assessment tools, and the predominance of cross-sectional designs, as well as some conflicting results. Overall, confidence in evidence is moderate, downgraded due to these limitations but strengthened by the number of studies and the overall consistency of the main findings.

3.4. Theory of Mind

Theory of mind was the most studied concept along with emotional processing, investigated in 50% (9) of the studies using five different assessment instruments. Dickhoff et al. (2021) found better performance in the hinting task (Corcoran et al., 1995; Gil et al., 2012) among participants with previous suicide attempts or current suicidal ideation (F (1,644) = 4.4, $p = 0.04$). Furthermore, participants with both conditions (suicide attempts and current suicidal ideation) performed better than those with only one condition. This finding was supported by Sastre-Buades et al. (2023), who observed the same trend with a small mean effect size (t = 2.04, d = 0.403), although their results did not reach statistical significance.

In contrast, using the FBT task (Frith & Corcoran, 1996), studies by Canal-Rivero et al. (2017) and Duñó et al. (2009) found worse performance in participants with a history of suicidal behavior for second-order tasks (X2 = 6.27, $p = 0.01$; X2 = 5.223, $p = 0.022$). The first study also reported worse performance for first-order tasks (X2 = 3.95, $p = 0.04$). Additionally, they identified both first-order (OR = 4.26, CI = 1.05–17.31, $p = 0.04$) and second-order (OR = 4.02, CI = 1.18–13.62, $p < 0.05$) task performance as potential predictors of increased suicidal behavior at 12-month follow-up.

On the other hand, using the IRI index (Davis, 1983; Pérez-Albéniz et al., 2003), we found significant results ($p = 0.002$) related to personal distress (F = 5.045, $p = 0.020$; t = −3.166, $p = 0.002$), defined as the anxiety and discomfort produced by observing negative experiences of others and considered part of affective empathy. Significant results were also found for fantasy (F = 10.445, $p = 0.001$), which represents the tendency to identify with others and is part of cognitive empathy) (Liu et al., 2023; Wang et al., 2020; Zhu & Zhang, 2024).

Finally, Abdo et al. (2021) found a deficit in the affective component of theory of mind as assessed by the RMET (Baron-Cohen et al., 2001; Fernández-Abascal et al., 2013), which correlated negatively with the hopelessness subdomain of suicidal risk (R = − 0.526, $p = 0.017$), although not with overall suicidal risk. In addition, Liu et al. (2023) and Wang et al. (2020) identified personal distress score, a component of affective empathy, as a predictor of suicide attempts and suicidal ideation (OR = 1.092, CI = 1.013–1.177, $p = 0.022$; OR = 1.076, CI = 1.013–1.142, $p = 0.017$).

Therefore, following Jarvis et al. (2024) and their division between cognitive and affective theory of mind, we observe that the method of assessment can significantly influence results for the cognitive component, as different findings were obtained depending on the instrument used (Canal-Rivero et al., 2017; Dickhoff et al., 2021; Duñó et al., 2009; Sastre-Buades et al., 2023). Concerning the affective component, the results are similar: all three studies that assessed this domain found that higher scores were related to suicidal behavior, although Abdo et al. (2021) found the opposite pattern with hopelessness related to suicide but not to suicidal behavior itself.

Theory of mind was investigated in nine studies using various assessment instruments, with mixed and sometimes conflicting results depending on the specific aspect and tool evaluated (cognitive vs. affective theory of mind). While some studies found better performance or higher empathy in individuals with suicidal behavior, others reported worse performance or no significant association, and findings often varied depending on the instrument and outcome. The certainty of the evidence is limited by methodological heterogeneity, inconsistency across studies, and the predominance of cross-sectional designs. Confidence in evidence is low to moderate, downgraded due to these limitations but strengthened by the number of studies and the exploration of both cognitive and affective components.

3.5. Attributional Style

Attributional style was studied in 16.6% (3) of the studies, using two different assessment instruments. Statistically significant results were found only with the AIHQ questionnaire (Combs et al., 2007), which showed a specific tendency to blame others in participants with suicidal ideation (p = 0.006, d = 0.599) (Depp et al., 2018). However, in the study by Chalker et al. (2022), this was observed only in the sample that had experienced emotional (t = 2.75, p = 0.007) or physical (t = 2.39, p = 0.019) abuse. Furthermore, Depp et al. (2018) identified a hyper attribution of blame to others, especially in participants with recurrent suicidal ideation present at two time points, as a predictor of greater future suicidal ideation (OR = 1.203, CI = 1.045–1.386, p = 0.010). In the study by Sastre-Buades et al. (2023), no statistically significant results were found, but a small effect size (t = 2.07, d = 0.482) indicated a tendency to make internal attributions for more negative events, similar to that associated with depressive disorders, i.e., a lower externalizing bias in participants with a history of suicide attempt.

The evidence for attributional style is based on three studies using two different assessment instruments. Significant results were mainly found with the AIHQ, indicating a tendency to blame others in participants with suicidal ideation and a lower externalizing bias in those with a history of suicide attempts. However, the strength of the evidence is limited by the small number of studies, variability in assessment tools, small to moderate effect sizes, predominance of cross-sectional designs, and lack of replication. Confidence in evidence is low, downgraded due to these limitations.

3.6. Social Perception

Social perception is the least studied domain within social cognition, being assessed in only one study, by Depp et al. (2018). In this study, participants with higher current ideation demonstrated greater normative unreliability in judging untrustworthy faces, as measured by the Trustworthiness Task (p = 0.042, d = 0.39) (Adolphs et al., 1998). The strength of evidence is limited, as only one study at level 3 evidence is available, with no replication, a small effect size, and possible methodological limitations. Therefore, confidence in the evidence is currently low.

3.7. Additional Analyses

Some of the 18 studies included in the final analysis examined additional variables that might mediate the relationship between social cognition and suicidal behavior in psychosis. Liu et al. (2023) noted that scores on positive and negative syndrome and general psychopathology, as assessed by the Positive and Negative Syndrome Scale for Schizophrenia (PANSS) (Kay et al., 1987; Peralta & Cuesta, 1994), might mediate the relationship between personal distress, as part of theory of mind, and suicidal ideation.

Something similar was found in Dickhoff et al. (2021), who also noted that the PANSS score (Kay et al., 1987; Peralta & Cuesta, 1994) could mediate between emotion recognition as part of emotional processing and the hinting task as part of theory of mind, and current ideation or past suicidal intent. Depp et al. (2018) identified another factor, the depression score, as a possible mediator in the relationship between negative biases—such as the tendency to blame others, greater unreliability in unreliable faces, and greater accuracy in rating negative affect— and suicidal ideation. Zhu and Zhang (2024) mentioned cognitive performance measured by the Mini-Mental State Examination (MMSE) (Folstein et al., 1983; Lobo et al., 1999) and gender as possible mediating factors in the relationship between empathy and suicidal ideation, finding greater empathy in men with cognitive dysfunction.

Finally, Chalker et al. (2022) identified emotional trauma, as measured by the Childhood Trauma Questionnaire (CTQ) (Bernstein et al., 1998; Hernandez et al., 2013), as a mediator between the tendency to blame others, as part of attributional style, and suicidal behavior.

4. Discussion

In this systematic review, we identified differences across social cognition domains that are related to increased suicidal behavior in individuals with psychotic disorders. Individuals with psychotic disorder and suicidal behavior showed better emotional processing in basic emotional recognition tasks, but poorer in more complex tasks, as well as greater empathy within the affective theory of mind. Cognitive biases, such as a tendency to blame others as part of attributional style, and greater distrust as part of social perception, were also found in patients with higher suicidal behavior.

Within emotional processing, we found complementary results. In studies where basic emotions recognition was assessed, better performance was observed, especially for negative emotions (Depp et al., 2018; Dickhoff et al., 2021). However, Harenski et al. (2017) report the opposite, indicating inconsistencies in the literature. Parrish et al. (2024) and Villa et al. (2018) observed an over-attribution of threat bias, which could be indirectly related to increased suicidal behavior, as it is associated with perceptions of being a burden to others, reduced social motivation, and increased social avoidance. Comparelli et al. (2018) found that poorer performance was related to greater severity of suicidal ideation; however, their measurement instrument was much more complex and extended beyond emotion recognition. Thus, individuals may perform better on basic affect ratings but worse in more complex tasks. These findings may be due to greater reactivity to and accuracy of negative stimuli as part of negative bias, and these affect recognition biases could contribute to increased perceptions of isolation and lack of support, concepts related to suicidal behavior (Depp et al., 2018). Additionally, it appears that individuals with higher suicidal behavior demonstrate a greater ability to detect negative social cues and exhibit a threat over-attribution bias, where negative emotions are misattributed to neutral faces (Dickhoff et al., 2021; Sastre-Buades et al., 2023).

We found the greatest discrepancies between studies regarding the theory of mind domain. Within the cognitive component, better performance was observed in the interpretation of hints during social interactions, particularly among individuals with more severe suicidal behavior (Dickhoff et al., 2021; Sastre-Buades et al., 2023). However, when theory of mind was assessed using tasks that involve both simple and a complex forms of interpersonal problem-solving, such as predicting false beliefs, the opposite pattern emerged (Canal-Rivero et al., 2017; Duñó et al., 2009). In contrast, when the affective component of theory of mind was examined, findings were more consistent across studies, although not entirely uniform. A higher score was observed, particularly in personal distress. which is a component of affective empathy defined as the emotional response of an individual who observes the affective state of others (Liu et al., 2023; Wang et al., 2020; Zhu & Zhang, 2024). However, Abdo et al. (2021), using a different measurement instrument that assess empathic accuracy, found poorer performance, although this was related only to hopelessness and not to suicidal behavior itself. Overall, our findings suggest that participants with higher suicidal behavior tend to show higher empathy, which may be explained by increased anxiety and discomfort when observing the negative experiences of others, or by heightened anxiety in stressful interpersonal environments. This heightened emotional reactivity may negatively affect their perception of support, thereby contributing to increased suicidal behavior (Liu et al., 2023; Wang et al., 2020).

For attributional style and social perception, we found few studies reporting statistically significant results. Greater unreliability and a tendency to blame others were observed in patients with higher suicidal behavior (Chalker et al., 2022; Depp et al., 2018). Depp et al. (2018) hypothesized that a negative attribution bias is linked to suicidal ideation.

Additionally, Sastre-Buades et al. (2023) observed a tendency to a very low externalizing bias in individuals with a history of suicide attempts.

In our approach to identifying possible variables that mediate this relationship, we found that psychopathology (including positive and negative syndrome, depression, and emotional trauma), cognitive performance, and gender could be involved. However, further studies are needed to clarify these associations (Chalker et al., 2022; Depp et al., 2018; Dickhoff et al., 2021; Liu et al., 2023; Zhu & Zhang, 2024).

Several strengths and limitations emerged throughout this systematic review. This review aimed to clarify whether social cognition is a risk factor for a major cause of mortality in these patients. Furthermore, differentiating between subdomains allows for better clinical application when considering this factor in treatment. Several limitations also emerged in this review. The main limitation is the difficulty in defining and measuring variables with no clear consensus (Gil-Sanz et al., 2019; Green et al., 2008; Pinkham, 2014) and the predominance of cross-sectional methodologies, with more than 60% of studies employing this design. There is also a tendency for research on social cognition to focus primarily on emotional processing and theory of mind (Healey et al., 2016).

Further research on social cognition in psychosis, and specifically on whether there is a determinant relationship with suicidal behavior, is important to clarify whether social cognition constitutes a risk factor for one of the main causes of mortality in these population, and to inform clinical applications focused on optimizing and individualizing treatment. More longitudinal studies and more comprehensive analyses assessing all domains, as well as possible mediating variables in this relationship are potential future lines of research.

5. Conclusions

Better emotional processing in simpler tasks, such as emotional recognition but poorer performance in more complex tasks, as well as greater empathy within the affective theory of mind, appear to be associated with increased suicidal behavior. Biases, such as a tendency to blame others as part of attributional style and greater distrust as part of social perception, are also observed in patients with higher suicidal behavior. Further studies are needed to clarify the relationship with the cognitive theory of mind, to integrate the four subdomains in more longitudinal studies, and to investigate the variables that influence these relationships.

Supplementary Materials: The following supporting information can be downloaded at: https://www.mdpi.com/article/10.3390/bs15060759/s1, Table S1: Quality assessment of studies using a tool designed by the NIH (2014) for longitudinal and cross-sectional observational designs.

Author Contributions: M.C.H.: Conceptualization, Methodology, Investigation, Formal Analysis, Writing—Original Draft Preparation; A.S.-B.: Writing—Review and Editing, Supervision; M.L.B.: Writing—Review and Editing, Supervision (CRediT author statement). All authors have read and agreed to the published version of the manuscript.

Funding: This research received no external funding.

Institutional Review Board Statement: Not applicable.

Informed Consent Statement: Not applicable.

Data Availability Statement: No new data were created or analyzed in this study. Data sharing is not applicable to this article.

Conflicts of Interest: The authors declare no conflicts of interest.

References

Abdo, M. M. M., Mohamed, A. S., Hammed, M. A. E., Hashem, R. E., & El Nagar, Z. M. (2021). Affective theory of the mind and suicide in women with borderline personality disorder and schizophrenia: A comparative study. *Middle East Current Psychiatry, 28*, 64. [CrossRef]

Addington, D., Addington, J., & Maticka-Tyndale, E. (1993). Assessing depression in schizophrenia: The Calgary depression scale. *The British Journal of Psychiatry, 163*(S22), 39–44. [CrossRef]

Adolphs, R., Tranel, D., & Damasio, A. R. (1998). The human amygdala in social judgment. *Nature, 393*(6684), 470–474. [CrossRef] [PubMed]

Al-Halabí, S., Sáiz, P. A., Burón, P., Garrido, M., Benabarre, A., Jiménez, E., Cervilla, J., Navarrete, M. I., Díaz-Mesa, E. M., García-Álvarez, L., & Muñiz, J. (2016). Validation of a Spanish version of the Columbia-suicide severity rating scale (C-SSRS). *Revista de Psiquiatría y Salud Mental, 9*(3), 134–142. [CrossRef]

Baron-Cohen, S., Wheelwright, S., Hill, J., Raste, Y., & Plumb, I. (2001). The "reading the mind in the eyes" test revised version: A study with normal adults, and adults with Asperger syndrome or high-functioning autism. *The Journal of Child Psychology and Psychiatry and Allied Disciplines, 42*(2), 241–251. [CrossRef]

Baron-Cohen, S., Wheelwright, S., & Jolliffe, A. T. (1997). Is there a" language of the eyes"? Evidence from normal adults, and adults with autism or Asperger syndrome. *Visual Cognition, 4*(3), 311–331. [CrossRef]

Beck, A. T., Ward, C. H., Mendelson, M., Mock, J., & Erbaugh, J. (1961). An inventory for measuring depression. *Archives of General Psychiatry, 4*(6), 561–571. [CrossRef]

Benton, A., Sivan, P. A., Hamsher, K., Varney, D., & Spreen, O. (1983). *Facial recognition: Stimulus and multiple choice pictures: Contributions to neuropsychological assessment*. Oxford University Press.

Bernstein, D. P., Fink, L., Handelsman, L., & Foote, J. (1998). *Childhood trauma questionnaire. Assessment of family violence: A handbook for researchers and practitioners*. APA PsycTests. [CrossRef]

Bora, E., & Pantelis, C. (2013). Theory of mind impairments in first-episode psychosis, individuals at ultra-high risk for psychosis and in first-degree relatives of schizophrenia: Systematic review and meta-analysis. *Schizophrenia Research, 144*(1–3), 31–36. [CrossRef]

Bryson, G., Bell, M., & Lysaker, P. (1997). Affect recognition in schizophrenia: A function of global impairment or a specific cognitive deficit. *Psychiatry Research, 71*(2), 105–113. [CrossRef]

Canal-Rivero, M., Lopez-Moriñigo, J. D., Barrigón, M. L., Perona-Garcelán, S., Jimenez-Casado, C., David, A. S., Obiols-Llandrich, J. E., & Ruiz-Veguilla, M. (2017). The role of premorbid personality and social cognition in suicidal behaviour in first-episode psychosis: A one-year follow-up study. *Psychiatry Research, 256*, 13–20. [CrossRef] [PubMed]

Cassidy, R. M., Yang, F., Kapczinski, F., & Passos, I. C. (2018). Risk factors for suicidality in patients with schizophrenia: A systematic review, meta-analysis, and meta-regression of 96 studies. *Schizophrenia Bulletin, 44*(4), 787–797. [CrossRef] [PubMed]

Chalker, S. A., Parrish, E. M., Cano, M., Kelsven, S., Moore, R. C., Granholm, E., Pinkham, A., Harvey, P. D., & Depp, C. A. (2022). Childhood trauma associations with the interpersonal psychological theory of suicide and social cognitive biases in psychotic disorders. *The Journal of Nervous and Mental Disease, 210*(6), 432–438. [CrossRef] [PubMed]

Chapman, C. L., Mullin, K., Ryan, C. J., Kuffel, A., Nielssen, O., & Large, M. M. (2015). Meta-analysis of the association between suicidal ideation and later suicide among patients with either a schizophrenia spectrum psychosis or a mood disorder. *Acta Psychiatrica Scandinavica, 131*(3), 162–173. [CrossRef]

Combs, D. R., Penn, D. L., Wicher, M., & Waldheter, E. (2007). The Ambiguous Intentions Hostility Questionnaire (AIHQ): A new measure for evaluating hostile social-cognitive biases in paranoia. *Cognitive Neuropsychiatry, 12*(2), 128–143. [CrossRef]

Comparelli, A., Corigliano, V., Lamis, D. A., De Carolis, A., Stampatore, L., De Pisa, E., Girardi, P., & Pompili, M. (2018). Positive symptoms and social cognition impairment affect severity of suicidal ideation in schizophrenia. *Schizophrenia Research, 193*, 470–471. [CrossRef]

Comparelli, A., Corigliano, V., Montalbani, B., Nardella, A., De Carolis, A., Stampatore, L., Bargagna, P., Forcina, F., Lamis, D., & Pompili, M. (2022). Building a neurocognitive profile of suicidal risk in severe mental disorders. *BMC Psychiatry, 22*(1), 628. [CrossRef]

Corcoran, R., Mercer, G., & Frith, C. D. (1995). Schizophrenia, symptomatology and social inference: Investigating "theory of mind" in people with schizophrenia. *Schizophrenia Research, 17*(1), 5–13. [CrossRef]

Correll, C. U., Solmi, M., Croatto, G., Schneider, L. K., Rohani-Montez, S. C., Fairley, L., Smith, N., Bitter, I., Gorwood, P., Taipale, H., & Tiihonen, J. (2022). Mortality in people with schizophrenia: A systematic review and meta-analysis of relative risk and aggravating or attenuating factors. *World Psychiatry, 21*(2), 248–271. [CrossRef]

Cuesta, M. J., Sánchez-Torres, A. M., Moreno-Izco, L., de Jalón, E. G., Gil-Berrozpe, G. J., Zarzuela, A., Peralta, V., Ballesteros, A., Fañanás, L., Hernández, R., & Janda, L. (2022). Neurocognitive correlates of the varied domains of outcomes at 20 year follow-up of first-episode psychosis. *Psychiatry Research, 318*, 114933. [CrossRef]

Cull, J. G., & Gill, W. S. (1982). *Suicide probability scale (SPS)*. APA PsycTests. [CrossRef]

Davis, M. H. (1983). Measuring individual differences in empathy: Evidence for a multidimensional approach. *Journal of Personality and Social Psychology, 44*(1), 113. [CrossRef]

Depp, C. A., Villa, J., Schembari, B. C., Harvey, P. D., & Pinkham, A. (2018). Social cognition and short-term prediction of suicidal ideation in schizophrenia. *Psychiatry Research, 270*, 13–19. [CrossRef] [PubMed]

Dickhoff, J., Opmeer, E. M., Heering, H. D., Bruggeman, R., van Amelsvoort, T., Bartels-Velthuis, A. A., Cahn, W., de Haan, L., Schirmbeck, F., Simons, C., van Os, J., Aleman, A., & van Tol, M. J. (2021). Relationship between social cognition, general cognition, and risk for suicide in individuals with a psychotic disorder. *Schizophrenia Research, 231*, 227–236. [CrossRef]

Duñó, R., Pousa, E., Miguélez, M., Montalvo, I., Suarez, D., & Tobeña, A. (2009). Suicidality connected with mentalizing anomalies in schizophrenia: A study with stabilized outpatients. *Annals of the New York Academy of Sciences, 1167*(1), 207–211. [CrossRef]

Extremera, N., Fernández-Berrocal, P., & Salovey, P. (2006). Spanish version of the Mayer-Salovey-Caruso Emotional Intelligence Test (MSCEIT). Version 2.0: Reliabilities, age and gender differences. *Psicothema, 18*, 42–48.

Fernández-Abascal, E. G., Cabello, R., Fernández-Berrocal, P., & Baron-Cohen, S. (2013). Test–retest reliability of the 'reading the mind in the eyes' test: A one-year follow-up study. *Molecular Autism, 4*, 33. [CrossRef]

Folstein, M. F., Robins, L. N., & Helzer, J. E. (1983). The mini-mental state examination. *Archives of General Psychiatry, 40*(7), 812. [CrossRef]

Fortuny, J. J., Navarra-Ventura, G., Fernández-Gonzalo, S., Tomàs, E. P., Armengol, J. M. C., Vidal, D. P., & Vicente, M. J. (2023). Social cognition in first-episode schizophrenia/schizoaffective disorder patients. *Spanish Journal of Psychiatry and Mental Health, 16*(3), 169–174. [CrossRef]

Frith, C. D., & Corcoran, R. (1996). Exploring 'theory of mind' in people with schizophrenia. *Psychological Medicine, 26*(3), 521–530. [CrossRef]

Fu, X. L., Qian, Y., Jin, X. H., Yu, H., Wu, H. R., Du, L., Chen, H., & Shi, Y. Q. (2023). Suicide rates among people with serious mental illness: A systematic review and meta-analysis. *Psychological Medicine, 53*(2), 351–361. [CrossRef] [PubMed]

Gil, D., Fernández-Modamio, M., Bengochea, R., & Arrieta, M. (2012). Adaptation of the Hinting Task theory of the mind test to Spanish. *Revista de Psiquiatría y Salud Mental, 5*(2), 79–88. [CrossRef]

Gil-Sanz, D., Bengochea-Seco, R., Arrieta-Rodríguez, M., Santacoloma-Cabero, I., & González-Fraile, E. (2019). ¿Cómo se evalúa la cognición social en esquizofrenia en España? *Informaciones Psiquiátricas, 236*, 9–28. Available online: https://dialnet.unirioja.es/servlet/articulo?codigo=7143289 (accessed on 20 April 2024).

Green, M. F., Penn, D. L., Bentall, R., Carpenter, W., Gaebel, W. T., Gur, R. C., Kring, A., Park, S., Silverstein, S., & Heinssen, R. (2008). Social cognition in schizophrenia: An NIMH workshop on definitions, assessment, and research opportunities. *Schizophrenia Bulletin, 34*(6), 1211–1220. [CrossRef] [PubMed]

Harenski, C. L., Brook, M., Kosson, D. S., Bustillo, J. R., Harenski, K. A., Caldwell, M. F., Van Rybroek, G. J., Koenigs, M., Decety, J., Thornton, D. M., & Calhoun, V. D. (2017). Socio-neuro risk factors for suicidal behavior in criminal offenders with psychotic disorders. *Social Cognitive and Affective Neuroscience, 12*(1), 70–80. [CrossRef]

Healey, K. M., Bartholomeusz, C. F., & Penn, D. L. (2016). Deficits in social cognition in first episode psychosis: A review of the literature. *Clinical Psychology Review, 50*, 108–137. [CrossRef]

Hernandez, A., Gallardo-Pujol, D., Pereda, N., Arntz, A., Bernstein, D. P., Gaviria, A. M., Labad, A., Valero, J., & Gutiérrez-Zotes, J. A. (2013). Initial validation of the Spanish childhood trauma questionnaire-short form: Factor structure, reliability and association with parenting. *Journal of Interpersonal Violence, 28*(7), 1498–1518. [CrossRef]

Hor, K., & Taylor, M. (2010). Review: Suicide and schizophrenia: A systematic review of rates and risk factors. *Journal of Psychopharmacology, 24*(Suppl. 4), 81–90. [CrossRef]

Huerta-Ramos, E., Ferrer-Quintero, M., Gómez-Benito, J., González-Higueras, F., Cuadras, D., del Rey-Mejías, Á. L., Usall, J., & Ochoa, S. (2021). Translation and validation of Baron Cohen's Face Test in a general population from Spain. *Actas Españolas de Psiquiatría, 49*(3), 106–113.

Instituto Nacional de Estadística. (2023). *Estadística de defunciones según la causa de muerte*. Available online: https://www.ine.es/jaxi/Datos.htm?tpx=72065 (accessed on 20 April 2024).

Jarvis, A. L., Keage, H. A., Wong, S., Weightman, M., & Stephens, R. G. (2024). Evidence for a multidimensional account of cognitive and affective theory of mind: A state-trace analysis. *Memory & Cognition, 52*(3), 525–535. [CrossRef]

Kay, S. R., Fiszbein, A., & Opler, L. A. (1987). The positive and negative syndrome scale (PANSS) for schizophrenia. *Schizophrenia Bulletin, 13*(2), 261–276. [CrossRef]

Keilp, J. G., Beers, S. R., Burke, A. K., Melhem, N. M., Oquendo, M. A., Brent, D. A., & Mann, J. J. (2014). Neuropsychological deficits in past suicide attempters with varying levels of depression severity. *Psychological Medicine, 44*(14), 2965–2974. [CrossRef] [PubMed]

Keilp, J. G., Gorlyn, M., Russell, M., Oquendo, M. A., Burke, A. K., Harkavy-Friedman, J., & Mann, J. J. (2013). Neuropsychological function and suicidal behavior: Attention control, memory and executive dysfunction in suicide attempt. *Psychological Medicine, 43*(3), 539–551. [CrossRef]

Kerr, S. L., & Neale, J. M. (1993). Emotion perception in schizophrenia: Specific deficit or further evidence of generalized poor performance? *Journal of Abnormal Psychology, 102*(2), 312–318. [CrossRef] [PubMed]

Kinderman, P., & Bentall, R. P. (1996). A new measure of causal locus: The internal, personal and situational attributions questionnaire. *Personality and Individual Differences, 20*, 261–264. [CrossRef]

Kohler, C. G., Turner, T. H., Bilker, W. B., Brensinger, C. M., Siegel, S. J., Kanes, S. J., Gur, R. E., & Gur, R. C. (2003). Facial emotion recognition in schizophrenia: Intensity effects and error pattern. *American Journal of Psychiatry, 160*(10), 1768–1774. [CrossRef]

Kohler, C. G., Walker, J. B., Martin, E. A., Healey, K. M., & Moberg, P. J. (2010). Facial emotion perception in schizophrenia: A meta-analytic review. *Schizophrenia Bulletin, 36*(5), 1009–1019. [CrossRef]

Lan, X., Zhou, Y., Zheng, W., Zhan, Y., Liu, W., Wang, C., Jiang, M., Yu, M., Zhang, B., & Ning, Y. (2020). Association between cognition and suicidal ideation in patients with major depressive disorder: A longitudinal study. *Journal of Affective Disorders, 272*, 146–151. [CrossRef]

Liu, J., Zhao, K., Zhou, S., Hong, L., Xu, Y., Sun, S., Tong, S., Huang, L., Liu, J., Wang, J., & Li, N. (2023). Suicidal ideation in Chinese adults with schizophrenia: Associations with neurocognitive function and empathy. *BMC Psychiatry, 23*(1), 311–322. [CrossRef]

Lobo, A., Saz, P., Marcos, G., Día, J. L., de la Cámara, C., Ventura, T., Morales Asín, F., Fernando Pascual, L., Montañés, J. Á., & Aznar, S. (1999). Revalidación y normalización del Mini-Examen Cognoscitivo (primera versión en castellano del Mini-Mental Status Examination) en la población general geriátrica. *Medicine Clínica (Barc), 112*(20), 767–774.

Lu, L., Dong, M., Zhang, L., Zhu, X. M., Ungvari, G., Ng, C., Wang, G., & Xiang, Y. T. (2019). Prevalence of suicide attempts in individuals with schizophrenia: A meta-analysis of observational studies. *Epidemiology and Psychiatric Sciences, 29*, e39. [CrossRef]

Martín, M. C., Secades, R., López-Goñi, J. J., & Tirapu, J. (2017). Empatía, cognición social y calidad de vida subjetiva en esquizofrenia. *Anales del Sistema Sanitario de Navarra, 40*(2), 211–219. [CrossRef]

Mayer, J. D., Salovey, P., & Caruso, D. (2002). *Mayer-Salovey-Caruso Emotional Intelligence Test (MSCEIT) item booklet* (Version 2.0). MHS Publishers.

Ma, Z., Tian, Y., Li, J., Liu, J., Wang, D., & Zhang, X. Y. (2024). Association of empathy with clinical symptoms and cognitive function in chronic schizophrenia patients with and without suicide attempts. *European Archives of Psychiatry and Clinical Neuroscience, 274*, 1395–1404. [CrossRef] [PubMed]

McDonald, S., Bornhofen, C., Shum, D., Long, E., Saunders, C., & Neulinger, K. (2006). Reliability and validity of The Awareness of Social Inference Test (TASIT): A clinical test of social perception. *Disability and Rehabilitation, 28*(24), 1529–1542. [CrossRef]

Miller, I. W., Norman, W. H., Bishop, S. B., & Dow, M. G. (1986). The modified scale for suicidal ideation: Reliability and validity. *Journal of Consulting and Clinical Psychology, 54*(5), 724–725. [CrossRef]

National Institutes of Health. (2014). *Quality assessment tool for observational cohort and cross-sectional studies*. Available online: https://www.nhlbi.nih.gov/health-topics/study-quality-assessment-tools (accessed on 20 October 2024).

OCEBM Levels of Evidence Working Group. (n.d.). *The Oxford 2011 levels of evidence. Oxford centre for evidence-based medicine*. Available online: http://www.cebm.net/index.aspx?o=5653 (accessed on 22 March 2025).

Page, M. J., McKenzie, J. E., Bossuyt, P. M., Boutron, I., Hoffmann, T. C., Mulrow, C. D., Shamseer, L., Tetzlaff, J. M., Akl, E. A., Brennan, S. E., & Chou, R. (2021). The PRISMA 2020 statement: An updated guideline for reporting systematic reviews. *Bmj, 71*, 372. [CrossRef]

Parrish, E. M., Pinkham, A., Moore, R. C., Harvey, P. D., Granholm, E., Roesch, S., Joiner, T., & Depp, C. A. (2024). An ecological momentary cognitive assessment study of over-attribution of threat and suicide risk factors in people with serious mental illness. *Schizophrenia Research, 266*, 136–144. [CrossRef]

Pelizza, L., Azzali, S., Garlassi, S., Scazza, I., Paterlini, F., Rocco Chiri, L., Poletti, M., Pupo, S., & Raballo, A. (2020). Un estudio longitudinal de 2 años sobre la experiencia subjetiva de la cognición social en jóvenes con primer episodio de psicosis. *Actas Españolas de Psiquiatria, 48*(6), 287–300.

Peralta, V., & Cuesta, M. J. (1994). Validación de la escala de los síndromes positivo y negativo (PANSS) en una muestra de esquizofrénicos españoles. *Actas Luso Españolas de Neurología Psiquiatría y Ciencias Afines, 22*(4), 171–177.

Pérez-Albéniz, A., De Paúl, J., Etxeberría, J., Montes, M. P., & Torres, E. (2003). Adaptación de interpersonal reactivity index (IRI) al español. *Psicothema, 15*, 267–272.

Phelan, M., Slade, M., Thornicroft, G., Dunn, G., Holloway, F., Wykes, T., Strathdee, G., Loftus, L., McCrone, P., & Hayward, P. (1995). The Camberwell Assessment of Need: The validity and reliability of an instrument to assess the needs of people with severe mental illness. *The British Journal of Psychiatry, 167*(5), 589–595. [CrossRef]

Pinkham, A. E. (2014). Social cognition in schizophrenia. *The Journal of Clinical Psychiatry, 75*(Suppl. 2), 14–19. [CrossRef] [PubMed]

Posner, K., Brown, G. K., Stanley, B., Brent, D. A., Yershova, K. V., Oquendo, M. A., Currier, G. W., Melvin, G. A., Greenhill, L., Shen, S., & Mann, J. J. (2011). The Columbia–Suicide Severity Rating Scale: Initial validity and internal consistency findings from three multisite studies with adolescents and adults. *American Journal of Psychiatry, 168*(12), 1266–1277. [CrossRef] [PubMed]

Premack, D., & Woodruff, G. (1978). Does the chimpanzee have a theory of mind? *Behavioral and Brain Sciences, 1*(4), 515–526. [CrossRef]

Roca, M., Del Amo, A. R.-L., Riera-Serra, P., Pérez-Ara, M. A., Castro, A., Roman Juan, J., García-Toro, M., García-Pazo, P., & Gili, M. (2019). Suicidal risk and executive functions in major depressive disorder: A study protocol. *BMC Psychiatry, 19*(1), 253. [CrossRef]

Rocca, P., Galderisi, S., Rossi, A., Bertolino, A., Rucci, P. A., Gibertoni, D. I., Montemagni, C., Sigaudo, M., Mucci, A., Bucci, P., & Acciavatti, T. (2016). Social cognition in people with schizophrenia: A cluster-analytic approach. *Psychological Medicine, 46*(13), 2717–2729. [CrossRef]

Rosales, C., Torres, F., Luna, J., Jiménez, J., & Martínez, G. (2002). Fiabilidad del instrumento de Evaluación de Necesidades de Camberwell (CAN)(Versión española del CAN Estudio de fiabilidad). *Actas Españolas de Psiquiatría, 30*(2), 99–105.

Sanz, J., Perdigón, A. L., & Vázquez, C. (2003). The Spanish adaptation of Beck's Depression Inventory-II (BDI-II): 2. Psychometric properties in the general population. *Clínica y Salud, 14*(3), 249–280.

Sarró, S., Dueñas, R. M., Ramírez, N., Arranz, B., Martínez, R., Sánchez, J. M., González, J. M., Saló, L., Miralles, L., & San, L. (2004). Cross-cultural adaptation and validation of the Spanish version of the Calgary Depression Scale for Schizophrenia. *Schizophrenia Research, 68*(2–3), 349–356. [CrossRef]

Sastre-Buades, A., Alacreu-Crespo, A., Courtet, P., Baca-Garcia, E., & Barrigon, M. L. (2021). Decision-making in suicidal behavior: A systematic review and meta-analysis. *Neuroscience and Biobehavioral Reviews, 131*, 642–662. [CrossRef]

Sastre-Buades, A., Caro-Cañizares, I., Ochoa, S., Lorente-Rovira, E., Barajas, A., Gutiérrez-Zotes, A., Sánchez-Alonso, S., López-Carrilero, R., Grasa, E., Pousa, E., Pélaez, T., Cid, J., González-Higueras, F., Ruiz-Delgado, I., Baca-Garcia, E., & Barrigon, M. L. (2023). Relationship between cognition and suicidal behavior in recent-onset psychosis. *Schizophrenia Research, 252*, 172–180. [CrossRef]

Savla, G. N., Vella, L., Armstrong, C. C., Penn, D. L., & Twamley, E. W. (2013). Deficits in domains of social cognition in schizophrenia: A meta-analysis of the empirical evidence. *Schizophrenia Bulletin, 39*(5), 979–992. [CrossRef]

Turecki, G., Brent, D. A., Gunnell, D., O'Connor, R. C., Oquendo, M. A., Pirkis, J., & Stanley, B. H. (2019). Suicide and suicide risk. *Nature Reviews Disease Primers, 5*(1), 74. [CrossRef] [PubMed]

Van't Wout, M., Aleman, A., Kessels, R. P., Larøi, F., & Kahn, R. S. (2004). Emotional processing in a non-clinical psychosis-prone sample. *Schizophrenia Research, 68*(2–3), 271–281. [CrossRef] [PubMed]

Vazquez-Barquero, J. L., Gaite, L., Arenal, A., Díez Manrique, J. F., Cuesta Núñez, M., & Higuera, A. (1994). Development and verification of the Spanish version of the" scanning system" psychiatric interview ("Questionnaires for clinical evaluation in neuropsychiatry". *Actas Luso-Españolas de Neurología, Psiquiatría y Ciencias Afines, 22*(3), 109–120. [PubMed]

Villa, J., Ehret, B. C., & Depp, C. A. (2019). Systematic review of the inclusion of people with psychosis in suicide-specific clinical trials. *Crisis, 41*(3), 233–236. [CrossRef]

Villa, J., Pinkham, A. E., Kaufmann, C. N., Granholm, E., Harvey, P. D., & Depp, C. A. (2018). Interpersonal beliefs related to suicide and facial emotion processing in psychotic disorders. *Journal of Psychiatric Research, 100*, 107–112. [CrossRef]

Wang, W., Zhou, Y., Wang, J., Xu, H., Wei, S., Wang, D., Wang, L., & Zhang, X. Y. (2020). Prevalence, clinical correlates of suicide attempt and its relationship with empathy in patients with schizophrenia. *Progress in Neuro-Psychopharmacology and Biological Psychiatry, 99*, 109863. [CrossRef]

Wastler, H. M., Moe, A. M., Pine, J. G., & Breitborde, N. J. (2022). Cognition and suicide risk among individuals with first-episode psychosis: A 6-month follow-up. *Psychiatric Rehabilitation Journal, 45*(1), 27–33. [CrossRef]

Westheide, J., Quednow, B. B., Kuhn, K.-U., Hoppe, C., Cooper-Mahkorn, D., Hawellek, B., Eichler, P., Maier, W., & Wagner, M. (2008). Executive performance of depressed suicide attempters: The role of suicidal ideation. *European Archives of Psychiatry and Clinical Neuroscience, 258*(7), 414–421. [CrossRef]

Wing, J. K., Babor, T., Brugha, T. S., Burke, J., Cooper, J. E., Giel, R., Jablenski, A., Regier, D., & Sartorius, N. (1990). SCAN: Schedules for clinical assessment in neuropsychiatry. *Archives of General Psychiatry, 47*(6), 589–593. [CrossRef]

World Health Organization. (2014). *Preventing suicide: A global imperative*. World Health Organization. Available online: https://iris.who.int/bitstream/handle/10665/131056/?sequence=1 (accessed on 20 October 2024).

World Health Organization. (2021). *Suicide worldwide in 2019: Global health estimates*. World Health Organization. Available online: https://iris.who.int/bitstream/handle/10665/341728/9789240026643-eng.pdf?sequence=1 (accessed on 20 October 2024).

Yin, Y., Tong, J., Huang, J., Tian, B., Chen, S., Cui, Y., An, H., Tan, S., Wang, Z., Yang, F., & Tian, L. (2020). Suicidal ideation, suicide attempts, and neurocognitive dysfunctions among patients with first-episode schizophrenia. *Suicide and Life-Threatening Behavior, 50*(6), 1181–1188. [CrossRef] [PubMed]

Yüksel, A., Yilmaz, E. B., & Dikmen, S. N. (2024). Suicide probability among patients with schizophrenia and bipolar disorder. *Journal of Psychosocial Nursing and Mental Health Services*, *62*(8), 37–45. [CrossRef] [PubMed]

Zhu, Q. Y., & Zhang, X. Y. (2024). Correlation analysis and gender differences of cognitive function based on mini-mental state examination (MMSE) and suicidal tendency in patients with schizophrenia. *BMC Psychiatry*, *24*(1), 24–32. [CrossRef] [PubMed]

behavioral sciences

MDPI

Systematic Review

Suicidal Ideation in Adolescents and Young Adults: The Role of Defeat, Entrapment, and Depressive Symptoms—From a Systematic Review to a Tentative Theoretical Model

Ana Huertes-del Arco [1,2], Eva Izquierdo-Sotorrío [2], Miguel A. Carrasco [1,*], Irene Caro-Cañizares [2] and Francisco Pablo Holgado-Tello [1]

1 Department of Personality, Assessment and Psychological Treatments, Faculty of Psychology, National University of Distance Educationa (UNED), 28040 Madrid, Spain; ahuertes3@alumno.uned.es (A.H.-d.A.); pfholgado@psi.uned.es (F.P.H.-T.)

2 School of Health Sciences and Education, Open University of Madrid (UDIMA), 28400 Madrid, Spain; eva.izquierdo@udima.es (E.I.-S.); irene.caro@udima.es (I.C.-C.)

* Correspondence: macarrasco@psi.uned.es

Abstract: Suicide stands as one of the leading causes of non-accidental death among adolescents and young adults. The Integrated Motivational–Volitional Model (IMV) of suicidal behavior identifies feelings of defeat and entrapment as pivotal factors in the complex dynamics underlying suicidal behaviors. Additionally, depressive symptomatology plays a crucial role in the development of these behaviors. The aim of this work was to provide a systematic review of the scientific literature on the association of three risk factors—entrapment, defeat, and depressive symptomatology—with suicidal ideation in the adolescent and young adult population and to test a tentative theoretical model. The databases used were PubMed, Web of Science, and ProQuest. Primary studies were selected that examined the role of entrapment, defeat, and depressive symptomatology in suicidal ideation among adolescents and young adults (ages 10–35). Additionally, a model based on structural equation modeling was analyzed to assess the relationships between entrapment, defeat, and depressive symptomatology and suicidal ideation. Eleven studies met the established inclusion criteria. The results showed defeat and entrapment to be associated with depressive symptomatology and suicidal ideation, regardless of the country studied. Additionally, the model indicates that entrapment and defeat lead to depressive symptomatology, which in turn contributes to the occurrence of suicidal ideation. These findings suggest that defeat and entrapment could be universal factors in explaining suicidal behavior in adolescents and young adults. Consequently, the results of this work may contribute to the development of strategies for preventing suicidal ideation in this population.

Keywords: entrapment; defeat; depressive symptoms; suicidal ideation; adolescents; young adults; systematic review

1. Introduction

According to the World Health Organization [1], approximately 703,000 people die by suicide each year, making suicidal behavior one of the leading causes of death worldwide. It has become the second leading cause of premature death among young people aged 15 to 29 [2].

Suicidal ideation and behaviors typically begin to emerge during preadolescence and become more pronounced during adolescence [3–5]. It is estimated that adolescents experiencing suicidal ideation are 12 times more likely than others to attempt suicide by the age of 30 [3–5]. Furthermore, suicidal ideation and attempts in adolescents are associated with a lower life satisfaction and reduced emotional well-being [6].

Suicidal behavior is a complex and multifaceted reality that appears to be influenced by numerous biopsychosocial factors [7]. Additionally, the existential and social nature of suicide complicates its reduction into discrete elements [8]. For this reason, new approaches to the study of suicide propose a shift in focus, from searching for the causes of suicide to understanding the reasons and processes involved, with the aim of developing effective prevention strategies [9].

The Integrated Motivational–Volitional (IMV) model is one of the current theoretical paradigms seeking to explain suicidal behavior [10,11]. According to this model, suicidal behavior begins and develops through three phases: the **premotivational phase** (i.e., dispositional factors and triggering events), **the motivational phase** (i.e., suicidal ideation and intent), and the **volitional phase** (i.e., suicidal action). Throughout these phases, various factors are considered to be responsible for the onset of suicidal ideation and its progression towards attempted and completed suicide. The IMV model considers the perception of feeling defeated combined with a sense of entrapment and a lack of available help as key factors in the progression from passive ideation, or the emergence of thoughts of ending one's life as a sole means of escape, to the transition to an attempt. Defeat has been defined [12] as feelings of helplessness and humiliation along with a perceived failure in a struggle following a loss of or change in a valuable status of the individual. Meanwhile, entrapment is characterized as the sensation of being unable to escape from painful or confining situations [13].

One of the main elements of interest in O'Connor's model [10,11] is its proposal of the mechanisms that contribute to the transition from suicidal ideation to lethal suicidal action (motivational–volitional phase). Three groups of moderators are identified in this transition. In the motivational phase, moderators include deficits in problem-solving, rumination, and biases in autobiographical memory, which catalyze the progression from defeat to entrapment. In the volitional phase, factors such as perceived burdensomenessand the perception of being a burden moderate the relationship between entrapment and suicidal ideation, influencing either the intensification of entrapment or the generation of more hopeful expectations. Within the motivational phase, depressive symptomatology is highly relevant [14–16]. Notably, cognitive biases, negative attributions about the future, and hopelessness are prominent variables in the processes of suicidal ideation and crisis.

Previous studies have demonstrated a strong association between depressive symptomatology and suicidal behavior [17,18]. Other research has provided evidence of the association between hopelessness—a motivational factor in the IMV model [10] as well as a central concept in the work of Beck et al. [19,20]—and suicidal ideation [21,22]. A positive and statistically significant association has also been found between the severity of depressive symptoms, hopelessness, and suicidal ideation e.g., [12,23–26].

Meanwhile, Griffiths et al. [27] noted that depressive symptoms and defeat–entrapment variables can mutually reinforce each other and that both defeat–entrapment and depressive symptomatology are predicted in both directions. There is significant empirical evidence showing that both defeat and entrapment are predictors of suicidal ideation [28–30] and suicide attempts [31]. Additionally, the meta-analysis by Siddaway et al. [26] revealed a robust relationship between entrapment, defeat, and suicidal risk.

Given the prominent role of these variables in suicidal ideation in the general population [32–38], review studies that analyze different findings on their contribution to the prediction and prevention of suicidal behavior in community and clinical populations will be useful for understanding the current state of the issue and the mechanisms leading to suicidal ideation and behavior. Additionally, exploring models of the relationship between entrapment, defeat, and depressive symptomatology with respect to suicidal ideation in the adolescent–young adult population may advance our understanding of suicidal behavior and guide more effective therapeutic strategies for its prevention.

The primary objective of this work is to explore the findings from empirical research on the role of entrapment and defeat in suicidal behavior among adolescents and young adults. A secondary aim, based on the data extracted from the review, is to investigate the potential mediating effect of depressive symptomatology in the relationship between defeat, entrapment, and suicidal ideation in this population.

2. Method

The search for studies was carried out in accordance with PRISMA-P (Preferred Reporting Items for Systematic Review and Meta-Analysis Protocols) [39,40].

The review protocol was registered in March 2024 with the International Prospective Register of Systematic Reviews (PROSPERO, registration number CRD42024525551) to ensure transparency in the review procedures undertaken [41].

The AMSTAR 2 [42] tool was used to assess the quality of the systematic review conducted.

2.1. Search Strategy

In March 2024, a systematic search was conducted using the electronic databases PubMed, Web of Science (Core Collection), and ProQuest. No limits were imposed on the publication date of the studies. The search was performed by two of the authors (A.H. and E.I.), who independently assessed the eligibility of each article. After an initial screening based on this criterion, the full texts of the remaining articles were examined to evaluate their potential inclusion.

The search strategy was conducted using a combination of the following terms: (1) "Entrapment" and "Defeat" and "Suicid*" and "adolescen*"; (2) "Entrapment" and "Defeat" and "Suicid*" and "young adults".

The search terms were grouped into four sets using the Boolean term AND. To select the primary original documents, the following search string was used across all fields: [("entrapment" AND "defeat" AND "suicid*" AND "adolescen*")]. Simultaneously, a second search string was used that modified the target population: [("entrapment" AND "defeat" AND "suicid*" AND "young adults")]. In ProQuest (Ann Arbor, MI, USA), without a restricted search, the results were unmanageable; therefore, the search was conducted using the same strings but selecting the "Abstract" field for each term.

The eligibility criteria for the studies analyzed were as follows. The inclusion criteria called for primary studies that (a) involved participants who were adolescents and young adults of both sexes, aged between 10 and 35 years, from both clinical and general populations; (b) investigated the relationship between defeat and/or entrapment variables and suicidal behavior; (c) used validated assessment instruments with evidence of reliability; and (d) were published in English. The exclusion criteria ruled out studies with samples of adults over 35 years old or mixed-age samples (including both young adults and adults); studies that omitted fundamental methodological information in the abstract, such as the number or ages of participants; and studies that did not provide differentiated data regarding the study variables, i.e., defeat or entrapment in relation to suicidal behavior. Review articles, trials, case studies, and qualitative studies were also excluded. Finally, articles written in languages other than English were excluded.

In longitudinal studies with multiple measurement points for the variables, only the measures from the first assessment point were considered in order to avoid overlap.

Figure 1 illustrates the sequence of the search and selection procedure for the studies. In total, 92% of the studies found were excluded after all titles and abstracts had been analyzed, leaving 11 studies that met the established eligibility criteria. It is important to note that the study by Tarsafi et al. [43] includes two samples, which were analyzed independently due to the presence of two distinct population groups (from Iran and the USA).

2.2. Data Extraction and Coding

In accordance with Lipsey and Wilson [44], a coding protocol and an Excel spreadsheet were designed to ensure both systematic data coding and replicability. The following categories were coded, beginning with bibliographic data (a–c), continuing with participant-related variables (d–e) and methodological variables (f), and ending with coding results (g) for (a) authorship; (b) publication year; (c) country where the study was conducted and where the sample was obtained; (d) number, mean and standard deviation of age, respective percentages of female and male participants; (e) sample type (adolescents vs.

young adults, general vs. clinical); (f) instruments used to assess defeat, entrapment, and depressive symptomatology; and finally (g) correlations between pairs of any of these variables: depressive symptomatology, entrapment, defeat, and suicidal ideation.

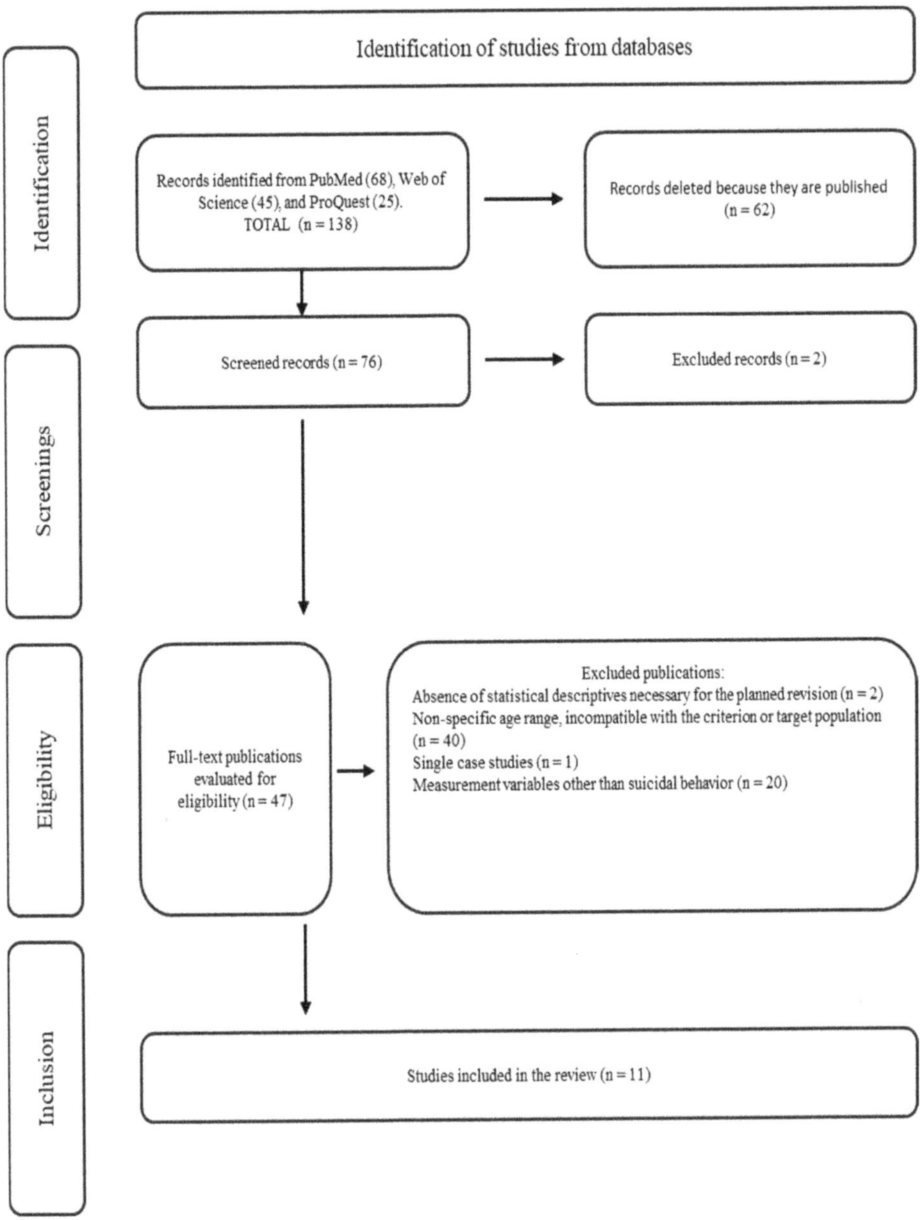

Figure 1. Flow diagram according to the PRISMA Model for Systematic Review.

2.3. Data Analysis

To be able to compare the correlations between the variables among the different studies, we first obtained the Fisher Z weighted by the sample size. Then, we transformed the Fisher Z to the correlations by Psychometrica [45]. To evaluate the mediational model, we used structural equation modeling with LISREL 9 and Maximum Likelihood (ML) as the estimation method.

For the mediation analyses, the measures from the cross-sectional studies and only the first measure from each one of the two longitudinal studies were included in this review.

3. Results

Following the process of searching for and selecting documents, 11 studies were included, all published between 2010 and 2022 (Table 1). Most of the selected studies (n = 81%) were cross-sectional, while two (n = 19%) were longitudinal.

The selected studies included a total of 25,638 participants aged between 10 and 35 years, with the mean age of participants in the included samples ranging from 13.6 to 23.6. Regarding gender, 10 studies provided detailed percentages; overall, the percentage of female participants was higher than that of male ones (55%). The sample size ranged from 74 to 11,393 participants.

Regarding the origins of the samples, four studies were from the United Kingdom, three from China, two from the United States, one from South Korea, one from Iran, and one from Spain. All the included studies employed non-probabilistic sampling in the selection of participants. Out of the total 25,638 participants, the samples were primarily composed of high school students (78.22%), young adults with unspecified occupations (17.23%), university students (3.37%), students with unspecified educational levels (0.87%), and, in one study, a community sample of adolescents (0.32%).

Regarding the instruments used to assess the variables of defeat, entrapment, depressive symptomatology, and suicidal ideation, it is notable that all studies employed self-report measures, with an average of 21 items per scale and response options of the Likert type. Tarsafi et al. [43] assessed the presence of suicidal ideation using a single ad hoc item: 'I have had thoughts of suicide in the past'. Similarly, Ren et al. [46] used the item 'Have you had suicidal ideation in the last 12 months?'. A 6-point scale was provided for the responses, from 1 = never through to 2 = once, 3 = twice, 4 = three times, 5 = four times, and 6 = five times or more.

To assess the reliability of the instruments used in the student sample for measuring defeat and entrapment, 10 studies (90%) employed the original Defeat and Entrapment Scale [12]. The Defeat Scale showed a Cronbach's alpha of 0.94, indicating strong internal consistency. The Internal Entrapment subscale reported Cronbach's alpha values ranging from 0.93 to 0.95, while the External Entrapment subscale ranged from 0.88 to 0.96, both reflecting high internal consistency. Pollak et al. [47] used the Short Defeat and Entrapment Scale (SDES) [48], a short version of the original scale, which showed excellent internal consistency in its original validation, with Cronbach's alpha values ranging from 0.88 to 0.94. However, the internal consistency for the sample in their study was not reported.

For the assessment of depressive symptomatology, four studies (36%) used the Beck scales: the Beck Depression Inventory (BDI) [49] and the Beck Depression Inventory-II (BDI-II) [50], both showing a good internal consistency. The authors reported a mean alpha coefficient of 0.87 for the BDI and 0.92 to 0.95 for the BDI-II [50] in their samples. Three studies (27%) used the Short Depression Anxiety Stress Scale (DASS-D) [51] and the 21-item Depression, Anxiety, and Stress Scale (DASS-21) [52], which are two versions of the original Depression, Anxiety, and Stress Scale (DASS) [53], with a Cronbach's alpha of 0.86 to 0.93 for the depression subscale in their samples. Lastly, Park et al. [54] used the Depression Scale (CES-D) [55], showing a Cronbach's alpha of 0.89 in its sample.

The reliability of the instruments used for assessing suicidal ideation was generally good, although the use of different assessment tools led to some variability. The Beck Scale for Suicidal Ideation (BSSI) [56] had a Cronbach's alpha of 0.86 in the study by Wetherall et al. [30], the Plutchik Suicide Risk Scale (PSRS) [57] had an alpha of 0.78 in the study by Ordóñez-Carrasco et al. [58], and the alpha for the Suicidal Behaviors Questionnaire Revised (SBQ-R) [59] ranged from 0.83 to 0.93 depending on the study.

The Suicidal Ideation Questionnaire (SIQ) [60] had an alpha of 0.97, while the Suicidal Ideation Attributes Scale (SIDAS) [61] and the Scale for Suicide Ideation (SSI) [62] both had alphas of 0.90.

A detailed outline of the specific instruments used in each study is provided in Table 1.

Table 1. Summary of the articles included in the systematic review.

Reference	Year	Country	Study Sample (N, Average Age, SD, Sex)	Sample Type	Study Variables	Instruments Used	Results
Bradford et al. [63]	2021	UK	N = 259; Mean Age = 21.15, SD = 2.11; Sex = 34.4% Men	Students and non-students	Depression symptoms, defeat, entrapment, and suicidal ideation	Defeat and Entrapment Scale, DASS-21, SIDAS	r DS/E = 0.69; r DS/D = 0.67; r DS/I = 0.53; r E/D = 0.67; r E/I = 0.55; r D/I = 0.54
Li et al. [64]	2020	China	N = 1239; Mean Age = 14.07, SD = 1.54; Sex = 45.2% Men	Students	Depression symptoms, defeat, entrapment, and suicidal ideation	Entrapment Scale, DASS-21	r DS/E = 0.54; r DS/D = 0.38; r DS/I = 0.34; r E/D = 0.31; r E/I = 0.39; r D/I = 0.19
Ordóñez-Carrasco et al. [58]	2021	Spain	N = 644; Mean Age = 25.91, SD = 5.14; Sex = 48.8% Men	General population	Defeat and entrapment, suicidal ideation, and depression	Defeat and Entrapment Scale, PSRS, BDI-II	r E/I = 0.52
Park et al. [54]	2010	Korea	N = 11,393; Mean Age = 14.62, SD = 1.50; Sex = 56.5% Men	Students	Depression symptoms, entrapment, and suicidal ideation	SSI, CES-D, Entrapment Scale	r DS/E = 0.71; r DS/I = 0.55; r E/I = 0.59
Pollak et al. [47]	2021	USA	N = 74, Mean age = 16.27, Sex = Men–Women, SD = 2.21	Non-clinical sample, general population	Defeat and entrapment, suicidal ideation and depression	SDES, SIQ, QIDS-SR	r DS/E = 0.77; r DS/D = 0.77; r DS/I = 0.60; r E/I = 0.71; r D/I = 0.71
Ren et al. [46]	2018	China	N = 1074; Mean Age = 13.83, SD = 1.53; Sex = 45.8% Men	Students	Depression symptoms, entrapment, and suicidal ideation	Entrapment Scale, DASS-D	r DS/E = 0.6; r DS/I = 0.44; r E/I = 0.38
Tarsafi et al. [43]	2015	USA/Iran	N = 194 (USA); Mean Age = 21.6, SD = 5.2 years; Sex = 23.20% Men N = 146 (Iran); Mean Age = 21, SD = 1.7 years; Sex = 28.08% Men	Students	Depression symptoms, defeat, entrapment, and suicidal ideation	Defeat and Entrapment Scale and BDI	N USA: r DS/E = 0.77; r DS/D = 0.7; r DS/I = 0.54; r E/D = 0.81; r E/I = 0.46; r D/I = 0.45 N Iran: r DS/E = 0.72; r DS/D = 0.72; r DS/I = 0.41; r E/D = 0.73; r E/I = 0.37; r D/I = 0.34
Taylor et al. [65]	2010	UK	N = 93; Mean Age = 23.45, SD = 7.06; Sex = 18.28% Men	University students	Defeat, entrapment, and suicidal ideation	Defeat and Entrapment Scale, SBQ-R	r E/D = 0.73; r E/I = 0.45; r D/I = 0.49
Taylor et al. [25]	2011	UK	N = 79; Mean Age = 19.61, SD = 4.45; Sex = 16.46% Men	University students	Depression symptoms, defeat, entrapment, and suicidal ideation	SBQ-R, BDI-II, Defeat and Entrapment Scale	r DS/E = 0.73; r DS/D = 0.73; r DS/I = 0.62; r E/D = 0.79; r E/I = 0.6; r D/I = 0.6
Yang et al. [66]	2022	China	N = 4515; Mean Age = 15.24, SD = 1.66; Sex = 50.23% Men	High school students	Defeat and suicidal ideation	DSI-SS, Defeat Scale	r D/I = 0.43
Wetherall et al. [30]	2022	Scotland	N = 3508	General population	Defeat and entrapment, suicidal ideation, and depression symptoms	BSSI, BDI-II, Defeat and Entrapment Scale	r DS/D = 0.84; r DS/I = 0.58; r D/I = 0.53

Note. SD: standard deviation; BDI: Beck Depression Inventory [49]; BDI-II: Beck Depression Inventory-II [50]; BSSI: Beck Scale for Suicidal Ideation [56]; CES-D: Depression Scale [55]; DASS-D: Short Depression Anxiety Stress Scale [51]; DASS-21: 21-item Depression, Anxiety, and Stress Scales [52,53]; D: Defeat; DS: Depressive Symptom; DSI-SS: Depressive Symptom Index-Suicidality Subscale [67]; E: Entrapment; I: Suicidal Ideation; PSRS: Plutchik Suicide Risk Scale [57]; QIDS-SR: Quick Inventory of Depressive Symptomatology-Self Report [68]; SBQ-R: Suicidal Behaviors Questionnaire Revised [59]; SIQ: Suicidal Ideation Questionnaire [60]; SDES: Short Defeat and Entrapment Scale [48]; SIDAS: Suicidal Ideation Attributes Scale [61]; SSI: Scale for Suicide Ideation [62].

An analysis of the (normalized) correlations between the variables across the selected studies is presented in Table 2. Although the effect size of these correlations is small, they are statistically significant. Beyond the quantitative value of the relationship, these results suggest the qualitative importance of these associations.

Table 2. Normalized correlations calculated from the selected studies.

	1	2	3	4
Ideation (1)	-			
Depressive symptomatology (2)	0.14	-		
Defeat (3)	0.05	0.14	-	
Entrapment (4)	0.12	0.13	0.09	-

In accordance with the second objective, the mediating effect of depressive symptomatology in the relationship between defeat, entrapment, and suicidal ideation was explored (see Figure 2).

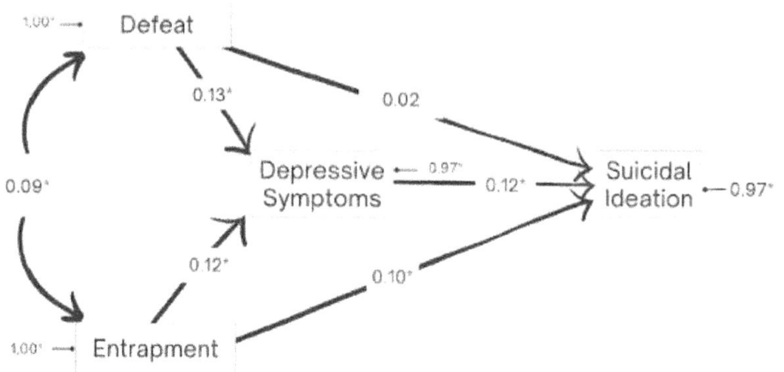

Figure 2. Standardized solution of the tentative model. Note. * $p < 0.05$.

The tested structural equation model showed an excellent fit: $\chi^2 = 0.42$ ($p = 0.93$; $df = 3$), GFI = 0.99, CFI = 1.00, ECVI = 0.006, RMSEA = 0.00 (90% CI [0.0; 0.008]), and SRMR = 0.005. This model is consistent with the idea that entrapment and defeat act as predictors of depressive symptomatology, which in turn contributes to the emergence of suicidal ideation in adolescents and young people. Suicidal ideation would thus be the result of both the direct effects of entrapment and depressive symptomatology and the indirect effects of entrapment (c = 0.015; CR = 4.79) and defeat (c = 0.016; CR = 4.59) through depressive symptomatology. This indicates a total mediating effect for the defeat variable and a partial mediating effect for entrapment.

4. Methodological Quality and Risk of Bias

4.1. Methodological Quality of the Analyzed Studies

For the analysis of methodological quality, the MINORS tool [69] was employed as the review included non-randomized and non-comparative studies. For all 11 of the studies included, the overall quality of the trials was considered, taking into account aspects such as randomization, participant dropout/attrition, selective reporting of results, and other potential sources of bias (e.g., sources of funding). The results of the complete checklist are presented in Table 3.

Table 3. The revised and validated version of MINORS.

Methodological Items for Non-Randomized Studies	Score †
1. A clearly stated aim: The question addressed should be precise and relevant in light of the available literature.	2
2. Inclusion of consecutive patients: All patients potentially fit for inclusion (satisfying the criteria for inclusion) should have been included in the study during the study period (there should be no exclusion or details about reasons for exclusion).	2

Table 3. *Cont.*

Methodological Items for Non-Randomized Studies	Score †
3. Prospective collection of data: The data should have been collected according to a protocol established before the beginning of the study.	2
4. Endpoints appropriate to the aim of the study: There should be an unambiguous explanation of the criteria used to evaluate the main outcome, which should be in accordance with the question addressed by the study. Also, the endpoints should be assessed on an intention-to-treat basis.	2
5. Unbiased assessment of the study endpoint: There should be blind evaluation of objective endpoints and double-blind evaluation of subjective endpoints. Otherwise, the reasons for not blinding should be stated.	not applicable
6. Follow-up period appropriate to the aim of the study: The follow-up should be sufficiently long to allow for assessment of the main endpoint and possible adverse events.	1
7. Loss to follow-up less than 5%: All patients should be included in the follow-up. Otherwise, the proportion lost to follow-up should not exceed the proportion experiencing the major endpoint.	not applicable
8. Prospective calculation of the study size: There should be information on the size of detectable difference in interest with a calculation of a 95% confidence interval, according to the expected incidence of the outcome event, and information about the level for statistical significance and estimates of power when comparing the outcomes.	0

† The items are scored 0 (not reported), 1 (reported but inadequate), or 2 (reported and adequate). The global ideal score is 16 for non-comparative studies and 24 for comparative studies. The total score obtained was 9 of out 16 points.

4.2. Methodological Quality of the Review

The systematic review adhered to PRISMA-P criteria [39,40] and followed the bias control guidelines recommended by AMSTAR 2 [42]. The methodological quality of the systematic review was assessed using the AMSTAR 2 tool [42], which evaluates confidence levels across 16 criteria. The overall confidence level was deemed to be moderate, with only a few limitations identified, such as the lack of a more comprehensive literature search method.

5. Discussion

This study conducted a systematic review of the literature investigating the association between the variables of defeat, entrapment, and depressive symptoms in relation to suicidal ideation in adolescents and young adults utilizing formal search strategies. The use of a comprehensive search strategy that is easily replicable in future research facilitated the thorough exploration of empirical findings on the role of defeat and entrapment in suicidal behavior within the child and adolescent population.

The most noteworthy result from the selected studies is the consistent association between the key variables highlighted in the Integrated Motivational–Volitional (IMV) model [10]. Specifically, the model underscores the role of defeat as a variable implicated in the formation of entrapment, which is, in turn, closely linked to the development of suicidal ideation in the general population [58].

This evidence supports the theoretical framework of the IMV model [10] and aligns with other studies that have tested the relationships among the different factors within the model [70]. It also supports models that focus on identifying psychological states preceding a suicide attempt and factors that elevate the risk of suicidal behavior, such as those proposed by Galynker et al. [71]. The contribution of defeat and entrapment as variables has also been confirmed in the review by Taylor et al. [13], which indicated that these factors were associated with an increased risk of suicide in both clinical and community populations.

Specifically, when analyzing the interplay between the three variables, several studies included in this review demonstrate that defeat and entrapment are robustly associated with measures of depressive symptoms and suicidal ideation, regardless of the country under study [43,47]. This suggests the universal presence of defeat and entrapment, independent of cultural context or age, as significant factors in explaining potential mechanisms behind suicidal behavior. These variables may also serve as relevant indicators of suicide risk.

Furthermore, as highlighted by various studies, both perceptions of defeat and entrapment are strongly associated with the risk of self-harm [72] and suicidal thoughts and behaviors [73].

This review is grounded in O'Connor's [10] Integrated Motivational–Volitional (IMV) model, which explores the variables of entrapment and defeat and their association with suicidal ideation in child and adolescent populations. The IMV model proposes that suicidal behavior results from dynamic and reciprocal interactions among various factors, some of which may act as mediators in the relationship between the core variables implicated in suicidal behavior. Studying the interaction between these variables can suggest mechanisms that can explain the dynamics of suicide in adolescents and young adults. Depressive symptomatology—particularly those components related to future expectations and hopelessness—has been interpreted as being directly linked to suicidal ideation, as argued by Beck et al. [20] from a cognitive perspective. It also acts as a potential mediating variable between the motivational and volitional phases of suicide risk. According to the IMV model [11], this depressive symptomatology may facilitate the transition from suicidal ideation to action. The findings of this review and the proposed model support these concepts in the child and adolescent population, contributing to a better understanding of the role of depressive symptoms in suicidal dynamics. Consequently, this contributes to early detection as well as the improvement of prevention and intervention strategies in clinical, educational, and other settings [33,74].

These results, when considered globally, provide evidence supporting both the IMV model [11], which posits a central role for perceived defeat and entrapment as key variables in the motivational phase of suicidal ideation development, and Beck et al.'s [20] model, where depressive symptomatology plays a crucial role as a precursor to suicidal thoughts. Together, these findings reinforce the understanding that both perceived defeat and depressive symptoms are pivotal factors in the trajectory toward suicidal ideation, emphasizing the need to address them in prevention and intervention efforts.

As for the methodological quality of the studies analyzed, the overall level of confidence is moderate since only a few critical weaknesses have been detected. An accurate summary is provided of the available state-of-the-art studies. The systematic review conducted followed the PRISMA-P criteria [39,40] and the guidelines for bias control indicated by AMSTAR 2 [42].

6. Limitations and Future Directions

Despite the strengths of this study, it is necessary to highlight some of its limitations. One of them, primarily methodological in nature, stems from the undefined number of studies that may have been excluded from the database search; specifically, in ProQuest, the search was limited to abstracts, whereas this restriction was not applied across the other databases, WoS and PubMed. A second limitation arises from the inclusion and exclusion criteria themselves, as studies that did not specify certain variables, such as the ages of the participants, were discarded. Additionally, it is important to emphasize that the published literature in this area remains scarce due to the ethical and legal requirements involved in studying suicidal behavior in minors. Furthermore, the limited availability of longitudinal studies constrains the capacity to establish causal inferences.

In light of all this and given the shortcomings of the review realized, the results suggest the need for further research in this field, including both cross-sectional studies with the general population and longitudinal studies in diverse cultural contexts as well as studies at different stages of adolescent development, that allow us to carry out meta-analysis using structural equation modeling to obtain more realistic empirical evidences about the tentative model proposed. This would help, firstly to properly stablish causal relationship, and consequently shed light on the processes involved in the transition from ideation to attempt and lethal suicidal action, clarifying the contributions of defeat and entrapment in this process.Despite the methodological limitations and the scarcity of longitudinal studies that examine the transition from suicidal ideation to attempt, the present work provides a solid foundation for future research and preventive actions. It is worth noting that research on suicide prevention has evolved from attempting to establish causal relationships to focusing on plausible explanatory models that enhance prevention efforts [9]. Thus, the consistent relationships found between defeat, entrapment, depressive symptoms, and suicidal ideation underscore the importance of addressing these variables in the early detection of and intervention in this issue, whose prevalence has been increasing in recent years [1,2]. Ultimately, addressing these factors comprehensively may significantly contribute to reducing the risk of suicide in the child and adolescent population, thus improving the effectiveness of prevention and treatment strategies in clinical and educational settings.

Author Contributions: Conceptualization, A.H.-d.A., M.A.C., E.I.-S. and I.C.-C.; methodology, A.H.-d.A. and F.P.H.-T.; formal analysis, A.H.-d.A. and F.P.H.-T.; investigation, A.H.-d.A., M.A.C., E.I.-S. and F.P.H.-T.; data curation, M.A.C., E.I.-S. and F.P.H.-T.; writing—original draft preparation, A.H.-d.A., M.A.C., E.I.-S. and I.C.-C.; writing—review and editing, A.H.-d.A., M.A.C., E.I.-S. and I.C.-C.; supervision, F.P.H.-T., M.A.C. and E.I.-S. All authors have read and agreed to the published version of the manuscript.

Funding: This research was funded by The Ministry of Science and Innovation of the Government of Spain, Project Reference: PID2020-114538RB-I00; AEI/10.13039/501100011033.

Conflicts of Interest: The authors declare no conflicts of interest.

References

1. Organización Mundial de la Salud. *Suicide Worldwide in 2019: Global Health Estimates*; Organización Mundial de la Salud: Geneva, Switzerland, 2021.
2. World Health Organization. WHO Media Centre. 2017. Available online: http://www.who.int/mediacentre/factsheets/fs398/en/ (accessed on 15 January 2024).
3. Cha, C.B.; Franz, P.J.; Guzmán, E.M.; Glenn, C.R.; Kleiman, E.M.; Nock, M.K. Annual research review: Suicide among youth—Epidemiology, (potential) etiology, and treatment. *J. Child Psychol. Psychiatry* **2018**, *59*, 460–482. [CrossRef] [PubMed]
4. Kessler, R.C.; Borges, G.; Walters, E.E. Prevalence of and risk factors for lifetime suicide attempts in the National Comorbidity Survey. *Arch. Gen. Psychiatry* **1999**, *56*, 617–626. [CrossRef] [PubMed]
5. Reinherz, H.Z.; Tanner, J.L.; Berger, S.R.; Beardslee, W.R.; Fitzmaurice, G.M. Adolescent suicidal ideation as predictive of psychopathology, suicidal behavior, and compromised functioning at age 30. *Am. J. Psychiatry* **2006**, *163*, 1226–1232. [CrossRef] [PubMed]
6. Fonseca-Pedrero, E. Análisis de redes en psicología. *Papeles Psicólogo* **2018**, *39*, 1–12. [CrossRef]
7. Tan, L.; Xia, T.; Reece, C. Social and individual risk factors for suicide ideation among Chinese children and adolescents: A multilevel analysis. *Int. J. Psychol.* **2018**, *53*, 117–125. [CrossRef] [PubMed]
8. Rudd, M.D. Fluid Vulnerability Theory: A Cognitive Approach to Understanding the Process of Acute and Chronic Suicide Risk. In *Cognition and Suicide: Theory, Research, and Therapy*; Ellis, T.E., Ed.; American Psychological Association: Washington, DC, USA, 2006; pp. 355–368. [CrossRef]
9. Al-Halabí, S.; Fonseca-Pedrero, E. *Manual de Psicología de la Conducta Suicida*; Pirámide: Madrid, Spain, 2023.
10. O'Connor, R.C. The integrated motivational-volitional model of suicidal behavior. *Crisis* **2011**, *32*, 295–298. [CrossRef]
11. O'Connor, R.C.; Kirtley, O.J. The integrated motivational-volitional model of suicidal behaviour. *Philos. Trans. R. Soc. B Biol. Sci.* **2018**, *373*, 20170268. [CrossRef]
12. Gilbert, P.; Allan, S. The role of defeat and entrapment (arrested flight) in depression: An exploration of an evolutionary view. *Psychol. Med.* **1998**, *28*, 585–598. [CrossRef]
13. Taylor, P.J.; Gooding, P.; Wood, A.M.; Tarrier, N. The role of defeat and entrapment in depression, anxiety, and suicide. *Psychol. Bull.* **2011**, *137*, 391–420. [CrossRef]
14. Brown, G.K.; Beck, A.T.; Steer, R.A.; Grisham, J.R. Risk factors for suicide in psychiatric outpatients: A 20-year prospective study. *J. Consult. Clin. Psychol.* **2000**, *68*, 371–377. [CrossRef]
15. Prinstein, M.J.; Nock, M.K.; Simon, V.; Aikins, J.W.; Cheah, C.S.; Spirito, A. Longitudinal trajectories and predictors of adolescent suicidal ideation and attempts following inpatient hospitalization. *J. Consult. Clin. Psychol.* **2008**, *76*, 92–103. [CrossRef] [PubMed]
16. Wenzel, A.; Beck, A.T. A cognitive model of suicidal behavior: Theory and treatment. *Appl. Prev. Psychol.* **2008**, *12*, 189–201. [CrossRef]
17. Brent, D.A.; Perper, J.A.; Moritz, G.; Allman, C.; Friend, A.; Roth, C.; Schweers, J.; Balach, L.; Baugher, M. Psychiatric risk factors for adolescent suicide: A case-control study. *J. Am. Acad. Child Adolesc. Psychiatry* **1993**, *32*, 521–529. [CrossRef]

18. Shaffer, D.; Gould, M.S.; Fisher, P.; Trautman, P.; Moreau, D.; Kleinman, M.; Flory, M. Psychiatric diagnosis in child and adolescent suicide. *Arch. Gen. Psychiatry* **1996**, *53*, 339–348. [CrossRef]
19. Beck, A.T.; Steer, R.A.; Kovacs, M.; Garrison, B. Hopelessness and eventual suicide: A 10-year prospective study of patients hospitalized with suicidal ideation. *Am. J. Psychiatry* **1985**, *142*, 559–563.
20. Beck, A.T.; Brown, G.; Berchick, R.J.; Stewart, B.L.; Steer, R.A. Relationship between hopelessness and ultimate suicide: A replication with psychiatric outpatients. *Am. J. Psychiatry* **1990**, *147*, 190–195. [CrossRef]
21. Beck, A.T.; Steer, R.A.; Beck, J.S.; Newman, C.F. Hopelessness, depression, suicidal ideation, and clinical diagnosis of depression. *Suicide Life Threat. Behav.* **1993**, *23*, 139–145. [CrossRef]
22. Wetzel, R.D. Hopelessness, depression, and suicide intent. *Arch. Gen. Psychiatry* **1976**, *33*, 1069–1073. [CrossRef]
23. Carvalho, S.; Pinto-Gouveia, J.; Pimentel, P.; Maia, D.; Gilbert, P.; Mota-Pereira, J. Entrapment and defeat perceptions in depressive symptomatology: Through an evolutionary approach. *Psychiatry* **2013**, *76*, 53–67. [CrossRef] [PubMed]
24. Panagioti, M.; Gooding, P.; Taylor, P.J.; Tarrier, N. A model of suicidal behavior in posttraumatic stress disorder (PTSD): The mediating role of defeat and entrapment. *Psychiatry Res.* **2013**, *209*, 55–59. [CrossRef] [PubMed]
25. Taylor, P.J.; Gooding, P.A.; Wood, A.M.; Johnson, J.; Tarrier, N. Prospective predictors of suicidality: Defeat and entrapment lead to changes in suicidal ideation over time. *Suicide Life Threat. Behav.* **2011**, *41*, 297–306. [CrossRef] [PubMed]
26. Siddaway, A.P.; Taylor, P.J.; Wood, A.M.; Schulz, J. A meta-analysis of perceptions of defeat and entrapment in depression, anxiety problems, posttraumatic stress disorder, and suicidality. *J. Affect. Disord.* **2015**, *184*, 149–159. [CrossRef]
27. Griffiths, A.W.; Wood, A.M.; Maltby, J.; Taylor, P.J.; Tai, S. The prospective role of defeat and entrapment in depression and anxiety: A 12-month longitudinal study. *Psychiatry Res.* **2014**, *216*, 52–59. [CrossRef]
28. O'Connor, R.C.; Portzky, G. Looking to the future: A synthesis of new developments and challenges in suicide research and prevention. *Front. Psychol.* **2018**, *9*, 2139. [CrossRef]
29. Rasmussen, S.A.; Fraser, L.; Gotz, M.; MacHale, S.; Mackie, R.; Masterton, G.; McConachie, S.; O'Connor, R.C. Elaborating the cry of pain model of suicidality: Testing a psychological model in a sample of first-time and repeat self-harm patients. *Br. J. Clin. Psychol.* **2010**, *49*, 15–30. [CrossRef]
30. Wetherall, K.; Cleare, S.; Eschle, S.; Ferguson, E.; O'Connor, D.B.; O'Carroll, R.E.; O'Connor, R.C. Predicting suicidal ideation in a nationally representative sample of young adults: A 12-month prospective study. *Psychol. Med.* **2022**, *52*, 3168–3175. [CrossRef]
31. O'Connor, R.C.; Smyth, R.; Ferguson, E.; Ryan, C.; Williams, J.M.G. Psychological processes and repeat suicidal behavior: A four-year prospective study. *J. Consult. Clin. Psychol.* **2013**, *81*, 1137–1143. [CrossRef]
32. Chiles, J.A.; Strosahl, K.D.; Roberts, L.W. *Clinical Manual for Assessment and Treatment of Suicidal Patients*, 2nd ed.; American Psychiatric Association: Arlington, VA, USA, 2019.
33. Franklin, J.C.; Ribeiro, J.D.; Fox, K.R.; Bentley, K.H.; Kleiman, E.M.; Huang, X.; Musacchio, K.M.; Jaroszewski, A.C.; Chang, B.P.; Nock, M.K. Risk factors for suicidal thoughts and behaviors: A meta-analysis of 50 years of research. *Psychol. Bull.* **2017**, *143*, 187–232. [CrossRef]
34. Large, M.; Galletly, C.; Myles, N.; Ryan, C.J.; Myles, H. Known unknowns and unknown unknowns in suicide risk assessment: Evidence from meta-analyses of aleatory and epistemic uncertainty. *BJPsych Bull.* **2017**, *41*, 160–163. [CrossRef] [PubMed]
35. McHugh, C.M.; Corderoy, A.; Ryan, C.J.; Hickie, I.B.; Large, M.M. Association between suicidal ideation and suicide: Meta-analyses of odds ratios, sensitivity, specificity and positive predictive value. *BJPsych Open* **2019**, *5*, e18. [CrossRef]
36. Mulder, R.; Newton-Howes, G.; Coid, J.W. The futility of risk prediction in psychiatry. *Br. J. Psychiatry* **2016**, *209*, 271–272. [CrossRef] [PubMed]
37. Runeson, B.; Odeberg, J.; Pettersson, A.; Edbom, T.; Jildevik Adamsson, I.; Waern, M. Instruments for the assessment of suicide risk: A systematic review evaluating the certainty of the evidence. *PLoS ONE* **2017**, *12*, e0180292. [CrossRef] [PubMed]
38. Steeg, S.; Quinlivan, L.; Nowland, R.; Carroll, R.; Casey, D.; Clements, C.; Cooper, J.; Davies, L.; Knipe, D.; Ness, J.; et al. Accuracy of risk scales for predicting repeat self-harm and suicide: A multicentre, population-level cohort study using routine clinical data. *BMC Psychiatry* **2018**, *18*, 113. [CrossRef]
39. Cajal, B.; Jiménez, R.; Gervilla, E.; Montaño, J.J. Doing a systematic review in health sciences. *Clínica Salud* **2020**, *31*, 77–83. [CrossRef]
40. Moher, D.; Shamseer, L.; Clarke, M.; Ghersi, D.; Liberati, A.; Petticrew, M.; Shekelle, P.; Stewart, L.A. Preferred reporting items for systematic review and meta-analysis protocols (PRISMA-P) 2015 statement. *Syst. Rev.* **2015**, *4*, 1. [CrossRef] [PubMed]
41. Pieper, D.; Rombey, T. Where to Prospectively Register a Systematic Review. *Syst. Rev.* **2022**, *11*, 8. [CrossRef]
42. Shea, B.J.; Reeves, B.C.; Wells, G.; Thuku, M.; Hamel, C.; Moran, J.; Moher, D.; Tugwell, P.; Welch, V.; Kristjansson, E.; et al. AMSTAR 2: A critical appraisal tool for systematic reviews that include randomised or non-randomised studies of healthcare interventions, or both. *BMJ* **2017**, *358*, j4008. [CrossRef]
43. Tarsafi, M.; Kalantarkousheh, S.M.; Lester, D. The defeat-entrapment theory versus Beck's hopelessness theory of depression and suicidality: A cross-national analysis in Iran and the United States. *Int. J. Soc. Psychiatry* **2015**, *61*, 777–780. [CrossRef]
44. Lipsey, M.W.; Wilson, D.B. *Practical Meta-Analysis*; Sage: Thousand Oaks, CA, USA, 2001.
45. Psychometrica. Online Calculator for Testing Correlations. Available online: https://www.psychometrica.de/correlation.html#fisher (accessed on 28 April 2024).

46. Ren, Y.; You, J.; Lin, M.P.; Xu, S. Low self-esteem, entrapment, and reason for living: A moderated mediation model of suicidal ideation. *Int. J. Psychol.* **2018**, *54*, 807–815. [CrossRef]
47. Pollak, O.H.; Guzmán, E.M.; Shin, K.E.; Cha, C.B. A dynamic systems perspective on suicidal behavior. *Front. Psychol.* **2021**, *12*, 590388. [CrossRef]
48. Griffiths, A.W.; Wood, A.M.; Maltby, J.; Taylor, P.J.; Tai, S. The development of the Short Defeat and Entrapment Scale (SDES). *Psychol. Assess.* **2015**, *27*, 1182–1194. [CrossRef] [PubMed]
49. Beck, A.T.; Ward, C.; Mendelson, M.; Mock, J.; Erbaugh, J. An inventory for measuring depression. *Arch. Gen. Psychiatry* **1961**, *4*, 561–571. [CrossRef] [PubMed]
50. Beck, A.T.; Steer, R.A.; Brown, G.K. *Manual for the Beck Depression Inventory-II*; Psychological Corporation: San Antonio, TX, USA, 1996.
51. Taouk, M.; Lovibond, P.F.; Laube, R. *Psychometric Properties of a Chinese Version of the 21-Item Depression Anxiety Stress Scales (DASS21)*; Transcultural Mental Health Centre, Cumberland Hospital: Sydney, NSW, Australia, 2001.
52. Henry, J.D.; Crawford, J.R. The short-form version of the Depression Anxiety Stress Scales (DASS-21): Construct validity and normative data in a large non-clinical sample. *Br. J. Clin. Psychol.* **2005**, *44*, 227–239. [CrossRef]
53. Lovibond, P.F.; Lovibond, S.H. The structure of negative emotional states: Comparison of the Depression Anxiety Stress Scales (DASS) with the Beck Depression and Anxiety Inventories. *Behav. Res. Ther.* **1995**, *33*, 335–343. [CrossRef]
54. Park, Y.J.; Ryu, H.; Han, K.; Kwon, J.H.; Kim, H.K.; Kang, H.C.; Yoon, J.W.; Cheon, S.H.; Shin, H. Suicidal ideation in adolescents: An explanatory model using LISREL. *West. J. Nurs. Res.* **2010**, *32*, 168–184. [CrossRef]
55. Chon, K.K.; Rhee, M.K. Preliminary development of Korean version of CES-D. *Korean J. Clin. Psychol.* **1992**, *11*, 65–76.
56. Beck, A.T.; Steer, R.A.; Ranieri, W.F. Scale for suicide ideation: Psychometric properties of a self-report version. *J. Clin. Psychol.* **1988**, *44*, 499–505. [CrossRef]
57. Plutchik, R.; van Praga, H.; Conte, H.; Picard, S. Correlates of suicide and violence risk 1: The Suicide Risk Measure. *Compr. Psychiatry* **1989**, *30*, 296–302. [CrossRef]
58. Ordóñez-Carrasco, J.L.; Cuadrado-Guirado, I.; Rojas-Tejada, A.J. Experiential avoidance in the context of the integrated motivational-volitional model of suicidal behavior. *Crisis* **2021**, *42*, 284–291. [CrossRef] [PubMed]
59. Osman, A.; Bagge, C.L.; Gutierrez, P.M.; Konick, L.C.; Kopper, B.A.; Barrios, F.X. The Suicidal Behaviors Questionnaire-Revised (SBQ-R): Validation with clinical and non-clinical samples. *Assessment* **2001**, *8*, 443–454. [CrossRef]
60. Reynolds, W.M. *Suicidal Ideation Questionnaire: Professional Manual*; Psychological Assessment Resources: Lutz, FL, USA, 1988.
61. van Spijker, B.A.J.; Batterham, P.J.; Calear, A.L.; Farrer, L.; Christensen, H.; Reynolds, J.; Kerkhof, A.J. The Suicidal Ideation Attributes Scale (SIDAS): Community-based validation study of a new scale for the measurement of suicidal ideation. *Suicide Life Threat. Behav.* **2014**, *44*, 408–419. [CrossRef] [PubMed]
62. Beck, A.T.; Kovacs, M.; Weissman, A. Assessment of suicidal intention: The Scale for Suicide Ideation. *J. Consult. Clin. Psychol.* **1979**, *42*, 343–352. [CrossRef]
63. Bradford, D.R.R.; Biello, S.M.; Russell, K. Defeat and entrapment mediate the relationship between insomnia symptoms and suicidal ideation in young adults. *Arch. Suicide Res.* **2021**, *26*, 1632–1643. [CrossRef] [PubMed]
64. Li, X.; Ren, Y.; Zhang, X.; Zhou, J.; Su, B.; Liu, S.; Cai, H.; Liu, J.; You, J. Testing the integrated motivational-volitional model of suicidal behavior in Chinese adolescents. *Arch. Suicide Res.* **2020**, *25*, 373–389. [CrossRef]
65. Taylor, P.J.; Wood, A.M.; Gooding, P.; Tarrier, N. Appraisals and suicidality: The mediating role of defeat and entrapment. *Arch. Suicide Res.* **2010**, *14*, 236–247. [CrossRef]
66. Yang, Q.; Hu, Y.Q.; Zeng, Z.H.; Liu, S.J.; Wu, T.; Zhang, G.H. The relationship of family functioning and suicidal ideation among adolescents: The mediating role of defeat and the moderating role of meaning in life. *Int. J. Environ. Res. Public Health* **2022**, *19*, 15895. [CrossRef]
67. Stanley, I.H.; Hom, M.A.; Christensen, K.; Keane, T.M.; Marx, B.P.; Björgvinsson, T. Psychometric properties of the Depressive Symptom Index-Suicidality Subscale (DSI-SS) in an adult psychiatric sample. *Psychol. Assess.* **2021**, *33*, 987–997. [CrossRef]
68. Rush, A.; Trivedi, M.H.; Ibrahim, H.M.; Carmody, T.J.; Arnow, B.; Klein, D.N.; Markowitz, J.C.; Ninan, P.T.; Kornstein, S.; Manber, R.; et al. The 16-item Quick Inventory of Depressive Symptomatology (QIDS), clinician rating (QIDS-C), and self-report (QIDS-SR): A psychometric evaluation in patients with chronic major depression. *Biol. Psychiatry* **2003**, *54*, 573–583. [CrossRef]
69. Slim, K.; Nini, E.; Forestier, D.; Kwiatkowski, F.; Panis, Y.; Chipponi, J. Methodological Index for Non-Randomized Studies (MINORS): Development and validation of a new instrument. *ANZ J. Surg.* **2003**, *73*, 712–716. [CrossRef]
70. Dhingra, K.; Boduszek, D.; O'Connor, R.C. A structural test of the Integrated Motivational-Volitional model of suicidal behaviour. *Psychiatry Res.* **2016**, *239*, 169–178. [CrossRef]
71. Galynker, I.; Yaseen, Z.S.; Cohen, A.; Benhamou, O.; Hawes, M.; Briggs, J. Prediction of suicidal behavior in high risk psychiatric patients using an assessment of acute suicidal state: The Suicide Crisis Inventory. *Depress. Anxiety* **2017**, *34*, 147–158. [CrossRef] [PubMed]
72. Russell, K.; Rasmussen, S.; Hunter, S.C. Insomnia and nightmares as markers of risk for suicidal ideation in young people: Investigating the role of defeat and entrapment. *J. Clin. Sleep Med.* **2018**, *14*, 775–784. [CrossRef]

73. Littlewood, D.L.; Gooding, P.A.; Panagioti, M.; Kyle, S.D. Nightmares and suicide in posttraumatic stress disorder: The mediating role of defeat, entrapment, and hopelessness. *J. Clin. Sleep Med.* **2016**, *12*, 393–399. [CrossRef]
74. Zuromski, K.L.; Bernecker, S.L.; Gutierrez, P.M.; Joiner, T.E.; King, A.J.; Liu, H.; Naifeh, J.A.; Nock, M.K.; Sampson, N.A.; Zaslavsky, A.M.; et al. Assessment of a risk index for suicide attempts among US Army soldiers with suicide ideation: Analysis of data from the Army Study to Assess Risk and Resilience in Servicemembers (Army STARRS). *JAMA Netw. Open* **2019**, *2*, e190766. [CrossRef] [PubMed]

MDPI AG
Grosspeteranlage 5
4052 Basel
Switzerland
Tel.: +41 61 683 77 34

Behavioral Sciences Editorial Office
E-mail: behavsci@mdpi.com
www.mdpi.com/journal/behavsci

www.ingramcontent.com/pod-product-compliance
Lightning Source LLC
Chambersburg PA
CBHW040834250926
51850CB00007BA/1311

* 9 7 8 3 7 2 5 8 6 9 9 8 5 *